BODY LOVE
EVERY DAY

KELLY LeVEQUE

WILLIAM MORROW
An Imprint of HarperCollins*Publishers*

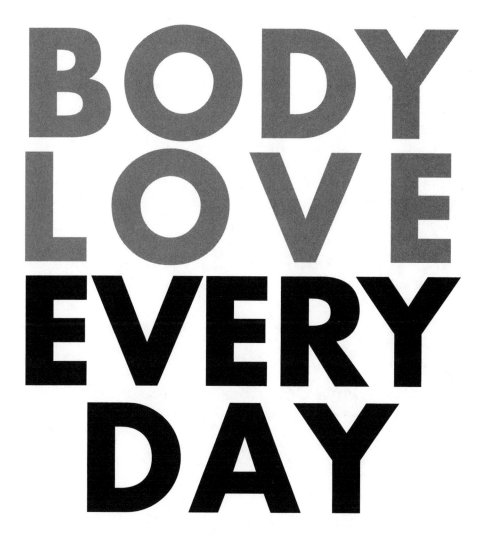

BODY LOVE EVERY DAY

CHOOSE YOUR LIFE-CHANGING 21-DAY PATH TO FOOD FREEDOM

BODY LOVE EVERY DAY. Copyright © 2019 by Kelly LeVeque. All rights reserved. Printed in the United States of America. No part of this book may be used or reproduced in any manner whatsoever without written permission except in the case of brief quotations embodied in critical articles and reviews. For information, address HarperCollins Publishers, 195 Broadway, New York, NY 10007.

HarperCollins books may be purchased for educational, business, or sales promotional use. For information, please email the Special Markets Department at SPsales@harpercollins.com.

FIRST EDITION

Designed by Bonni Leon-Berman

Photography by Matthew Morgan and Vanessa Tierney

Graphics by Amber Moon

Library of Congress Cataloging-in-Publication Data has been applied for.

ISBN 978-0-06-287080-3

19 20 21 22 23   LSC   10 9 8 7 6 5 4 3 2 1

To Sebastian Dume

CONTENTS

FOREWORD
By Emmy Rossum

I MET KELLY IN 2016 at the start of my health journey. The word *journey* suggests an epic tale. Imagine a young woman on an adventurous quest, beginning with struggle, resulting in glory, and finding true love along the way. That's what it's like to meet Kelly and have her change your life.

In the years pre-Kelly, I'd never been busier, happier, or more creatively excited. But my schedule was grueling. Filming fourteen-hour days, I often found myself sleeping on airplanes and cramming in interviews, talk shows, and photo shoots. I was exhausted. Trying to cope and looking to food to soothe my stress, I'd fallen into a cycle of caffeine, crash, sugar, crash, sugar, crash. Sound familiar? This pattern left me feeling stagnant, anxious, and often reaching for dietary Band-Aids. I yearned for an easy, comprehensive, holistic approach to health and nutrition and help dealing with my polycystic ovary syndrome (PCOS).

PCOS is a condition of chronic ovarian cysts. Besides monthly discomfort and pain, it can affect fertility and prevent eggs from maturing. Since my early twenties, I had been plagued by these little monsters. My cysts felt like heavy, stabbing pains in my abdomen. They left me swollen, massively bloated, and sometimes in the emergency room for pain management. Needless to say, it took a mental and emotional toll.

For years, my doctors tried to manage my PCOS with birth control, a common treatment. But it really wasn't working. I was still suffering flare-ups and I didn't want to be on birth control anymore. PCOS was just a microcosm of how I'd been dealing with my health in general—or, rather, how my health had been dealing with me. I didn't feel like I was in charge. My intuition told me it was time to get back in the driver's seat.

In many ways in my life, I've taken the road less traveled to pursue a goal. I've always followed my gut (no pun intended, unless you like bad jokes, in which case we can be friends), tireless and determined to find solutions. I take pride in my work and career, in navigating the challenging and mostly male world of Hollywood, standing up for women, equal pay, and what I believe in. I wanted that same sense of action, direction, and purpose with my health.

Enter Kelly. Meeting Kelly was the turning point in this epic tale on my road to glory.

Kelly was instrumental in helping me find a better way. From the moment we met, she was an advocate, ally, and friend. Deeply educated in science, Kelly focused on nutrition, which hadn't been on my doctor's radar. I learned that many women with PCOS are often insulin resistant. When we analyzed my diet, we saw signs that I might be, too. Every day, I was processing the stress and demands of my profession with sugar, caffeine, and carbs. My system was likely flooded with insulin and inflammation as a result.

Kelly gave me a manageable plan. For breakfast, I blended up a Fab Four Smoothie and cut back on sugary lattes, toast, and fruit. This set me up for balance during the day. With lunch, we hit the Fab Four again: protein, fat, fiber, and greens. After a nourishing dinner, I made a concerted effort not to snack or eat chocolate. This would help clear excess insulin from my bloodstream while I slept.

Kelly's approach to nutrition had radical, positive changes on my health. In time, my ovarian cysts were under control, without birth control or other drugs.

My blood sugar was more stable. I had more sustained energy without dips during the day. I had a lot less anxiety. A nice bonus? My jeans were fitting better than ever. I have followed this plan happily for years, liberated from the old cycles I once felt captive to. I feel optimistic and empowered.

Kelly stokes my curiosity. She sweet-talks me with science. She helps me believe in myself and listen to my body. She is my cheerleader. Over the years we've worked together, she has held my hand and helped me prepare for countless photo shoots, films, and—most important—my wedding day.

Kelly is a know-it. She's not a know-it-all. If she doesn't know the answer, she goes in search of it. She wants to know the *why*, just like me. One of the biggest takeaways from my experience with Kelly: I've learned how to truly take ownership of my health.

Ultimately, I make up my own mind. I take what Kelly says and decide how to incorporate it into *my* lifestyle. I don't feel the pressure to make it my whole entire life. Because it's my body, my choice, and my health. I have a foundation, but I also have flexibility and independence. The Fab Four isn't a diet in the way we have been taught to fear, dread, and loathe diets. It's not something to break or cheat. It's not a set of handcuffs. It's a key.

This is the turning point in your journey, on your road to glory and the true love of your body. This is where it starts.

FOREWORD

By Jennifer Garner

I WAS INTRODUCED TO Kelly in late 2017 by my friend and fitness coach, Simone de la Rue. I had heard about Kelly and her approach and knew she had devoted fans in several of my girlfriends. I needed to change my body for a new movie, and I had about eight weeks to do it.

Peppermint was going to be a physically demanding shoot. The script was full of stunts, action scenes, and a boxing match or two with the bad guys. I needed to be strong, fit, and lean. I was going to be training, lifting, and rehearsing every day, so I needed to keep my body fueled and help it recover at night. I didn't want a diet; I wanted a healthy plan to hit my deadline.

When I sat down with Kelly, it clicked. The way she explained the science of blood sugar, the simplicity of prioritizing the Fab Four, her sunny attitude—it gave me this feeling of "Oh, this makes sense, I can do this." She gave me the right amount of information to know what to do, without overloading me. Kelly is really good at that—a little of her "why" goes a long way.

We started each day with a Fab Four Smoothie. From there, Kelly let me be me.

Foreword

I love to cook and bake. There are few places I'd rather be than in my kitchen, making a little something for my family. Nine times out of ten (okay, maybe eight), I try to make the healthy decision. But I'm not immune to the calls of a slice of pizza, a glass of wine, a little bite of chocolate. What I really want is balance. I want to live a healthy life, but I also want the freedom to live in the moment.

I thought carbs would definitely be off the menu. Wine, too. But they weren't. Kelly just shifted my focus to cleaner vino (who knew this existed?!) and more nutrient-dense carb options. And on harder workout days when my muscles needed more fuel, we actually added a serving of carbs. The trade-off was that those were nights without my beloved glass of Cab. I had my goal and I had my fun, too. I had balance.

But on my next project, my circadian rhythm quickly became circadian chaos. Filming until 2 or 3 A.M.—way past my bedtime—meant sleeping less and sleeping worse. During the day, I was tired and having all sorts of cravings. Kelly explained how the sleep disruption was affecting my insulin sensitivity and my body's ability to do its normal detox. We added a protein-based snack and pulled back on a few inflammatory treats. Within a few days, I felt much better. Balance was restored.

I like food. And food likes me. We've always had a pretty solid relationship. But I know what it's like to be nitpicked, judged, and overanalyzed. It's hard not to let the "bad guy," whether it's you or someone else, put a dent in your self-confidence and make you question everything you eat. Life is challenging enough without having to battle your plate. With Kelly, you don't.

I hope you learn as much from *Body Love Every Day* as I have from Kelly.

INTRODUCTION

WELCOME TO *BODY LOVE EVERY DAY!* My name is Kelly LeVeque and I'm a holistic nutritionist, celebrity health coach, and wellness expert based in Los Angeles, California. Whether you're just starting your body love journey or already on your way, I'm thrilled and honored to be working with you.

In my first book, *Body Love*, I shared my science-based approach to clean eating, health, and wellness. At its heart, my approach is about how eating the Fab Four (protein, fat, fiber, and greens) at every meal balances your blood sugar, helps you eat to satiety, and naturally balances your hunger hormones. The result is a realistic, sustainable way to get results, whether it's a weight or body composition goal, addressing a lingering health issue, or simply living a healthier lifestyle. The Fab Four lifestyle works because it's based on how our bodies metabolize food. It's rooted in the science of human nutrition, it's backed by research, and it follows our biological blueprint. It gives your body exactly what it needs at every meal.

It also leads to a more positive relationship with food because it makes you feel good about your choices. The Fab Four grew out of my own need for positive reinforcement. Growing up, I always studied longer for teachers who believed in me and trained harder for coaches who cheered me on. My parents raised me to believe that it was never about being perfect; it was about trying my best. I needed that from my plate, too. I needed to feel positive about the choices I was making, not try to be perfect at every meal. As it turns out, a lot of you needed that, too.

The response to *Body Love* has been nothing short of amazing. It's incredibly humbling to hear all the success stories and inspiring messages from readers who are making the Fab Four their own. And it fills my heart that people are improving their relationship with food and themselves through the book. We all need a healthy dose of body love, and I'm glad the underlying theme of body positivity has resonated so strongly with people.

I love my job and feel so grateful for the opportunity to help people. But I know I can always improve and do more, which is why I've been listening closely to all of the feedback and questions I've received in response to *Body Love*. If I could sum it all up and distill it into one big-picture question, it would be this:

How do I live the Fab Four lifestyle every day?

I'm a choose-your-own-adventure type of nutritionist. I want to help my clients live the lifestyle of their choice while still helping them reach their goals. I work with all types of people, from meat eaters and raw vegans to pescatarians and vegetarians. I teach them the science behind the Fab Four, give them the tools to apply it, and empower them to choose the right path for their body and personal preference. In *Body Love*, I called this light structure. Interestingly, I've found that many of you, in one form or another, actually want a little more structure. Like in the medium-plus range.

Many of you have adopted the Fab Four lifestyle and want a more specific, daily program to aspire to and follow. In addition, you want more practical guidance on how to apply the Fab Four and execute on what *Body Love* teaches. *How do I choose a protein powder? How can I add fiber to a salad? What if I'm vegetarian or vegan? Should I eat before or after I work out? More Fab Four recipes, please!* People want to know what

I recommend, what I shop for, order, and cook, and what my typical day looks like. In essence, they want a deeper dive into the Fab Four lifestyle, one that helps answer the question of how to truly live it, day in and day out. Whether they're already on their Fab Four journey or about to embark on one, they want a more practical, hands-on guide to carry with them.

I wrote *Body Love Every Day* to be that guide.

We'll start with a quick trip back to school. In **Blood Sugar 101,** I'll give you a brief and powerful refresher of the Fab Four and the science behind it. I'll reintroduce the concept of blood sugar balance, explain why it's so important, and show you how the Fab Four supports it.

Then, in **Part One: The Fab Four Every Day,** you'll learn how to put the Fab Four into practice at breakfast, lunch, and dinner. We'll go through each macronutrient one by one, and you'll learn exactly what to eat, no matter your lifestyle preference. Whether you're a meat eater or a vegetarian, the guiding principle is the same. The key is to eat protein, fat, fiber, and greens at every meal. All of these essential macronutrients should be included in every dish, on every plate, and in every Fab Four Smoothie you consume.

That's how simple it is.

You'll learn the specific sources of protein, fat, fiber, and greens I prefer and why. I'll give you daily goals, highlight foods with the highest nutrient density, show you ways to increase the bioavailability of those nutrients, and teach you simple calculations such as net carbohydrates and carbohydrate density. I'll name some names and list specific brands and products I use and prefer. I'll also do my best to answer many of the real-world questions I've received from readers, clients, and followers. I'll touch on some clean cooking and preparation techniques, offer shopping tips, and provide charts with valuable nutritional information. I'll teach you why eating certain vegetables can activate genes that help us detoxify, fight inflammation, and promote longevity. I'll also explain why overeating processed, sugary, certain starchy, and liquid carbohydrates—what I call the "Not So Fab" Four—at every meal is not part of my approach and can be detrimental to your goals and overall health. Notice that I said "at every meal." You don't need to banish these foods from your life forever. In my experience, doing so gives them power over you. That's not the kind of relationship I want you to have with food. I don't want you to swear off these foods or beat yourself up when you eat them. Instead, I want you to prioritize and feel good about yourself when you eat the Fab Four—it breeds confidence, positivity, and ultimately body love.

My goal in Part One is to give you the practical guidance you need to apply the Fab Four to your daily life. I want to show you how to execute on what *Body Love* teaches, every day. In the process, you'll learn what some of the latest research is saying and how different foods affect brain, gut, and skin health. You'll also learn a variety of new Fab Four strategies, tips, and hacks. My hope is that you will feel inspired and empowered to make healthier decisions on your own, and always remember to pat yourself on the back when you do.

Next, in **Part Two: The Body Love Archetypes and Fab Four Plans**, I'll share four different examples of how you can live the Fab Four lifestyle, every day, for three weeks. Using the Fab Four as the foundation, I've created detailed 21-day plans for four different archetypal women. So more structure, yes, but my version of it—the body-loving version—because I haven't changed. I'm not an all-or-nothing nutritionist, I don't demand perfection from myself or my clients, and the Fab Four isn't a fad diet. None of that is changing. So don't mistake daily macronutrient recommendations, a 21-day time period, or the word "plan" for any of those things. I want you to live the version of the Fab Four lifestyle that's right for *you.* There are an infinite number of ways to make it your own. The plans are merely four examples that you can aspire to and follow—if you want to. They're a guide to reference, an expert to learn from, a companion to lean on, and a coach to help you reach your goals.

An archetype is a typical example of a certain type of person. My hope is that you'll be able to identify with at least one of the archetypes I've written about. This is not to discount the importance of your bio-individuality, which was (and still is) a central principle of *Body Love*. Rather, it's to recognize that many of us are on similar journeys, and that we can identify with and see ourselves through certain universal archetypes. Call it our bio-commonality—our shared aspirations, struggles, and characteristics. I see women like this every day in my practice. By creating a 21-day Fab Four plan for four common archetypes, I hope to give each of you some measure of the personalized, one-on-one attention I give my clients. And as you change and evolve, I hope to be there for the future you, too.

Depending on where we're at in life, we might be . . .

The **Girl on the Go**, who wants to find balance and consistency amid a hectic or demanding schedule. She might be in her twenties at her first job, or higher up the corporate ladder and feeling the pressure that comes with it, or a mom being pulled in all different directions. She might work late, be an entrepreneur, take night classes, eat out or order takeout rather than cook at home, have to squeeze in workouts, travel and entertain for work, and have a full social calendar on top of all that. She needs a Fab Four plan that will help anchor her but be flexible enough to adapt to her busy, unpredictable life. I want stability and calm to be her new normal.

- Annie, age thirty-eight, the owner of a national beauty chain and mother of two, used the Fab Four amid constant work travel and lost eighteen pounds in three months.
- Brooke, age twenty-six, was challenged by emotional eating and food anxiety in times of work stress. She relied on the Fab Four to gain confidence in herself, and over the course of a year she lost thirteen inches and thirty pounds.

The **Domestic Goddess,** who wants to create a true home base for clean eating, health, and wellness. Whether she lives in the suburbs or the city, home is her sanctuary and the kitchen is her happy place. She loves to cook, doesn't mind meal prep, is conscientious about food quality, and wants to source the best ingredients for her refrigerator and pantry. She might want to shed a few pounds, instill better habits in her family and kids, or simply live the healthiest life she can. She needs a Fab Four plan that gives her the recipe to do it. I want to give her the tools to build her healthy dream house. (This is who I aspire to be, but in reality I'm a Girl on the Go.)

- Dawn, age thirty-two, a mother of two young kids, loved to cook and bake for her family but was unhappy with her weight and dealing with constipation.

Once she started using the Fab Four as her recipe guideline, her digestion improved, she lost eight pounds, and she found that her kids were happier and calmer.

- Jeana, age fifty-seven, a mom and cancer survivor, used the light structure of the Fab Four to celebrate life while still nourishing her body, strengthening her gut microbiome, and eating anti-inflammatory foods. Her goal was to thrive and stay strong without overthinking every decision.

The **Plant-Based Devotee**, who wants to live the Fab Four lifestyle but without consuming meat or animal products. She's committed to a vegetarian or vegan diet and needs a Fab Four plan that gives her enough plant-based sources of protein and key nutrients to stay healthy and nourished and still hit her goals. Here I welcome her to the *Body Love* family, offer her a bunch of new plant-based Fab Four recipes, and help her thrive and reduce nutrient deficiencies.

- Annaliese, age twenty-five, a publicist, learned how to add protein and fat to her plate to regulate her hunger hormones and prevent office snacking. She lost six pounds in one month.
- Marin, age thirty-four, an office administrator, didn't realize she was undereating key macronutrients during the day. She added a Fab Four Smoothie as an afternoon bridge snack to up her protein and fat consumption, and in the process stopped an eight-year struggle with late-night binge eating.

And depending on our calendar, we might need to get . . .

Red-Carpet Ready, so we look and feel our best for an upcoming vacation, wedding, reunion, or other big occasion. Or we may just want to commit to achieving a goal by a definitive deadline. As a result, this archetype is willing to follow a Fab Four plan that's a bit more regimented. She wants a healthy kick in the booty so she can rock that dress or bikini. But even though she has a shorter-term goal, the plan will set her up for long-term, sustainable success. It will break bad habits, breed new confidence, and show the power of eating the Fab Four. It will empower her, not starve her, so she can build on her lifestyle changes and prevent backsliding. I want the whole person in the after photo—not just the body—to be the new her.

- Jennifer Garner, age forty-five, actress and mother, used the Fab Four to prepare for the physical demands of her role in the action film *Peppermint,* which required her to be both lean and strong. She got to be creative and decide what she wanted to eat while she hit her body composition goal.
- Emmy Rossum, age thirty-two, actress, writer, and director, always has a red carpet to walk and makes nourishing her body a priority by meal-prepping Fab Four recipes.

In addition to identifying with one of these four archetypes, there might be a part of you that's battling perfectionist thoughts—your **Inner Perfectionist**—and wants to stop chasing the unattainable and start a new relationship with food. We've all been there. On the diet roller coaster, beating ourselves up, dreading the mirror, feeling ashamed and out of control, letting one "mistake" ruin an entire day. She needs a dose of body love and a mind-set reset. I want to redefine the meaning of a good day, redirect her pursuit of size 0, and recast her inner villain as Wonder Woman. I want to help her ditch the unattainable ideal of perfection and accept herself. I've dedicated a chapter to this aspect of your journey and included some simple but powerful tools I call on every day for myself and with my clients.

As a holistic nutritionist, I strive to treat and counsel the whole person. This means I try to take into account more than just my clients' physical condition. I ask them what's going on at home, at work, and in their relationships. I try to understand their mental and emotional state, social factors at play in their life, and what's motivating them and why. All of it has an impact on reaching your goals, improving your health, and successfully adopting lifestyle changes. The plans reflect this philosophy. They're holistic programs that touch on different aspects of the body, mind, and soul and include the following elements:

- Fab Four meals or smoothies for every breakfast, lunch, and dinner.
- Exercise, fitness, and movement.
- Wind-down and recharge techniques for nights and weekends.
- Tools for alleviating stress, anxiety, and negative thoughts.
- Emotional support for rough patches.
- Simple ways to build self-confidence and resilience.
- Success stories to inspire, motivate, and spark the fire within.

My goal is to help you build a clean, healthy lifestyle. Food and nutrition form the foundation, but it goes beyond that. These other factors should be taken into account as well so that we can nurture and nourish the whole you. Hopefully, by doing so, you'll develop a stronger connection to the authentic you and start to heal what might need repair. From a place of self-love, your daily decisions will take on a deeper meaning and your goals will always be within reach.

How should you use the Fab Four plans? In the way that's best suited to you and your health, wellness, weight, and lifestyle goals. Here are a few options to consider:

YOU CAN LITERALLY GO BY THE BOOK AND FOLLOW ONE PLAN TO A T. If one archetype really speaks to you and you want that level of structure, go for it. Just remember, the Fab Four lifestyle isn't all-or-nothing. It isn't about perfection. Neither are the plans. There's no starting over if you miss a meal, skip a day, or eat something that isn't on the plan. One decision—your next—is all that matters. Just pick up where you left off or move forward to the next meal or day.

YOU CAN PICK AND CHOOSE FROM MULTIPLE PLANS TO CREATE YOUR OWN UNIQUE VERSION OF THE FAB FOUR LIFESTYLE. You can pick Monday from one plan, Tuesday from another, do your own thing on Wednesday, go back to the first plan on Thursday, and so on. You might love five days of a particular plan and just do those on repeat. Or depending on the day, you might be one archetype at breakfast, another at lunch, and a third at dinner. The point is that all of the plans are rooted in the Fab Four, so if you want to use them interchangeably, you can.

YOU CAN USE THE PLANS AS INSPIRATION, TO LEARN SOMETHING NEW, OR TO GIVE YOURSELF A FRESH PERSPECTIVE. In other words, feel free not to follow them as plans for every day. But I do highly recommend that you read (or browse) through all of them. They're a valuable resource and come jam-packed with more than fifty new Fab Four recipes, contain a variety of practical tips, and are filled with insight and inspiration. In particular, the Girl on the Go plan is a great place to start and see the Fab Four in action—literally. It's filled with useful strategies for home and travel, accessible recipes that take minutes and taste amazing, and it embodies my realistic approach to eating clean and finding balance. For example, if you can add four quick Girl on the Go recipes to your repertoire, that's four nights you're not ordering takeout. Plus, who knows what life will throw at you? You'll be better prepared having read how the Fab Four can work under different circumstances.

I speak from personal experience. I'm constantly on the go and traveling for work. There are always events and occasions I want to look my best for. Perfectionist thoughts are still a challenge for me. And now I'm a mom of a one-year-old boy, which has inspired me to create the healthiest, most loving home I can. (When I was writing portions of this book, I was in my third trimester of pregnancy, which also inspired cravings for pizza, cottage cheese, and peaches.) Through it all, I've relied on the Fab Four, a livable framework that can adapt to fit wherever you are in life. The plans can show you how, and no matter how you use them, they'll help further your journey.

Each plan begins on a Monday (Day 1) and ends on a Sunday (Day 21). If that setup doesn't work for you, feel free to modify the days as you see fit. For example, if you want to start on a Wednesday, you could treat that as Day 1 (which would result in your weekend days falling during the week on Mondays and Tuesdays) or you could treat it as Day 3 (and add Days 1 and 2 at the end of the plan, after Day 21). It's up to you.

As we go, I'll introduce delicious new Fab Four Smoothie recipes with a functional boost. The functional food movement is based on the idea that we can use food as a form of medicine to help improve overall health and reduce the risk of disease. I'll show you how to incorporate many of the trending herbs and adaptogens in the functional space into great-tasting flavors like Triple Chocolate Crunch, Sweet Spiced Carrot Cake, Detox Winter Mint, Ginger Lemonade, and Sweet and Savory Basil. In addition, I'll share new recipes for Fab Four meals, soups, dressings, and desserts. They'll be accessible enough for anyone to make, not just my Domestic Goddesses. And I'll include plenty of vegetarian and vegan options for my Plant-Based Devotees.

Throughout the book, I've included practical strategies you can realistically execute and repeat. I've created simple, healthy hacks that save time, money, and stress. And I've proposed solutions to a host of real-life situations and what-ifs. Use these tools, modify them, make them your own. It's about being proactive and, if need be, reactive, while always moving toward your goals. Also, as noted earlier, throughout the book I've named some of the specific brands I use and prefer. My opinion on any food product is always driven by its nutrient density, ingredients, quality, form (cellular versus acellular), and other attributes that are important to me. Over time I've organically developed relationships with a small number of my favorite brands, including NOW Foods and Primal Kitchen. For full disclosure, I wanted to note these paid brand relationships.

Body Love, my first book, is the foundation of the Fab Four lifestyle. As you move through this book, I'll refer back to many of *Body Love*'s key concepts, discussions, and charts. Although it's not essential, I encourage you to read and consult it as part of your journey. It lays out in detail the science of blood sugar balance, which led me to create the Fab Four in the first place. It also contains a wealth of other valuable information, including recipes, clean food swaps, and tips for vibrancy and beauty.

The Fab Four lifestyle is about balance, body love, and sustainability. It's not about deprivation, perfection, or a quick fix. It's about feeling empowered, not overwhelmed, by food and nutrition. It's the end of yo-yo dieting and the beginning of a new relationship with food. When you nourish your body with protein, fat, fiber, and greens, you're giving it the essential micro- and macronutrients it needs to function optimally. You're giving it the nourishment and love it deserves. The science in *Body Love* sets you free, and the practical guidance in *Body Love Every Day* will set you up for more everyday success. It will help you eat clean, find balance, and love your healthy lifestyle.

We all need body love. We need it every day.

So let's get started!

STAY CONNECTED

As you read *Body Love Every Day* and embark on your body love journey, there are other ways to have me at your side! You can follow me on Instagram (@bewellbykelly), where I keep it real, share what I'm up to and what I'm eating, and show you what the Fab Four lifestyle looks like for a true Girl on the Go. (Use #Fab4Smoothie to share your favorite smoothies with me!) You can listen to me on the *Be Well By Kelly* podcast, which delves into all things health, nutrition, and wellness. My guests run the gamut . . . doctors, chefs, authors, scientists, industry leaders, entrepreneurs, health bloggers, fitness experts, and more. You'll learn about current trends in health and wellness, go more in-depth on the Fab Four, and hear some amazing stories. Finally, you can also go on my website (www.bewellbykelly.com) to find new recipes, take my course "Fab Four Fundamentals" video, read articles I've written on a variety of topics, and get more inspiration for your healthy lifestyle.

BLOOD SUGAR 101

THE FAB FOUR IS based on the biochemistry of controlling and maintaining optimal blood sugar balance. *Blood sugar is another name for glucose,* a type of sugar found in certain foods. When we eat and break these foods down, the glucose enters our bloodstream. That's why it's called blood sugar.

Blood sugar is fuel for our cells. It powers our brain, organs, muscles, and all sorts of bodily functions, and some is needed in the bloodstream at all times. What you don't want is too much or too little. Generally speaking, *the healthy range is between 70 mg/dl and 120 mg/dl (or milligrams per deciliter, the typical measure of blood sugar).* The body is constantly working to maintain blood sugar homeostasis, so that it has the daily energy it needs.

TOO MUCH OR TOO LITTLE

When you have too much glucose in your bloodstream, you may feel sluggish and sleepy. You may also crave sugary foods right after a meal. When you have too little glucose in your bloodstream, you may feel weak, jittery, light-headed, and hungry.

When there is excess blood sugar in the bloodstream, the body stores it for future use. Cue insulin, a hormone made in the pancreas. Its job is to transport unneeded glucose from the bloodstream and store it in the liver and muscles, and then fat cells (after it has been converted into a triglyceride). Think of your liver and muscles as spare gas tanks and your fat cells as the trunk. The liver can store between 200 and 500 calories of glucose. The muscles can store between 800 and 2,000 calories of glucose. Once those two tanks are full, glucose will (1) be converted into suboptimal free fatty acids (triglycerides) and stored as fat, and/or (2) linger in the bloodstream, resulting in elevated insulin levels (hyperinsulinemia), which increases the likelihood that other triglycerides, regardless of why they are elevated or where they originate from (converted fructose, elevated alcohol consumption, dietary fat, or another source), will be stored as fat. (See The Effect of Insulin on Fat on page 20.) Either way, fat cells don't have a maximum limit.

You can see the issue here. *When glucose stops being used as fuel, the body shifts into storage mode. If our gas tanks are full, triglycerides will get stuffed in the trunk.*

When there isn't enough blood sugar in the bloodstream for its energy needs, the body will dip into its reserves. It will access the liver tank first. Cue glucagon, another hormone made in the pancreas. Its job is to take glycogen in the liver and convert it back into glucose. (Technically, the storage form of glucose is called glycogen. Glycogen is basically a long chain of glucose molecules.) Once the glucose reenters the bloodstream, the body can use it as energy. The liver can be accessed for any energy need, and its stored glucose can be used to power any bodily function.

The muscle tanks work differently. They can only be accessed for one specific energy need, and their stored glucose can be used to power just one specific bodily function—muscle movement. The only way to access and use the glucose stored in the muscles is through muscle movement—in other words, physical activity and exercise. Perhaps this is an evolutionary safeguard to make sure the body always has some stored energy reserved exclusively for mobility. After all, our ancestors might have needed to run from predators and travel long distances to hunt and gather. This would guarantee there was stored energy on hand for the muscles if blood sugar levels were too low. Today, it's a safeguard to make sure you don't just sit on your tush! *If you aren't physically active and don't regularly exercise, your muscle tanks will stay full of glucose. This means the next time your body shifts into storage mode, triglycerides will be stored as fat.* So you have to exercise, work out, and move. There's no other way to make room in your muscles for more glucose. You must use what's stored first. You gotta burn it.

When insulin gets to a muscle cell, it signals for the cell to accept its delivery of glucose. Normally, the cell responds to the signal and accepts the glucose. However, when insulin levels are continuously high, muscle cells may stop responding. They might become "resistant" to the signal and therefore not accept the glucose. This is known as insulin resistance. The result is that glucose doesn't get stored in the muscles. Instead, it is converted into a triglyceride and stored as fat, and/or it lingers in the bloodstream, resulting in elevated insulin levels that increase the likelihood that other triglycerides will be stored as fat.

After insulin has done its job, it lingers in the bloodstream. *When you have excess insulin in your bloodstream, you don't burn fat. The presence of excess insulin shuts down the fat-burning process.* Remember that it's a storage hormone, and as long as it's there, it tells the body you're in storage mode. Why would the body burn fat in that state? It won't. Insulin makes it think you need to be storing, not burning. Depending on your body, diet, and health, insulin might stay in your bloodstream for six to eight hours, and in some cases longer. That's a lot of time you could be burning fat and losing weight.

So how does this all tie back to what you eat? What breaks down into glucose and raises your blood sugar? What causes the release of insulin, turns off fat burning, and results in more fat storage? And what causes insulin levels to be continuously high and puts you at risk of developing insulin resistance?

The answer is eating unbalanced meals. Specifically, overeating processed, sugary, certain starchy, and liquid carbohydrates at every meal. Here's why.

INSULIN SENSITIVITY

Insulin sensitivity sounds bad, but it's actually good. Being insulin sensitive means that your muscle cells properly respond to the signal from insulin and accept deliveries of glucose and that you need less insulin overall to transfer glucose out of your bloodstream. You can strengthen your insulin sensitivity through regular exercise and by eating the Fab Four. Low or weak insulin sensitivity sounds bad, and it actually *is* bad. It means you're insulin resistant and thus need more insulin overall to transfer glucose out of your bloodstream. The result is you store more fat and burn less. Your insulin sensitivity weakens when you don't exercise regularly and when you overeat processed, sugary, certain starchy, and liquid carbohydrates at every meal.

GLUCONEOGENESIS

Carbohydrates are not your body's only source of glucose. You can produce glucose from noncarbohydrates through a process called gluconeogenesis. For example, the stress hormone cortisol can release protein from your muscles and convert it into glucose in your liver.

KETONES: FAT-BASED FUEL

Carbohydrates are not your body's only source of energy, and glucose is not the only type of fuel your body can run on. It can also run on fat-based fuel called ketones. To run exclusively on ketones, your body needs to be in a state called nutritional ketosis. Although healthy when done correctly, this can be a difficult state to maintain. Eating the Fab Four gives you the metabolic flexibility to be fueled by glucose or ketones, allowing you to flow in and out of ketosis naturally depending on your carbohydrate intake. But my point is this: fat is fuel, too. See page 84 for more information.

Carbohydrates break down into glucose and raise your blood sugar. In response, the body releases insulin. Insulin stores excess glucose in your liver and muscles, thereby lowering your blood sugar and restoring balance. Overeating processed, sugary, certain starchy, and liquid carbohydrates at every meal disrupts this process. These types of carbohydrates break down into larger amounts of glucose and cause a more aggressive spike in blood sugar. As a result, the body has to release larger amounts of insulin. If your liver and muscles are already full (because you overate these foods at your previous meal), the glucose will be converted into a triglyceride and stored as fat, and/or linger in the bloodstream, resulting in elevated insulin levels that increase the likelihood that other triglycerides will be stored as fat. Meanwhile, you're now full of a larger amount of insulin, which shuts down fat burning for an even longer period of time.

But that's not the end of it.

What goes up must come down. The same is true for your blood sugar. The flip side of a spike is a crash. Depending on your insulin sensitivity, health, and other factors, your blood sugar might decline more abruptly or more slowly. Regardless of the speed, the fact that (1) your blood sugar is dropping and (2) you're still full of insulin will result in (3) an unwelcome side effect: you'll actually crave *more* carbohydrates. Why? Because eating carbohydrates represents the fastest and most direct way to get more glucose into your bloodstream and raise your blood sugar. When your body thinks it might be starving or running low on blood sugar, your hormones make you crave foods that provide the quickest fix. It doesn't matter if your blood sugar is still within the healthy range. It doesn't matter if you just ate ninety minutes ago. When your blood sugar is dropping and you have excess insulin in your bloodstream, it will trigger carbohydrate cravings. The reality is that you're not physically hungry. You're hormonally hungry and full of insulin.

You see where this can lead. If you act on the cravings and eat more carbohydrates, your body will release even more insulin, and the spike-crash-crave cycle will start all over again.

BLOOD SUGAR IMBALANCE

Blood sugar imbalance provokes hormone imbalance, lack of satiety, more immediate hunger, steep drops in energy, and cravings. It results in a shorter, more erratic blood sugar curve.

BLOOD SUGAR CHART

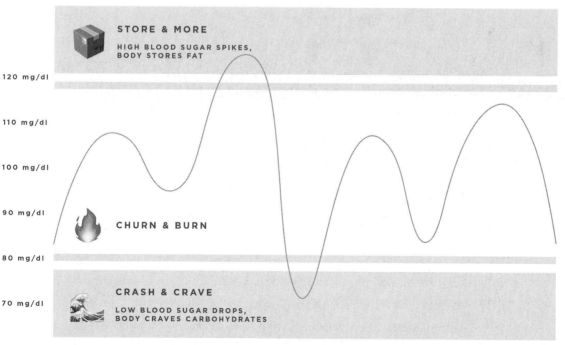

STORE & MORE
HIGH BLOOD SUGAR SPIKES, BODY STORES FAT

120 mg/dl

110 mg/dl

100 mg/dl

90 mg/dl

CHURN & BURN

80 mg/dl

CRASH & CRAVE
LOW BLOOD SUGAR DROPS, BODY CRAVES CARBOHYDRATES

70 mg/dl

HOW TO TEST YOUR BLOOD SUGAR

One way to understand how your body responds to the food you eat is to test your blood sugar with a glucometer, a small handheld device you can buy online or at the drugstore. Below is a simple protocol you can follow if you want to see how your diet is affecting your blood sugar and what your blood sugar curve looks like.

1. Test your glucose first thing in the morning before eating any food or doing any exercise, ideally after a twelve-hour fast. This is your *fasting glucose level,* and ideally you want it to be less than 85 mg/dl.

2. Eat a complete meal and then test your glucose three times: at one hour, two hours, and three hours after the meal. Don't eat anything else during this three-hour time period. Write down what you ate in a food journal and chart your glucose levels. Ideally, you want your post-meal glucose levels to average the following:

   - One hour after eating—less than 120 mg/dl

   - Two hours after eating—less than 100 mg/dl

   - Three hours after eating—less than 85 mg/dl

3. Repeat the testing process after every meal for three to five days. Your glucose chart/graph will show you the shape and range of your blood sugar curve. Together with your food journal, you can see how specific dietary choices affected you.

What do you do if your results aren't ideal? Adjust with the Fab Four, which will help balance, elongate, and smooth out your blood sugar curve. *Spiking too high?* Increase fiber intake and decrease carbohydrate density. For example, add a cup of broccoli to your meal. (Yes, I am asking you to eat more.) Or swap your pasta for whole food replacements like chickpeas, sweet potato noodles, or zucchini zoodles. (More on carbohydrate density on page 123) *Crashing too fast?* Add healthy fat and up the fiber. For example, add avocado to your Fab Four Smoothie so you're satisfied until lunch. *Erratic curve?* Poor food choices can lead to dehydration, inflammation, hormonal imbalance, and an unhealthy gut microbiome. Get back to the Fab Four, eat nutrient-dense foods, and drink more water.

The purpose of this protocol is to show you how the foods you eat at each meal affect your blood sugar and to give you a more detailed picture of your blood sugar curve over a three- to five-day period. It can be a helpful way to understand your body's reaction to food as you embark on a lifestyle change. However, long-term, I don't want you to obsessively check your blood sugar all day, every day.

One way to keep an eye on your blood sugar, but not go overboard, is to test your fasting blood sugar once per day first thing in the morning. This is simply step 1 in the protocol on page 18. Ideally, you want your fasting blood sugar first thing in the morning to be in the 70s or 80s mg/dl. If you aren't currently in that range, the goal is to see your fasting blood sugar come down over time. Don't fret—depending on your health this could take a few weeks to a few months. But eating the Fab Four will help you get there!

So how do you break the cycle? Or better yet, stop it before it starts? How do you balance your blood sugar and avoid spikes and crashes? How do you reduce the amount of insulin in your bloodstream and keep carbohydrate cravings at bay? How can you burn fat and support healthy weight loss?

By eating balanced meals consisting of protein, fat, fiber, and greens (the Fab Four) and not overeating processed, sugary, certain starchy, and liquid carbohydrates at every meal. It's as simple as that.

The body is designed to function optimally when it receives a balanced mix of these essential macronutrients. Protein breaks down into amino acids, which enable muscles and other tissues to build and stay strong. Fat breaks down into fatty

THE INSULIN TRAP

The insulin trap is when your blood sugar crashes just a few hours after eating, but you're still full of insulin for several hours longer than that. The time gap is the trap, when your blood sugar curve doesn't track or match your insulin levels. During the mismatch, you're not burning fat, but you're driven to eat more carbohydrates, releasing even more insulin. Soon enough, there will be another mismatch, which will cause more carbohydrate cravings, and so on. That's why it's called a trap.

acids, which enable hormone production, cell development and growth, and brain functioning. Fiber is important for gut health, healthy gut bacteria, and digestion. And greens and vegetables that are deep in color are a source of energy, vitamins, minerals, phytochemicals, and water. *All of these essential micro- and macronutrients should be included in every meal you eat.* They're not just food! They're information to your body and communication on a cellular and genetic level that you're being healthily fed, fueled, and nourished so you can thrive and be well.

THE EFFECT OF INSULIN ON FAT

Elevated insulin levels (hyperinsulinemia) not only prime the body to store fat, but also affect how the body uses fat. For example, the dietary fat you consume is typically utilized for a variety of beneficial purposes, including those listed above and in chapter 2. However, in the presence of excess insulin, it may instead be stored as fat. Remember, insulin is a storage hormone. It causes the increased release of lipoprotein lipase (LPL), an enzyme that supports the absorption of triglycerides by fat cells. In addition, insulin decreases the production of hormone-sensitive lipase (HSL), an enzyme that helps the body break down and use stored fat for energy. Essentially, insulin tells your fat cells to store and hold on to fat.

Fat stored in the body can start as excess glucose or fructose that has been converted into triglycerides. It can also originate from dietary fat if insulin levels in the bloodstream are elevated. However, as long as insulin is being consistently cleared from the bloodstream, a diet including a mix of healthy fats shouldn't result in high body fat. In my practice, I tend to see more satiety and weight loss with clients who eat a moderate-fat diet and who prioritize foods that do not cause a large release of less insulin. Party animal beware—your triglycerides will be elevated due to demands on your liver caused by excessive alcohol consumption.

Moreover, when you eat balanced meals with clean, nutrient-dense forms of these macronutrients, you will keep your blood sugar in balance, for the following reasons:

1. Protein and fat don't break down into glucose, so they don't directly raise your blood sugar. In fact, they slow digestion as a whole, which helps you feel satiated (full) for a longer period of time.
2. Fibrous and green vegetables break down into smaller amounts of glucose and therefore cause much smaller increases in blood sugar.
3. Fiber slows down the digestion of the glucose, meaning your blood sugar will rise more slowly and gently. It won't spike aggressively, and it won't go as high.
4. Since there is less glucose in your bloodstream, your body has to release less insulin. And since your blood sugar is rising more slowly, the insulin is released more slowly.

The result is that your blood sugar will stay within the healthy range, you'll have fewer ups and downs, and the fluctuations will be less dramatic (no steep spikes or crashes). This sets you up for success *because you burn fat and lose weight when your blood sugar is balanced and you don't have excess insulin in your bloodstream.*

Satiety means feeling full and satisfied. The Fab Four helps you eat to satiety by balancing your hunger hormones. In *Body Love*, I discussed the various hunger-related hormones in your body and how the Fab Four regulates them and supports their proper functioning. Each one of the Fab Four is specifically recommended for a reason. Here are a few examples:

- Protein causes the release of glucagon-like peptide-1 (GLP-1), which signals that we're full, and peptide YY (PYY), which controls appetite. Lack of protein causes the release of neuropeptide Y (NPY), which stimulates carbohydrate cravings.
- Fat causes the release of two satiety hormones, leptin and cholecystokinin (CCK). It also lowers fasting insulin levels and slows digestion as a whole.
- Fiber increases PYY levels and can double the production of the satiety hor-

mone CCK. Fiber also physically stretches your stomach lining, which calms the hunger hormone ghrelin.

- Green vegetables increase GLP-1 levels, help calm the hunger hormone ghrelin, and reduce insulin levels.

By supporting your hormones and bringing them into balance, the Fab Four help you feel full and satisfied. Depending on your unique body chemistry, this feeling of satiety can last for four to six hours after eating. Further, by giving your body the essential macronutrients it needs and slowing digestion as a whole, the Fab Four allows you to stay properly fueled during that time. *The result is an elongated blood sugar curve—you're satisfied, fueled, and have balanced blood sugar for a longer period of time.* If you plotted your blood sugar curve on a graph, it would look smoother and longer, slowly rising and falling like a gentle wave.

When you're balanced and fed, hunger isn't immediate. This type of blood sugar curve gives you the energy to maintain a four- to six-hour window between meals

BLOOD SUGAR CHART

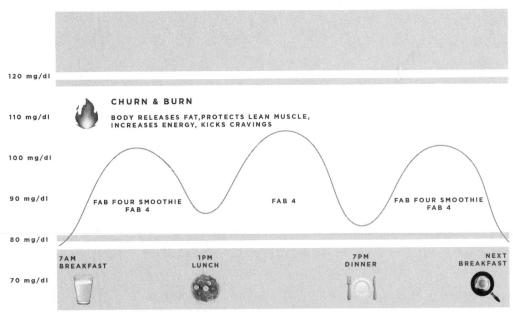

without the urge to snack. This window will allow your body to properly digest your food, cause a surge in human growth hormone, and reduce insulin levels in your bloodstream. It sets you up for more success *because it enables you to burn fat in between meals.* When your blood sugar is balanced and you don't have excess insulin in your bloodstream, you can stay out of storage mode. Over time, you sustain a healthy weight when your body receives the inputs it needs to maintain muscle mass, produce and balance your hormones, and support your gut microbiome every day. The Fab Four helps remind you to do this at every meal.

HOW DO CARBOHYDRATES FACTOR INTO THE FAB FOUR?
The Fab Four lifestyle isn't a no-carb diet. It simply emphasizes complex carbohydrates that are wrapped in fiber, or cellular carbohydrates. These are your fibrous and green vegetables—unprocessed, whole foods that are rich in fiber, vitamins, minerals, phytochemicals, and water. The Fab Four shifts the focus away from overeating processed, sugary, certain starchy, and liquid carbohydrates—what I call the "Not So Fab" Four.

As with the rest of my approach, this shift in focus is driven by science and the biochemical effect these foods have on our body. Fibrous and green vegetables continuously feed your gut microbiome, which reduces inflammation, produces healthy fatty acids, and protects our bodies from toxins and chemicals. Greens are nutrient-dense, break down into less glucose, don't raise your blood sugar as high or as fast, and release less insulin. As you've learned, the result is blood sugar balance, satiety, and hormonal balance, which results in an elongated blood sugar curve. By contrast, overeating processed, sugary, certain starchy, and liquid carbohydrates at every meal will have

SNACKING

Digestion is the process of breaking down food into usable forms so it can be absorbed and used by the body. Complete digestion can take up to six hours. It's work for the body and requires a lot of energy. When you eat snacks all day, or eat five or six meals per day, you're asking your body to restart a process it hasn't completed yet. This taxes your body and is a drain on your energy levels. Also, if you snack on processed, sugary, or starchy carbohydrates, you will spike your blood sugar and release more insulin. This can turn off fat burning, lead to fat storage, and make you crave more snacks. Some of my clients need a bridge snack between lunch and dinner, which I'm okay with if it's based on the Fab Four. But I don't recommend snacking all day or eating five or six meals per day. It disrupts digestion and can be detrimental to your health and weight loss goals.

WHAT ABOUT FRUIT?

I'm not antifruit, and I'm not here to demonize it. There are just a few key facts that I want you to be aware of. First, fruit has an immediate impact on your blood sugar. Fruit contains healthy nutrients such as fiber, vitamins, and phytochemicals, but it's also full of sugar—namely, glucose and fructose. Even these naturally occurring sugars will spike your blood sugar and can cause subsequent sugar cravings. Second, eating excessive amounts of fruit can be taxing on your liver. This is because fructose is metabolized in the liver just like alcohol. (Fructose also turns into fat more quickly than glucose.) Third, fruit at the grocery store is larger than what grew originally in nature. (Honestly, how did bananas get so big?!) If your goal is weight loss, I would keep your fruit to a single serving per day (about ¼ to ½ cup). The point of this benchmark is to help you get the nutritional benefits of fruit but in nature's traditional serving size. Our bodies were made to eat fruit seasonally and occasionally, not in jumbo sizes and not at every single meal year-round. You don't have to ditch all your fruit. In the chart on pages 99–101 I highlight a bunch of fruits that are nutrient-dense and high in antioxidants and are what's known as low-glycemic (having a low effect on blood sugar).

the opposite effect. They lack the full range of nutrients your body needs to function optimally and don't support optimal blood sugar balance. As a result, they shouldn't be the everyday foundation of your meals or overall diet.

This doesn't mean you can never, ever eat these foods. It just means you shouldn't overeat them at every single meal, especially if your goal is weight loss or improved body composition. You should always prioritize the Fab Four. We need to eat carbohydrates, but knowing how they will affect your blood sugar and hunger hormones is a powerful tool. I also don't want you going into what I call Low-Carb Purgatory (see page 122).

In chapter 5, I'll discuss the "Not So Fab" Four in greater detail. I'll teach you useful concepts like net carbohydrates, carbohydrate density, and the difference between cellular and acellular carbohydrates. Then I'll give you a few simple guidelines to follow depending on your specific goal. You'll see my approach to foods like pasta, bread, rice, grains, potatoes, and more. The beauty of prioritizing the Fab Four is that it empowers your food choices. If you know how to bring yourself back into balance, you give yourself the flexibility and freedom to live how you want.

In the chapters to come, I'll teach you how to put the Fab Four into practice at breakfast, lunch, and dinner. We'll go through protein, fat, fiber, and greens one by one, and you'll learn exactly how to incorporate them into every meal and Fab Four Smoothie. The Fab Four Smoothie is one of my favorite body-loving tools.

It balances blood sugar and primes your body chemistry and metabolism for the rest of the day. I think it's a wonderfully effective and simple tool to use as you build a healthy, active lifestyle, and I provide lots of recipes both in this book and in *Body Love.*

The power of blood sugar balance cannot be overstated. Using the Fab Four is how you can achieve it. It's beautifully simple science.

FOR MORE INFORMATION

This chapter contains simplified and condensed versions of the scientific discussions in *Body Love.* It's meant as a high-level summary of certain key concepts. If you want a more complete and nuanced understanding of blood sugar and the Fab Four, I recommend reading chapters 1 through 4 of *Body Love.* They contain in-depth explanations, address a variety of related concepts and topics, offer specific diet and lifestyle recommendations, and share inspiring client success stories. They also contain easy-to-understand and informative charts and graphs.

PART ONE

THE FAB FOUR EVERY DAY

1

PROTEIN

BUILDS LEAN MUSCLE AND
CURBS CRAVINGS

THE FIRST PILLAR OF the Fab Four is protein. Protein breaks down into amino acids, the building blocks for every cell in the body. They enable muscles, organs, and other tissues to build and stay strong. They also support the production of certain enzymes, hormones, and neurotransmitters, as well as antibodies in the immune system. Protein really is a pillar. Without this essential macronutrient or the amino acids it contains, our bodies and muscles would break down and deteriorate.

Protein supports blood sugar balance, satiety, and hunger hormones. As stated in Blood Sugar 101, protein doesn't break down into glucose, so it doesn't directly raise your blood sugar or cause a large surge of insulin. Amino acids don't directly raise blood sugar or insulin levels. (Technically, when amino acids enter the bloodstream, the body releases glucagon, a hormone that triggers the release of a small amount of stored glucose from the liver, which in turn triggers the release

THE PROS OF PROTEIN

Protein can boost your metabolic rate, reduce appetite, support blood sugar balance, and induce thermogenesis, a state in which the body uses calories to produce heat, benefiting weight loss efforts. One study found that eating 25 percent of your diet as protein led to increased satiety, decreased late-night appetite, and resulted in fewer obsessive thoughts regarding food. In another study, women who increased their protein intake to 30 percent (up from 15 percent) of their diet lost an average of eleven pounds in twelve weeks. Even a small increase in protein can help you sustain weight loss. One study found that weight regain rates went down by 50 percent when protein intake increased from 15 percent to 18 percent. Beyond the satiety and body composition benefits, higher protein intake has been shown to support a healthy cholesterol ratio and decrease triglycerides and the inflammatory marker C-reactive protein. Like a salmon swimming upstream against the current wave of antiprotein information, I not only give my clients permission to eat more protein—I encourage it.

of a minimal amount of insulin. This normal hormonal process supports and facilitates the uptake of amino acids into the muscles. This release of glucose and insulin isn't something to worry about because the levels aren't high and it's the body's normal and natural process of supporting the uptake of amino acids.)

Protein is the most satiating macronutrient and helps slow digestion as a whole. It takes time and energy to break down and helps you feel satiated (full) for a longer period of time. Protein also regulates certain hunger hormones. It causes the release of glucagon-like peptide-1 (GLP-1), which signals that we're full, and peptide YY (PYY), which reduces appetite. It also calms the release of neuropeptide Y (NPY), thereby reducing carbohydrate and sugar cravings. By having a neutral effect on blood sugar, slowing digestion, and supporting these hormones, protein helps you eat to satiety and elongates your blood sugar curve. If your goal is weight loss or improved body composition, adequate protein consumption is vital.

How much protein should you eat per day and meal? Everyone has different protein needs. The minimum daily amount recommended by the Food and Nutrition Board at the National Academy of Sciences is 0.36 gram per pound of body weight, but this is intended to prevent a protein deficiency, and I wouldn't consider it optimal. In my practice, I aim for a higher amount per day. Depending on the client, *I generally prefer 0.75 gram per pound of body weight per day.* For example, if you weigh 140 pounds, I would aim for about 100 grams of protein per day. *At a minimum, I recommend 0.5 gram per pound of body weight per day.* Again, if you weigh 140 pounds, this means eating a minimum of 70 grams of protein per day. Protein should comprise about 25 percent of the food you eat every day. For the majority of my clients, meals should average between 20 and 40 grams of protein. Between a Fab Four Smoothie, 3 to 4 ounces of chicken or salmon on a salad for lunch, and even a plant-based dinner, this is attainable. You don't need to measure or weigh your food to the ounce with a food scale, but try to get into the above range—at least 0.5 and ideally 0.75 gram per pound of body weight—so you garner the benefits.

Some bodybuilding websites say daily protein intake should be a minimum of 1.5 grams per pound of body weight. Others say upward of 2 grams per pound, even for women. (Picture me eating six and a half chicken breasts per day!) You need protein to build and maintain lean muscle mass, but not that much. One study found that people doing heavy strength training for ninety minutes didn't benefit from more than 0.75 gram of protein per pound of body weight. Another study in the *Journal of Sports Science* found that between 0.8 and 0.9 gram per pound was ideal for muscle building. Other studies have shown that 0.4 to 0.5 gram per pound can be sufficient to maintain muscle mass in active adults.

Again, I generally prefer a daily average of 0.75 gram per pound of body weight with meals averaging 20 to 40 grams for most of my clients. (One exception might be for more serious athletes or weight lifters who might need more based on how much they train or lift. But generally speaking, I would tell them to keep their per-meal protein intake to 40 to 50 grams, maximum.)

Next, let's discuss the specific types and sources of protein I prefer and why. I'll go through animal- and plant-based options separately. For many people, animal protein is still the centerpiece of every meal. For example, eggs and bacon at breakfast, chicken

PROTEIN GOAL FOR A FAB FOUR SMOOTHIE

The goal is to get 20 to 30 grams of protein in a Fab Four Smoothie. Different protein powders have different serving sizes, different amounts of protein per serving, and different-size scoops in the canister, jug, or bag. As a result, you might have to use more than one scoop of your specific protein powder. Read the nutrition facts on the label: the serving size and scoop equivalent will be listed at the very top, and the protein per serving will be listed in its usual spot down below. In the Fab Four Smoothie recipes in this book, the first ingredient listed is always protein powder, but I don't give the exact amount—you'll need to calculate it based on your particular brand.

NONESSENTIAL AMINO ACIDS

Don't let the term "non-essential" fool you. The eleven nonessential amino acids are critical for our health and serve important purposes in the body. For example, glycine supports lean muscle mass and protein synthesis, increases human growth hormone, and decreases inflammation. Tyrosine is another great example because it's the precursor for dopamine, our happy "reward" hormone. For other examples, see the chart on page 63.

or turkey at lunch, and then steak, fish, or more chicken at dinner. On the other hand, many people are vegetarian or vegan and choose not to eat animal protein at all, for reasons of animal rights, environmental impact, opposition to industrial food production methods, or simply personal preference. Wherever you land, the Fab Four can work for you. The guiding principles are the same.

Two quick notes before we dive in.

First, very few foods contain just one macronutrient. For example, meat and eggs contain both protein and fat. With a few exceptions, I will categorize foods by their predominant macronutrient. The exceptions are the plant-based protein sources. Many nuts and seeds contain mostly fat and many beans/legumes are mostly carbohydrates, but they all contain protein as well. In an effort to provide my Plant-Based Devotees (and anyone else who wants to eat a plant-based meal) with protein options, I've included them in this chapter. If you use nuts or seeds as your Fab Four protein, I would recommend using a different food from chapter 2 as your Fab Four fat. For example, if you use hemp hearts as the protein in a salad, you could use olive oil in the dressing or add avocado as your fat. The reason is so that you don't rely too heavily on a limited number of foods. Mixing it up will increase the type and range of other micronutrients you consume.

Second, it's important to mention amino acids again. As you may recall, protein breaks down into amino acids. There are twenty key amino acids. The body can synthesize eleven of them, but it must get the other nine—called *essential amino acids*—directly from our food. (In turn, these twenty amino acids are used by the body to make other amino acids.) *Complete* proteins contain all nine essential amino acids; proteins that are missing one or more of the nine are called *incomplete*. These can still have high nutritional value; they just lack all nine essential amino acids. See the chart beginning on page 63 for a list of the twenty key amino acids and their animal- and plant-based protein sources.

All animal protein sources are complete proteins containing all nine essential amino acids. This includes poultry, eggs, beef, game meats, fish, seafood, and pork. With a few caveats and conditions, I consider all of these foods to be body-loving choices as the protein base for any Fab Four meal. Dairy is also a complete protein, but it's not something I recommend eating at every meal and shouldn't be the primary protein base of a Fab Four meal. I discuss each of these food sources in more detail in the following pages.

ORGANIC CERTIFICATION

In general, I prefer food that is certified organic. In order to use the certified organic label, a farm or producer must be certified by the U.S. Department of Agriculture and meet strict standards regarding how its animals were raised or crops were grown.

Animals must have access to environments that accommodate their natural behavior, such as pasture grazing. In addition, they can't be given drugs or antibiotics unless they're sick. They must also be fed 100 percent organic food sources. This means their food must be grown on a certified organic farm and can't contain growth hormones, animal by-products, or genetically engineered grains. However, one caveat is that it doesn't matter what type of organic food the animal is fed. It could be grass, grains, or another type of feed. I prefer animals that eat the food their bodies are naturally adapted to digest. This is why I prefer pasture-raised, or pastured, poultry and pork, and grass-fed and grass-finished beef and game meats.

For crops, the use of synthetic pesticides, chemical fertilizers, industrial solvents, other synthetic additives, and irradiation is either limited or prohibited. These chemicals and agents can be toxic and may pose health risks. In addition, they can be bad for the environment, cause pollution, and contaminate the water and soil. However, even organic crops aren't always 100 percent clean; they can be grown with commercial pesticides as long as they're naturally occurring. *(continued)*

There has been debate in the scientific community regarding the nutritional value of organic versus conventionally raised/grown animals and crops. Some studies have concluded that there isn't an advantage to organic, while others have found that there is. At the end of the day, buying organic is a personal decision. Organic food is more expensive, but I personally believe that the benefits justify the cost. To know you're buying certified organic, look for the "USDA Organic" label on the packaging.

Two newly proposed organic certifications that have recently gained traction are Regenerative Organic Certified (ROC) and the Real Organic Project (ROP). Both aim to set a higher standard than the current U.S. Department of Agriculture certification. Among other things, they propose to take into account soil health, land management, animal welfare, and other social factors. They propose USDA Organic as the baseline requirement, then farms could earn ROC or ROP certification in addition. The goal is to encourage farmers to improve their techniques and growing practices beyond current government standards. ROC standards are currently being tested in a pilot program, and the certification is expected to launch in 2019. The ROP is in the process of finalizing its standards, and an anticipated launch date has not been specified. Whether and to what extent either or both of these certifications will be adopted by farmers and the marketplace is an open question.

Regenerative farming is a huge initiative that benefits the health of our entire planet. It seeks to protect and improve the entire agroecosystem by grazing multiple species of animals, growing perennial plants, composting, farmscaping, and implementing other holistic land management practices. This type of farming increases organic matter and microorganism diversity in the soil and improves the health of watersheds. It also helps offset carbon emissions by pulling carbon out of the air and putting it back into the soil, which improves soil health and increases the nutrient density of produce. When we support this balanced exchange of energy, the health of the entire planet improves. A 2019 Life Cycle Assessment of White Oak Pastures in Georgia showed that their regenerative farming efforts sequestered more carbon into the soil than was being emitted from their grass-fed cattle. Regenerative farming can improve the health of our soil, plants, and animals, and thus our own health. If you're interested in learning more, check out *The Soil Story* by Kiss the Ground (on YouTube), or follow the initiative through Kiss the Ground (www.kisstheground.com) or the Savory Institute (www.savory.global), or watch the documentary *The Sacred Cow* (expected summer 2020).

BODY-LOVING POULTRY OPTIONS:
Chicken, Eggs, Turkey, Duck, and Bone Broth

In addition to certified organic, I prefer pasture-raised, or pastured, poultry and eggs.

Pasture-raised refers to an animal that's free to roam a natural outdoor pasture environment and to eat wild grasses, plants, seeds, insects, and other foods their bodies are naturally adapted to digest. The opposite of pasture-raised would be animals confined indoors or raised on industrial farms or feedlots. Though there isn't a separate pasture-raised certification, poultry and eggs with the USDA Organic label must have been given access to pasture or rangeland that accommodates the animal's natural behavior.

Two other terms to know are *free-range* and *cage-free*. Free-range birds must be allowed to range freely "outdoors" at least 51 percent of the time. The caveat is that "outdoors" doesn't have to be a natural pasture environment. It can be a plot of barren dirt or a concrete slab. As a result, free-range doesn't necessarily mean the bird had access to grass or that it ate organic feed.

Cage-free birds must be free to roam and not caged. The caveat is that this doesn't mean they were ever actually outdoors. Birds can be cage-free indoors in

BONE BROTH

Bone broth is an excellent source of protein that is easy to digest. Depending on the brand, 1 cup (8 fluid ounces) can provide between 6 and 12 grams of protein. Heat a cup or two of chicken or beef bone broth for a warming Fab Four bridge snack. It can also easily become the base of a Fab Four soup, stew, or smoothie (see page 59). A few frozen options I like are Osso Good and Bonafide Provisions, and a few shelf-stable options I love are Thrive Market and Kettle & Fire (frozen is generally more expensive than shelf-stable boxes). They all have delicious flavors with no added sugar. For a homemade recipe, see page 107 of *Body Love*. Bone broth is also rich in glycine, a beautifying amino acid that promotes the synthesis of collagen. Collagen is good for skin health, complexion, and skin tone.

an industrial barn or warehouse. The bottom line: the free-range and cage-free labels are important but not the only factor to consider for poultry and eggs. I would prioritize the USDA Organic and pasture-raised, or pastured, labels.

In terms of protein content, 3 to 4 ounces of cooked, pasture-raised chicken can provide up to 25 grams of protein. One pasture-raised egg can provide 6 grams of protein, so if eggs are your main protein at breakfast I would eat three or four. Pasture-raised chicken and eggs also contain higher amounts of healthy omega-3 fats than caged alternatives. Specifically, pasture-raised chicken and eggs are higher in EPA and DHA, which are long-chain anti-inflammatory omega-3 fatty acids. These are "good" fats that have been linked to reduced heart disease, improved cognitive function and immunological response, and lower levels of depression. Also, don't skip the egg yolk. It's a superfood that contains up to thirteen essential nutrients, including B vitamins, vitamins A and E, and selenium.

BODY-LOVING BEEF AND GAME MEAT OPTIONS: Steak, Ground Beef, Ribs, Bison, Lamb, Venison, and Bone Broth

For the reasons listed on page 32, I prefer certified organic, pasture-raised, grass-fed, and grass-finished options. For beef, the cleanest, healthiest food source is grass. Grass is a cow's natural diet. Grains (such as corn) and soybeans are not. It doesn't matter if they're organic. The protein in grass-fed beef is healthier and more nutritious than that found in grain- or soybean-fed beef. To make things trickier, a cow can be referred to as grass-fed even when it's fed corn or another grain (or even soybeans) toward the end of its life. This is called "finishing," and it's done to fatten the cow up. The result is something closer to conventional feedlot beef. When beef is grass-finished, the cow was raised to maturity on grass and wasn't finished or fattened up with any corn or other grains. Grass-fed, grass-finished cows take twenty-four to thirty-six months to reach maturity. Industrially raised or conventional feedlot cows take only eighteen to twenty months. By going grass-fed and grass-finished, you'll reap the benefits of a mature, pasture-raised animal.

The American Grassfed Association certifies 100 percent grass-fed and grass-finished producers. Animals must be fed a lifetime of 100 percent grass or forage, raised on pasture and not in confinement, and never treated with antibiotics or hormones. Producers are audited annually by independent third parties to ensure compliance with the standards. You can look for their "American Grassfed" label on beef, lamb, bison, goat, and sheep.

Grass-fed beef packs an efficient punch: 4 to 6 ounces can provide between 22 and 32 grams of protein (5.25 grams per ounce). In addition to protein, grass-fed beef is a great source of other nutrients. As compared with chicken, grass-fed beef is a more nutrient-dense option. It contains vitamin A, vitamin D, and high levels of B vitamins, including B_{12}. It has minerals such as iron, zinc, selenium, magnesium, and potassium and the antioxidants lutein and zeaxanthin. It contains conjugated linoleic acid (CLA), the only healthy naturally occurring trans fat. CLA is an anti-inflammatory antioxidant that can reduce the risk of heart disease and type 2 diabetes, increase insulin sensitivity, and support your metabolism. Grass-fed beef contains higher amounts of the healthy omega-3 fats EPA and DHA. It also has a healthier ratio of omega-3 and omega-6 fats than conventionally raised beef.

One of the best and most affordable ways to source quality meats is through an online delivery program. My favorites include Thrive Market, US Wellness Meats, and ButcherBox.

PROTEIN EFFICIENCY AND NUTRIENT DENSITY

I like the idea of being able to get as much protein and nutrition per ounce of food as possible. We obviously need the protein and nutrients, but maximizing density aids in digestion, helps your body be more efficient, and conserves energy. Grass-fed beef and wild salmon are very protein-efficient and nutrient-dense. Chicken and pork have a good amount of protein but aren't as nutrient-dense. Recent food documentaries have made some people scared to eat red meat. They choose chicken or eggs because they think these are cleaner options. But don't let the fearmongering or headlines scare you! The difference in nutrient density is a real factor.

Further, in general, animal proteins are more protein-efficient and nutrient-dense than plant-based sources. For example, beans are an important source of protein for vegetarians and vegans, yet on average, beans contain 2.5 grams of protein per ounce, which is about one-third less than grass-fed beef. Another example is the branched-chain amino acid leucine, which is much higher in animal proteins. Leucine helps regulate blood sugar, energy, and stamina, and helps the growth and repair of skin, bone, and skeletal muscle. Ideally, my Plant-Based Devotees should always soak and/or sprout nuts, seeds, beans/legumes, and grains. It makes the nutrients more bioavailable, thereby increasing protein efficiency and nutrient density. More on this on page 51.

ORGAN MEATS

Animal organ meat can be a highly nutritious food source, providing B vitamins (including B_{12}, riboflavin, and folate), vitamin A, iron, copper, and choline. Organ meats include liver, kidney, spleen, heart, and brain. They can come from cows, pork, lamb, and other animals. US Wellness Meats sells two entry-level options online (both of which are grass-fed) if you're interested in trying organ meats:

(1) liverwurst, a seasoned paste containing beef trim, liver, heart, and kidney; and (2) braunschweiger, a type of sausage that contains beef trim and liver. Both liverwurst and braunschweiger are already cooked, so all you have to do is slice off a piece. Try it with a little mustard on a Jilz cracker. Another way to incorporate organ meats is to mix a small amount into the ground beef you use for burger patties or taco meat. For example, you could mix 2 tablespoons (or more for a gamy flavor) of finely chopped liver into 1 pound of ground beef.

Of note: "sweetbreads" are meat from the pancreas and thymus gland, typically from veal (a cow calf).

In terms of cooking techniques, baking and roasting are optimal. You can also grill and barbecue over an open flame, but you should be careful not to char, burn, or cook the meat too well done. Cooking at a high heat over an open flame can create toxic and carcinogenic compounds known as heterocyclic amines (HCAs), so use medium heat and don't overdo it. Marinating your meat beforehand and using a lot of spices can also help limit your exposure to HCAs and other bad compounds (just don't use a sugary marinade). Marinades that contain onion, garlic, and lemon juice, or a marinade rich in rosemary, can decrease HCAs by more than 75 percent. Another way to reduce exposure is by eating greens and vegetables. Cruciferous vegetables and salad greens can help counteract the damage from HCAs formed during grilling. Check out my new functional rubs at Williams-Sonoma, they are rich in HCA-fighting ingredients.

Dehydrated beef or game meat (aka jerky) is a popular food. Dehydration is actually a preservation technique. By extracting the moisture from food, you inhibit the growth

AGES: ADVANCED GLYCATION END PRODUCTS

Advanced glycation end products (AGES) are harmful compounds that deplete antioxidants and cause other negative health effects. AGES are produced when protein or fat combines with sugar. (That's why I don't suggest a sugary marinade for your meat.) But before you blame it on the meat, the majority of AGES are created in our body after we consume sugar, because our body is made up primarily of protein. The best way to keep AGES low is to maintain balanced blood sugar and avoid foods with added sugar.

of microorganisms and help preserve it for longer. Food dehydrators generally remove 75 to 80 percent of a food's moisture. The result is a concentrated version of the fresh counterpart, with many (but not all) of the nutrients, vitamins, and minerals still present. When you buy jerky, read the label carefully. Many brands and flavors are loaded with excess sugar, syrups, and additives. Ideally, you want minimal ingredients; no added, refined, or processed sugar (such as high-fructose corn syrup); and low sodium. Look for options that use coconut aminos instead of soy sauce or teriyaki. And just like fresh meat, ideally you want jerky to be made from organic, pasture-raised, grass-fed, and grass-finished animals.

DIY JERKY

If you own a food dehydrator, try making your own jerky. You'll be able to ensure that it's made with body-loving ingredients and no excess sugar. Here are a few quick tips.

- As a general rule, it's better to slightly overdehydrate than to underdehydrate. This helps inhibit the growth of microorganisms, and, in my opinion, the jerky tastes better.

- Always choose fresh, lean cuts of meat. The healthiest options are organic, pasture-raised, grass-fed, and grass-finished.

- Cut the meat into slices no thicker than ¼ inch.

- Cutting with the grain will make the jerky chewier. Cutting against the grain will make it more crisp and tender.

- Trim away the fat. It doesn't dehydrate well and can cause the jerky to go rancid more quickly.

- For more flavor and tenderness, you can marinate the meat beforehand. I like using coconut aminos. This is a soy-free, gluten-free, and low-sodium alternative to soy sauce and teriyaki. Don't add sugar to your marinade.

BODY-LOVING FISH AND SEAFOOD OPTIONS: Salmon, Halibut, Shrimp, Scallops, Mussels, Oysters, Canned Light Tuna, Sole, Sardines, Herring, Mackerel (Chub or Atlantic), Crab, and Lobster

Wild fish is generally the cleanest, most nutrient-dense option. I look for the Marine Stewardship Council's blue fish label. MSC-certified fish and seafood are wild, traceable, and sustainable. Their entire life cycle takes place in their natural habitat. They spawn naturally in the wild, live in the wild, and are caught in the wild. There are several affordable online stores that offer wild fish, including Vital Choice, Sizzlefish, and Thrive Market. Personally, my favorite fish is salmon. I even eat it from a BPA-free can (it will say BPA-free on the label). My favorite brands are Safe Catch and Wild Planet, and I opt for Alaska or sockeye (both of which are less likely to be farmed). When possible, go for wild over "wild-caught" fish. Wild-caught fish might only have been *caught* in the wild. They might have been spawned on a fish farm or lived on one for some portion of their life before being returned to their natural habitat.

A large number of fish today come from commercial fish farms or fisheries, where they are spawned and/or kept in pens, tanks, or ponds. Some fish farms operate at an industrial-level scale, with thousands of fish living, eating, and defecating in the same confined water space. This can create a higher risk of pollution and disease in the fish. As a result, some fish farms have been known to use antibiotics and even pesticides. The consequence is lower nutritional value and potential exposure to harmful chemi-

MERCURY

Mercury is a neurotoxin that interferes with the brain, nervous system, fertility, and fetal development. Swordfish, ahi tuna, bigeye tuna, king mackerel, tilefish, and shark have some of the highest mercury content and should be avoided. Sea bass, grouper, albacore tuna, and yellowfin tuna have high mercury content and should be limited. Halibut, canned light tuna, cod, lobster, mahi-mahi, trout, and whitefish generally have moderate to low mercury content. Salmon, shrimp, scallops, mussels, oysters, sole, sardines, herring, mackerel (chub or Atlantic), crab, lobster, anchovies, clams, crawfish, tilapia, and squid generally have low mercury content. See *Body Love* for more information on mercury and also selenium, another element present in fish that can bind to mercury and prevent its absorption.

FISH OIL

A lot of people (and husbands) don't love fish as much as I do. If you don't eat fish on a weekly basis, one supplement to explore is fish oil or another omega-3 source like krill or algae oil. It's loaded with EPA and DHA, two long-chain anti-inflammatory omega-3 fatty acids with numerous health benefits. Plus, fish oil has no mercury content, algae is great for vegetarians and krill is extremely bioavailable due to its phospholipid form. Three brands that I have used are Omega3 Innovations (Omega Cure Extra Strength), Nordic Naturals, and NOW Foods. I generally don't take (or recommend) many supplements, but omega-3 is one that I take every day.

cals, such as polychlorinated biphenyls (PCBs). This is, unsurprisingly, one of the reasons I prefer wild fish.

Fish and seafood are a great source of protein; 3 to 4 ounces of wild salmon can provide between 19 and 22 grams. Equally important, fish and seafood are an excellent source of the omega-3 fatty acids EPA and DHA, two of the "good" fats. EPA and DHA are anti-inflammatory, reduce levels of "bad" triglycerides (fats), and have been linked to numerous health benefits, such as reduced risk of heart disease, improved cognitive function, improved immunological response, improved fetal development, type 2 diabetes prevention, and even lower levels of anxiety and depression. DHA also supports the growth of new brain cells (neurogenesis) by increasing the brain's supply of brain-derived neurotrophic factor (BDNF). There is a growing body of research showing the positive effects of omega-3s on brain health, including their ability to improve brain function and longevity, and to help prevent Alzheimer's, dementia, and other neurodegenerative conditions. For more on the science behind these developments, a good resource is *Genius Foods*, written by my friend Max Lugavere. Also, *Body Love* describes many of the health benefits of fish and seafood in detail.

BODY-LOVING PORK OPTIONS: Pork Chops, Pork Tenderloin, and Ribs

Pork is not my go-to, everyday protein, but I like adding some variety to our diet with a roasted rosemary pork tenderloin or a baked rack of ribs for my husband. For the reasons listed on page 32, I prefer certified organic and pastured options.

To the surprise of some of my clients, I'm not strictly opposed to bacon and sausage. They're sources of protein and, from the standpoint of blood sugar, won't throw you off-balance like other breakfast foods such as a croissant, bagel, muffin, cereal, fruit bowl, toast, pancakes, or waffles. However, I would keep it to one or occasionally two servings per week maximum. (Check the serving size on the package. Usually, there are two to three slices of bacon per serving.) Also, I would prefer uncured bacon and sausage with no added nitrates and no added, refined, or processed sugar. This means they won't have added synthetic chemicals, won't spike your blood sugar, and won't produce AGES (see page 39).

DAIRY PROTEIN

Last on the animal-based side is dairy. Even though dairy is a complete protein with all nine essential amino acids, it's not something I recommend eating at every meal and shouldn't be the primary protein or base of a Fab Four meal. With a few exceptions, I eat a mostly dairy-free diet. One dairy product I do eat and cook with regularly is ghee, or clarified butter, which is 100 percent fat (I discuss it further on page 75). I also eat and cook with butter if it's from a grass-fed and pasture-raised cow.

I generally go dairy-free because dairy is one of the foods most commonly associated with food allergies, intolerances, and sensitivities. Many people are allergic or intolerant to lactose, the sugar found in dairy. Further, because of pasteurization, dairy products like butter, cheese, and yogurt may lack certain enzymes. This can make them potential allergens. Also, many cows in North America have a protein called beta-casein A1, which can trigger food aller-

DELI MEATS

Even though I ate more turkey sandwiches than I can count when I was growing up, nowadays I'm not the biggest eater of deli meats, mostly because of the additives. When I do buy deli meats, I go for unprocessed, uncured, and nitrate-free options. One thing I enjoy on occasion is a good charcuterie platter with some salami and prosciutto next to raw cheese and nuts. Again, for salami and prosciutto, I always try to go for uncured options with no added nitrates. Also, I would avoid hot dogs unless they're pasture-raised, uncured, and nitrate-free. All of these terms should be listed on the product label or packaging. Thank goodness for the generation of folks demanding better! I feel like cleaner options (and more of them) are available all the time.

ALLERGENS

Food allergens, including gluten and pasteurized dairy, may increase the risk of developing other health issues. The proteins in these allergens may leak through the gut lining and intestinal walls (intestinal permeability) and end up in the bloodstream. This can increase inflammation and, if the proteins end up in the brain, can act like an opioid drug.

gies. Dairy can contribute to gut and digestive issues, including leaky gut syndrome and irritable bowel syndrome, and other health issues such as eczema.

Pasteurization is the process of heating dairy to eliminate microbes and other potentially harmful bacteria. For example, pasteurized milk is heated to 160°F for fifteen seconds. Pasteurization may kill helpful enzymes, result in nutrient loss, and cause the dairy to be harder to digest. "Raw," or unpasteurized, dairy is not heated other than by the animal's natural body temperature, which is typically around 100°F. Unpasteurized dairy has a higher risk of bad bacteria and the potential for foodborne illness, especially in pregnant or immune-compromised people and the very young or old. Ultimately it's a personal decision, but if I eat dairy (and I'm not pregnant or breastfeeding), I typically try to go with unpasteurized.

I think cheese should be eaten only occasionally and thought of as a condiment, treat, or way to add flavor to a specific dish—for example, as part of Taco Tuesday, on a charcuterie plate during a date or nice dinner out, or to spruce up your salad a few times per month. I prefer goat or sheep cheese over cow cheese, and as noted above, raw cheese over pasteurized cheese. If you buy cow cheese, try to source from certified organic, pasture-raised, grass-fed, and grass-finished producers. Just like beef, the cheese from these cows is healthier and more nutrient-dense. For example, grass-fed dairy contains higher amounts of conjugated linoleic acid (CLA), the only healthy, naturally occurring trans fat. CLA is an antioxidant that has anti-inflammatory and other health benefits.

I tell my clients to eat cottage cheese as an occasional treat and to seek out options that are grass-fed, plain or unflavored, and with ingredients limited to live cultures and organic milk or cream. One such brand is Good Culture. I recommend the same approach with yogurt. Yogurt is high in lactose and full of added sugar, so I tell clients to eat it occasionally with no fruit or flavoring. This includes Greek yogurt. Finally, I generally avoid milk and cream because of the lactose and casein (see page 43). Some of my clients like a splash of dairy in their morning coffee. I try to encourage them to use a clean, plant-based alternative instead. But if I had to choose between milk and cream, my preference would be to use cream, which contains less lactose and casein and is mostly fat.

PLANT-BASED PROTEIN

Next, for all the Plant-Based Devotees out there, let's turn to plant-based protein sources.

As you may recall from page 32, *complete* proteins contain all nine essential amino acids. There are fewer complete proteins on the plant-based side. Quinoa, buckwheat, and amaranth are all complete proteins; however, like dairy, I think of them as add-ons or supplements, not the primary base of a plant-based Fab Four meal.

The reason is that despite their protein content (6 to 8 grams per cup), they contain large amounts of starchy carbohydrates. If you eat them at every single meal, you will continuously spike your blood sugar and buy yourself a ticket on the blood sugar roller coaster discussed in Blood Sugar 101. As discussed further in chapter 8, my opinion is that Plant-Based Devotees should keep grains to ¼ to ½ cup per meal. If your goal is weight loss or improved body composition, I would also keep grain con-

---

TMAO: TRIMETHYLAMINE N-OXIDE

There's been a lot of talk recently about how you shouldn't eat animal protein because of TMAO. TMAO is an organic compound made by your gut bacteria when you eat meat, fish, eggs, and dairy. These foods contain choline, lecithin, and L-carnitine, and when your gut bacteria ferment them (break them down), TMAO is produced. Recent research has linked elevated TMAO to heart disease, diabetes, and colon cancer. However, TMAO production depends on the type, health, and strength of the bacteria in your gut microbiome. The healthier your gut microbiome, the less TMAO is produced. Several studies have found that increasing consumption of greens and vegetables, even while still eating meat and fish, can limit TMAO production and blunt the TMAO marker. The reason is the fiber in greens and vegetables, which feeds the good bacteria in your gut microbiome. In fact, soluble fiber had the ability to reduce TMAO markers in mice that ate red meat by more than 60 percent. Other studies have found that healthy levels of vitamin B, vitamin D, and polyphenol all reduced TMAO levels, and that an increase in consumption of pistachios and Brussels sprouts does the same. The bottom line: I don't want you to banish choline-rich animal protein from your diet, you just need to eat adequate amounts of fiber and greens . . . aka the Fab Four.

sumption to once per day. This will keep your meals and days—and thus you—more balanced.

Soybeans are also a complete protein, but I generally don't recommend soy products or tofu as part of a Fab Four lifestyle. The isoflavones and phytoestrogens in soy products are endocrine disruptors and have been linked with thyroid disease, hypothyroidism, fatigue, weight gain, reproductive and ovulation problems, skin breakouts and blemishes, and cancerous tumor growth. Further, soy has been known to be treated with the pesticide glyphosate, and 90 percent of the soy in the United States is GMO, or genetically modified. I know tofu is traditionally one of the mainstays of a vegetarian diet, but for me the health risks and growing practices of soybeans outweigh the protein content. My recommendation is that soy be consumed minimally and occasionally in an organic, gluten-free, and fermented form, such as tamari or miso.

ENDOCRINE-DISRUPTING CHEMICALS

Endocrine-disrupting chemicals (EDCs) interfere with the endocrine system and can result in serious health issues (including cancerous tumor growth and birth defects), as well as weight gain and obesity. For example, perfluoroalkyl acid has been linked with increased weight regain after weight loss. Below are a few tips to limit your exposure. To learn more about EDCs, check out the book *Sicker, Fatter, Poorer* by Dr. Leonardo Trasande, M.D., M.P.P.

- Eat organic: it reduces your intake of chemical pesticides and has been shown to lower organophosphate metabolite output in the urine (from insecticides).
- Reduce plastic use: this can help reduce exposure to phthalates. Discard used food containers, never microwave them, and hand wash plastic containers.
- Go BPA-free: BPA is a synthetic estrogen found in plastic, the lining of canned food, beverages, thermal paper receipts, and other packaging. Look for products that say BPA-free or that come in glass or Tetra Pak.
- Check the Healthy Living app: it lists clean personal care products free of phthalates, paraben, triclosan, and benzophenones.

So what do I prefer as options for vegetarians and vegans? With a few caveats and conditions, I consider nuts, seeds, and legumes/beans to be body-loving choices as the protein base for a plant-based Fab Four meal. They're *incomplete* proteins because they don't contain all nine essential amino acids, but they contain protein, won't spike your blood sugar, and aren't linked to the health issues associated with soy products.

BODY-LOVING PLANT-BASED NUT OPTIONS: Almonds, Cashews, Pecans, Walnuts, Macadamia Nuts, Brazil Nuts, Pistachios, and Barùkas Nuts

Nuts are a great Fab Four food. They contain protein, fat, and fiber in every bite. They also travel light and are an easy add to your purse, bag, carry-on, or desk drawer. Nuts have other nutritional benefits as well. For example: almonds are high in calcium and support bone health; Brazil nuts are a good source of selenium, which supports thyroid health; pistachios serve up lutein, zeaxanthin, and beta-carotene, which support eyesight; and Barùkas nuts are a complete protein containing all essential amino acids.

I prefer raw and certified organic nuts. Raw nuts are in their natural state. They're what you would get if you picked the nut right off the tree and shelled it. I generally don't recommend roasted nuts. Most roasted nuts are roasted in man-made industrial seed oils, which oxidize quickly and essentially turn into (bad-for-you) free radicals. One exception is *dry-roasted* nuts, which are not roasted in industrial seed oils and are only lightly toasted with or without salt. Essentially, dry roasting brings out or uses only the nut's natural oils. The bottom line is that packaged nuts should contain only three

PROCESSED PLANT-BASED PROTEINS

If you often eat a lot of processed plant-based proteins like soy or pea fillings, bean-based pasta, or fermented nut cheese or dairy alternatives, you may also be ingesting a lot of acellular carbohydrates, emulsifiers, and gums. In excess, these can overfeed your bad gut bacteria (candida and yeast) and lead to an inflammatory gut microbiome. In turn, this can lead to poor skin health and possibly weight gain. Read the nutrition facts carefully and opt for products with limited ingredients as often as possible.

BUY NUTS IN BULK AND FREEZE

A great way to save money on nuts is to buy them in bulk, then pull out what you need each week and store the rest in your freezer. This helps prevent them from oxidizing and going bad. Nuts stored in your freezer may last up to a year, depending on the specific nut.

NUT AND SEED BUTTERS

Nut and seed butters are used in many Fab Four Smoothie recipes and can be part of a Fab Four bridge snack. For people other than Plant-Based Devotees, I consider nuts and seeds (and their respective butters) part of the fat category. In general, the same guidelines for nuts and seeds discussed in this chapter also apply to nut and seed butters. One exciting development to share: I've partnered with Wild Friends to develop a new line of nut and seed butters. We've created some really fun, clean, and delicious blends that can be added to any Fab Four Smoothie or eaten as a bridge snack, like a rich, creamy almond and macadamia nut blend and a crunchy super seed blend with chia, flax, and almonds. See them all at www.wildfriends.com.

ingredients, maximum: nuts, salt, and maybe organic spices. If you see any of the bad oils on page 82 listed in the ingredients, steer clear. These man-made industrial seed and vegetable oils are unhealthy for many reasons. Also, I would avoid any added, refined, and processed sugars (such as high-fructose corn syrup).

BODY-LOVING PLANT-BASED SEED OPTIONS:
Hemp Seeds, Hemp Hearts, Sunflower Seeds, Pumpkin Seeds, Pepitas, and Watermelon Seeds

Hemp seeds and hemp hearts pack a solid protein punch: 9 grams per ounce. The seeds are crunchy and best used as a salad topping. The hemp heart is the inside of the seed and has a much softer texture, which makes it a more versatile topping for smoothies, desserts, and hot and cold dishes. Sunflower seeds provide 5.5 grams of protein per ounce. Pepitas are green seeds without hulls found inside certain types of pumpkins (oilseed and Styrian); other pumpkins contain seeds with hulls. Both are good sources of protein and average 5 to 7 grams of protein per ounce. Watermelon seeds contain 5 grams of protein per ounce. As usual, I prefer raw and certified organic seeds. If you're wondering about chia or flaxseeds, I consider them part of the fiber category and discuss them in chapter 3.

A word of caution: don't mistake seed oils for seeds. They're not the same thing. Man-made industrial seed and vegetable oils are inflammatory omega-6s and not good for you. They oxidize quickly and turn into harmful free radicals. If you see any of the following on the list of ingredients, steer clear: peanut oil, cottonseed oil, grapeseed oil, canola oil, vegetable oil, safflower oil, sunflower oil, corn oil, soybean oil, palm oil, and anything hydrogenated or partially hydrogenated. Another word of caution: many of these oils are used and then reused in the preparation of deep-fried fast food. A 2019 study published in the journal *Cancer Prevention Research* found that mice who were fed reused soybean oil had four times the metastatic growth of breast cancer cells compared with mice who were fed fresh soybean oil. Another reason to skip the drive-through!

BODY-LOVING PLANT-BASED BEAN/ LEGUME OPTIONS: Lentils, Black Beans, Cannellini (White) Beans, Chickpeas, Navy Beans, Kidney Beans, and Pinto Beans

If you're vegetarian or vegan, you're probably familiar with the concept of pairing or combining incomplete proteins as a way to create a complete protein meal. For example: rice and black beans; hummus (chickpeas and sesame seeds); a nut mix that contains peanuts (which is a legume); or lentil soup thickened with cashew cream. However, I wouldn't stress about trying to create a complete protein meal for every single meal of the day. Your liver absorbs essential amino acids, and as long as you're eating a mix of plant-based proteins throughout the day, studies have shown that you don't need to pair at every single meal; your body has the ability to pair internally. The key is to eat a mix of plant-based proteins throughout the day (as usual, I prefer certified organic bean/legume options). The amino acid chart on pages 63–66 will give you some ideas on how to do this.

One potential downside of pairing plant-based proteins at every meal is that it may cause you to overconsume grains, which will raise your blood sugar. If your goal is weight loss or improved body composition, I would limit grains to ¼ to ½ cup per meal and preferably once per day. Jenny, age thirty-one, a stylist who had initially lost weight by eliminating meat from her diet, came to me confused by some sudden weight gain and inflammation. I quickly discovered she was relying too heavily on pairing quinoa and rice with her beans to create a complete protein. I told her to reduce her grain intake to once per day maximum and up her intake of nuts, seeds, and beans for more protein. With that quick adjustment, Jenny was down six pounds in a week.

Bioavailability refers to the degree and rate at which a nutrient can be absorbed. Nutrients that can be quickly and easily absorbed into the body are more bioavailable. Those that take longer or are more difficult are less bioavailable. Bioavailability is just as, if not more, important than nutritional density. The reason is that you can absorb and use only what is bioavailable. On page 114 I discuss the use of digestive enzymes as a way to increase the bioavailability of the nutrients in your food.

In a study in *The American Journal of Clinical Nutrition*, two groups of participants ate the same amount of protein. The difference was their diet. One group ate an animal-based diet, and the other group was placed on a vegetarian diet consisting of plants, grains, dairy, and eggs. The study found that participants in the animal-based group gained more lean muscle mass than the vegetarian group. Many have pointed to this study as showing that the bioavailability of nutrients from plant sources is lower than animal sources.

Two easy methods to increase the bioavailability of nutrients in plant-based sources are soaking and sprouting, simple techniques that unlock the enzymes and nutrients in nuts, seeds, beans/legumes, and grains. These foods contain natural agents whose job is to prevent premature germination or growth. The problem is that these agents prevent access to vitamins and minerals. In addition, they can cause digestive problems. Take phytic acid, for example. This enzyme inhibitor is known as an "antinutrient" because it can block the absorption of minerals. By soaking and sprouting, you can naturally neutralize and eliminate it from the plant. In the process, you unlock vitamins and minerals. You also support the growth of digestive enzymes that increase bioavailability even more.

SOAKING AND SPROUTING

Soaking is as easy as it gets. After a quick rinse, you can soak nuts, seeds, beans/legumes, or grains in three simple steps:

1. Place the item to be soaked in a glass jar or bowl. Add room temperature filtered water (enough to cover) and ½ teaspoon pink Himalayan salt. Cover with a mesh lid or cloth.

2. Let soak. A good rule of thumb is about 8 hours, but you can go as long as 12 hours (overnight) or as few as 4 hours.

3. Drain and discard the soaking water and thoroughly rinse the food.

After soaking, you have 24 hours to consume, cook, or dehydrate the activated "nonsprouts." To save nuts for snacking, you need to completely dry them out, otherwise they will grow mold. Place the nuts on a baking sheet in your oven at 150°F for 24 hours, or if your oven doesn't go that low, 350°F for 10 to 12 minutes. You can also use a food dehydrator at 115°F for 12 to 24 hours. (The lower temperatures are better at helping keep enzymes alive.) Dried nuts should be sealed in a glass container or jar and then stored in your refrigerator. Also, soaked grains need a 1:1 grain-to-water ratio to cook because they contain water from soaking.

Sprouting is nearly as easy. There are just a few extra steps, and the main difference is time—it takes two to three days. Most people sprout seeds, beans/legumes, and grains. Not all nuts will sprout, and if they do, the sprouts may end up more like nubs. Below are general instructions for sprouting seeds, beans/legumes, and grains:

1. Start by soaking. Follow the three-step soaking process above.

2. Place the item to be sprouted in a glass sprouting jar, preferably one with a wide mouth and a breathable mesh lid.

3. Add room temperature filtered water (enough to cover). Screw the lid in place.

(continued)

> Gently shake the jar. Drain and discard the water through the mesh lid. Invert the jar and lay it at an angle so that air can circulate and excess water can fully drain out. Then place the jar upright. Repeat this step three or four times per day for two to three days.
>
> 4. Within a day or two, sprouts should begin to form. The longer you let the sprouts grow, the more enzyme activity there will be. The goal is for the sprouts to be at least ¼ inch long. That's when you'll really start to unlock vitamins and minerals. Some sprouts may grow as long as 2 inches.
>
> 5. Thoroughly rinse the sprouts and refrigerate them in an airtight jar with a solid lid. Enjoy within two to three days. You can eat the whole thing—the seed, bean/legume, grain, and the sprout.

Without soaking and sprouting, vitamins and minerals are not as bioavailable and enzyme inhibitors will impair their absorption. But the good news is that enzyme inhibitors shouldn't affect your future meals. If you don't have the time to soak and sprout (or just don't want to), you can always buy presoaked or presprouted nuts, seeds, beans/legumes, or grains.

Canned beans cannot be soaked and sprouted, but they're a fast alternative that still gives you protein. Just make sure the canned beans you buy have four ingredients maximum: beans, water, possibly salt, and maybe organic spices. If you're committed to a plant-based lifestyle, then long term I would try to make your own beans in bulk instead of buying them in cans.

As for refried beans, skip the canned version. It's really easy to make them at home with clean, healthy oils. All you need is cooked or canned pinto or black beans, 1 to 2 tablespoons of avocado oil, and the taco mix on page 183 of *Body Love*. Add the avocado oil and seasoning to the beans, then just smash and cook them in a pan.

Of note: if a nut is pasteurized (heated to kill bacteria), it won't be able to sprout. By law, all California almonds must be pasteurized. This is the result of several salmonella outbreaks. California accounts for the majority of the country's almond supply, so this is a big deal. However, soaking your almonds can still help neutralize and eliminate enzyme inhibitors and make nutrients more bioavailable.

CHOOSING A PROTEIN POWDER

The Fab Four Smoothie is one of my favorite body-loving tools. It's a quick, easy, and effective way to nourish and fuel your body with the Fab Four, balance your blood sugar, and set yourself up for everyday success. I want you to truly love and enjoy drinking your smoothies, which is why I've created more than eighty delicious recipes for your taste buds here and in *Body Love*. It starts with your protein powder—if you love your protein powder, you're going to love your Fab Four Smoothies. Thankfully, the days of having to force down chalky, lumpy protein powders that taste like medicine are gone. Today there are smooth, flavorful options that all taste phenomenal. You won't even notice they're there—all you'll say is yum.

But before we dive into it, let me reiterate a key point from *Body Love*: the Fab Four Smoothie is not a blanket substitute for eating regular meals and whole foods.

FAB FOUR SMOOTHIE FORMULA

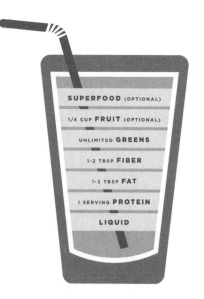

SUPERFOOD (OPTIONAL)

1/4 CUP FRUIT (OPTIONAL)

UNLIMITED GREENS

1-2 TBSP FIBER

1-2 TBSP FAT

1 SERVING PROTEIN

LIQUID

The Fab Four lifestyle is not a smoothie diet. It's about eating balanced meals consisting of real, anti-inflammatory, and whole foods that contain the four essential macronutrients our body needs. The Fab Four Smoothie is a tool to help you do that. Every single Fab Four Smoothie recipe includes whole foods. Take a look and you'll see: leafy greens like spinach, kale, and micro- greens; chia seeds and flaxseeds; avocado; lemon and lime; cucumber; herbs like mint, basil, and parsley; hemp hearts; cacao nibs; almond butter and peanut

> ## FAB FOUR HACK: PRESPROUTED DRY GOODS
>
> If you don't have the time to soak and sprout your own dry goods, I would consider buying presprouted products. Check your local health food store or go online to Thrive Market or Amazon and look for these brands: NOW Foods, Thrive Market, Go Raw, Lundberg, and TrūRoots. You can find almost everything under the sun, including sprouted sunflower seeds, pumpkin seeds, beans, lentils, quinoa, and rice (brown, basmati, red, short-grain).

butter; shredded coconut and coconut yogurt; slivered almonds and chopped walnuts; seasonal fruit like apple or peach; fiber and phytochemical-rich raspberries, blueberries, blackberries, and strawberries; and spices like cinnamon, nutmeg, and ginger.

Why am I reiterating this? Because the way I look at it, *your protein powder should simply be protein*, not an excessively fortified supplement that's stuffed with ingredients and trying to replicate every whole food under the sun. That's my starting point for choosing a protein powder.

So how do you find the one that's right for you? It can be a challenge, with so many different types and brands out there to choose from. For starters, it's important to realize that there's no such thing as a perfect protein powder. There are benefits and drawbacks to every type and every brand. As a result, you might have to make certain trade-offs, depending on what's most important to you.

Further, it's important to remember that research is always ongoing and our knowledge landscape is constantly evolving. What we accept today might be called into question tomorrow. As you know, this is true of nearly everything in health, food, and nutrition, not just protein powders. The key is to stay open-minded, listen to what the latest research says, and be willing to adapt. As new studies are published and more research is completed, my thinking and opinions might change and evolve, just like yours.

CHOOSING A PLANT-BASED MILK

I use a plant-based milk as the liquid base for my Fab Four Smoothies. With so many options on the market, it can be hard to decide what type and brand to use. Here are a few pointers. First, I don't look to my plant-based milk to add significant nutritional value. It's there primarily as a creamy flavored base. And even that isn't mandatory—you can always use filtered water in place of the milk in any Fab Four Smoothie. Second, I look for brands with minimal ingredients, ideally just the source (nut, seed, or grain) and water. Many brands add a thickener or emulsifier for consistency and to prevent separation. These will be listed in the ingredients and are typically a type of gum, lecithin, or fiber. I opt for brands that use two thickeners or emulsifiers maximum. Third, avoid milks that have added sugar or oils (prevalent in oat milk), or that are fortified with added vitamins, minerals, or protein. Just like my advice regarding protein powders, I believe that less is more. Beware of "barista blends," which might foam up for a latte but contain lots of added sugar. Fourth, as usual, I prefer certified organic options.

I recommend that my clients use nut- and seed-based milks like almond, cashew, coconut, walnut, hemp, or flax. Most of the recipes in this book and in *Body Love* use unsweetened almond or coconut milk, but you can swap for another option if you prefer. Just follow the pointers here. For a homemade formula, see the Domestic Goddess plan, page 205. I'm not opposed to grain-based milks like rice and oat, but they're not my first choice because they're less nutrient-dense. Don't use cow milk or any other dairy-based liquid.

My goal is to offer some simple guidance and basic knowledge, so you feel more empowered to choose what's right for you and your lifestyle. First, I'll walk you through some of the factors I consider when selecting a protein powder. Then, I'll discuss several animal- and plant-based options. On the animal side, I'll cover collagen, bone broth, beef, and whey. On the plant-based side, I'll cover certified organic pea protein and minimal plant-based blends. For each type, I'll highlight some key characteristics and pros and cons to be aware of. Then I'll share a few brands I've used and recommended to my clients.

Here are some of the main factors I consider when selecting a protein powder:

WHAT'S THE SOURCE? Where does this protein come from—what kind of animal or what type of plant? There are many different sources out there. Currently, my favorite six are collagen, bone broth, beef, whey, pea, and minimal plant-based blends. Together, they provide a range of options for different lifestyles, including vegetarian and vegan. My current second team would include egg white, brown rice, and hemp hearts (not hemp protein powder). Finally, two protein powders that I don't recommend are soy and casein.

WHAT ARE THE OTHER INGREDIENTS? Always read the list of ingredients (this applies to all the foods you buy, not just protein powder). It's impossible to go through every single ingredient you might ever see, but here are a few tips. (1) The first ingredient listed should always be the protein. After all, if you're buying collagen protein powder, you want the main ingredient to be collagen, not something else. (2) You don't want any added, refined, or processed sugars. Be on the lookout and avoid the following: fructose, cane sugar, cocoa sugar, maltodextrin, and sneaky names for sugar like "juice," "syrup," and "concentrate." Ideally, look for options that use monk fruit or stevia as the sweetener. (3) When in doubt, research it. A few people with online resources are Dr. Mark Hyman and Chris Kresser.

HOW MANY INGREDIENTS ARE THERE? In my opinion, the fewer the better. Some of the cleanest, most nutritious, and best-tasting options have as few as five or six ingredients. I've seen some protein powders that contain thirty or forty ingredients, which is too many in my opinion. The more ingredients, the greater the chance of contamination, and the protein powder is more likely to include unnecessary additives, fillers, and fortifiers.

FOR BLENDS, HOW MANY PROTEINS ARE USED? Some protein powders contain a blend of proteins. For example, a plant-based blend might have pea protein and brown rice protein. I'm okay with blends, but prefer four proteins maximum. I think more than that is unnecessary.

WHAT IS THE AMINO ACID PROFILE? Does it match your needs? This will depend on your specific body and health goals. If you want to go to this level of detail and analysis, you should consult with a functional medical doctor or a doctor with a fellowship in functional medicine. In the meantime, the chart on pages 63–66 can be a helpful place to start learning about the different amino acids.

HOW BIOAVAILABLE IS THE PROTEIN? In other words, how easily and quickly can it be digested and absorbed into the body for utilization? Some types of protein are more bioavailable than others. There are two bioavailability scales you can reference. Neither is perfect, but they offer another data input to consider. One is biological value (BV), which has a scale of 0 to 100, with 100 being ideal. Another is the protein digestibility–corrected amino acid score (PDCAAS), which has a scale of 0 to 1.0, with 1.0 being ideal.

HOW WAS THE PROTEIN EXTRACTED? There are multiple methods to extract the protein from an animal or plant source. Enzymatic processing involves the use of naturally occurring enzymes. Microfiltration and nanofiltration are cold, cross-flow processes. Some protein powders use a chemical to extract the protein. Many plant-based protein powders are processed with hexane, a chemical neurotoxin derived from petroleum. Others use sodium hydroxide, which is seen as less toxic than hexane. There are also methods that involve high heat, which is problematic for several reasons. High heat oxidizes cholesterol and fat and can lead to the denaturation (breakdown) of the protein. When protein is denatured, amino acids and nutrients are destroyed. For instance, one potential casualty can be glutamylcysteine, a precursor to the antioxidant glutathione.

HOW CLEAN ARE THE INGREDIENTS, AND COULD TOXINS BE PRESENT? No protein powder is perfect. For example, according to the Clean Label Project, some plant-based and certified organic protein powders may contain higher levels of heavy metals (lead, cadmium, and arsenic) than animal or nonorganic options. What's in the soil ends up in the plant, and buying organic won't prevent heavy metal absorption. It's important to be aware of the potential risks, so you can make a more fully informed decision. For more information, see the Clean Label Project

UNDENATURED WHEY

Some whey protein powders will say they're undenatured on their packaging or website. This means that the whey was pasteurized at a lower temperature. As you may recall, pasteurization is the process of heating a food to eliminate microbes and other potentially harmful bacteria. Typically, it's done at 160°F. Undenatured whey is pasteurized at about 145°F, and this lower heat results in less denaturation. One hundred percent undenatured dairy would be raw milk straight from the cow's udder.

(www.cleanlabelproject.org) or the NSF International's Certified for Sport certification program (www.nsfsport.com/our-mark.php).

WHO MAKES IT? I try to buy from reputable companies with good manufacturing practices, high quality-control standards, and a good history in terms of contamination and health issues. NOW Foods and Primal Kitchen stand out, which is one of the main reasons I partnered with them.

HOW MUCH DOES IT COST? Protein powder can range anywhere from twenty to eighty dollars per 24 ounces, depending on the type, brand, and quality. Most of the brands I've named (see pages 57 to 62) fall somewhere in the middle, between forty and sixty dollars.

HOW DOES IT TASTE, AND WHAT IS THE TEXTURE AND CONSISTENCY? Over the years, I've tried countless protein powders. The brands I recommend have some of the best flavor, smoothest texture, and nicest consistency in my opinion.

Now let's go through a few animal-based options:

COLLAGEN protein powder is primarily derived from the collagen protein found in cows and fish. In cows, it comes from around bones, ligaments, tendons, and other body parts. I prefer grass-fed if I'm buying a cow/bovine collagen. In fish, it comes from bones and skin. Collagen can also be derived from chicken and pork, though it's less prevalent. There is no vegan collagen.

Collagen is a good source of the amino acids glycine, hydroxyproline, and proline. Among other things, these amino acids support tissue repair, joints, ligaments, tendons, hair, skin, nails, and gut health. Also, our gut bacteria can ferment collagen into butyric acid, which supports our intestinal cells.

One drawback of collagen is that it doesn't contain the essential amino acid tryptophan, which is a precursor to the neurotransmitter serotonin. Serotonin helps regulate a variety of things, including mood, happiness, anxiety, sleep, memory, and appetite. Lack of tryptophan is cited as one main reason for collagen having a PDCAAS of 0. Factors within your body that could limit the bioavailability of collagen include vitamin C deficiency or a lack of stomach acid and digestive enzymes.

There are five main types of collagen. They all contain a beneficial blend of amino acids, but each is most supportive of the specific organs from which the type is derived. The majority of collagen protein powders are type I, which is derived from and supports bones, ligaments, tendons, organs, and skin. Type II supports joint health and cartilage. If you have rheumatoid arthritis or osteoarthritis, you want a mixed collagen blend with both type I and type II. Type III is found in the liver, bone marrow, and lymph (the fluid in the lymph system). Type IV is found in the respiratory and intestinal tract. Type V is found in your hair and on cell surfaces.

Below are two brands I have used and the types of collagen they contain:

- Primal Kitchen Collagen Fuel (types I and III)
- Dr. Axe Multi-Collagen Protein (types I through V)

BONE BROTH protein powder hasn't been around for very long, so the data regarding its benefits, bioavailability, and amino acid profile is based on bone broth itself. One of the reasons I like it is that the processing is straightforward and clean—it's simply dehydrated bone broth. Unlike the meat of an animal, the bone broth isn't a complete protein on its own. However, it still comes with cysteine, glutamic acid, and glycine, the amino acids needed to produce glutathione, our most potent antioxidant. If you want to try bone broth protein powder, I would try to source grass-fed beef or pasture-raised chicken options. (I have had a small number of clients who want to avoid powders altogether. If you fall into this camp, you can replace the liquid in your smoothie with 2 cups of regular bone broth; just realize that it will take on the flavor!)

- NOW Sports (beef or chicken powder)
- Thrive Market Organic Bone Broth Protein (beef)
- Ancient Nutrition Bone Broth Protein (chicken)

BEEF protein isolate is derived from cow flesh and is a dairy-, nut-, and legume-free option for those with tolerability issues. The processing is relatively straightforward: the beef is boiled down into a nutrient-rich liquid and then the carbohydrate and fat content is skimmed and discarded. After drying, the result is protein that is rich in essential and branched-chain amino acids. In terms of bioavailability, it scores well: 80 on the BV scale and a 0.92 PDCAAS.

Below are two brands I have used:

- Fab Four Protein by Kelly Leveque
- PaleoPro Paleo Protein Powder (contains a small amount of egg white protein as well)

WHEY protein is derived from cow dairy and is a by-product of making cheese. Sometimes it gets a bad rap, but whey can be a clean and nutritious option for people without dairy allergies. Whey is antimicrobial, supports the immune system, and has a great amino acid profile, including branched-chain amino acids. In terms of bioavailability, it scores very high: 104 on the BV scale and a 1.0 PDCAAS. I prefer whey from grass-fed cows. In terms of processing, I try to source brands that use microfiltration or nanofiltration. These cold, cross-flow processes preserve amino acids and prevent the denaturation of the protein via heat. (Remember, high heat can break the protein down and destroy amino acids.)

There are several types of whey. Whey concentrate is 80 percent protein, contains branched-chain amino acids and glutamine, and has minimal fat and lactose. Whey isolate must be 90 percent protein or more. There's additional filtration involved, so there's even less fat and lactose. It depends on your specific body and condition, but some people with a lactose sensitivity or intolerance may be able to tolerate whey isolate. Whey protein hydrolysate (WPH) is whey isolate that has been "predigested" by enzymes and not something I recommend. The thinking behind doing this is that smaller peptides result in faster absorption by the body. One downside is that some nutrients are lost in the predigestion. In addition, it can result in a flood of protein into your bloodstream. Your body might respond like you just ingested a starchy carbohydrate, releasing large amounts of insulin and storing the protein, not using it to build or repair muscle. (Remember, insulin is a storage hormone.) Also, it's not my first choice, but if you're adamantly against powders, you can use a plain grass-fed Greek yogurt in place of a whey protein powder; just recognize that you will be ingesting more allergens and carbohydrates.

Below are five options I have used and the type of whey they contain:

- NOW Sports Grass-Fed Whey Protein (vanilla or unflavored; concentrate)
- Tera's Whey Organic Whey Protein (concentrate)
- Natural Force Organic Whey (concentrate)
- Tera's Whey Simply Pure Whey Protein (isolate)
- Biochem 100% Whey Protein (isolate)

Do you love (or miss) cereal? Try Magic Spoon, a whey protein cereal that checks all the boxes: it's high in protein, low in net carbohydrates, and tastes amazing. It can be a fun topping for a Fab Four Smoothie Bowl or eaten as a bridge snack post-workout. (Use the code BEWELLBYKELLY on their website, www.magic spoon.com, for a discount.)

Next, let's go through the plant-based options I prefer: certified organic pea protein and minimal plant-based blends.

PEA protein is derived from peas and is naturally soy-, gluten-, and dairy-free. It has branched-chain amino acids but isn't a complete protein with all nine essential amino acids. In terms of bioavailability, it scores 65 on the BV scale and a 0.893 PDCAAS. One study found that pea protein may help eliminate free radicals and heavy metals and may stop the oxidation of linoleic acid. Another study found that pea protein was comparable to dairy protein in releasing satiety hormones such as CCK, GLP-1, and PYY. However, pea protein may contain phytic acid and oligosaccharides, which could block the absorption of nutrients and cause bloating.

Below are two brands I use and like:

- NOW Sports Organic Pea Protein

PLANT-BASED BLENDS are just what they sound like: blends of two or more plant proteins. As I mentioned on page 56, I'm okay with blends, but prefer if they contain no more than four proteins.

Below are two brands I have used and the proteins they contain:

- NOW Sports Organic Plant Protein (pea and brown rice)
- Tone It Up Organic Protein (pea and pumpkin seed)
- Truvani Certified Organic Plant-Based Protein

OTHER PROTEIN POWDERS. What about my second team? **Egg white protein** scores well in terms of bioavailability, but it's not a main go-to for me because you miss out on the B vitamins, choline, and healthy fat in the egg yolk and also because of the allergen risk. **Brown rice protein** is an incomplete protein and low in the essential amino acid lysine. However, some research has suggested it can help regulate glucose levels, aid in weight loss, and have similar effectiveness to whey. You'll find brown rice protein in a lot of plant-based blends. It's a tier-two option for me because it can be higher in heavy metals than pea or other plant sources, which is also why I don't recommend it for women who are pregnant or breastfeeding. Though hemp is anti-inflammatory and full of fiber, **hemp protein powder** can be low in protein compared with other vegan options. As an alternative, try using 3 tablespoons of hemp hearts, which will give you more protein as well as fat. Also, while **spirulina** and **chlorella** are great additions to a smoothie, I wouldn't use these detoxifying algae superfoods as a primary source of protein. They have been studied only in small doses, and their capacity to bind to chemicals (like chemotherapy agents) and heavy metals make them a poor choice for daily consumption, especially if your body doesn't do a good job of eliminating them. Other sources have higher protein density.

Finally, I would skip **soy and casein protein powders**. As I mentioned on page 45, I generally don't recommend soy products as part of the Fab Four lifestyle. This includes **soy protein powder**. Soy is an endocrine disruptor and has been linked to a number of health issues. It's also genetically modified and known to be treated with the pesticide glyphosate. Casein is another protein derived from dairy. A-1 casein has been linked to type 2 diabetes and heart disease. A few studies have also linked casein supplementation to the spread of prostate cancer cells. It's also a potential allergen. For these reasons, it's not one I prefer at this time.

In the chart that follows, I've summarized the key twenty amino acids and highlighted body-loving animal- and plant-based protein sources for each.

Amino Acid	Type	Benefits	Animal Sources	Plant Sources
Isoleucine	Essential Branched-chain	Aids muscle recovery; stimulates release of human growth hormone (HGH); helps regulate blood sugar levels; helps in formation of hemoglobin and the body's coagulation efforts	All animal protein sources*	Almonds, cashews, lentils
Leucine	Essential Branched-chain	Regulates blood sugar levels; increases energy and stamina; promotes growth and repair of skin, bones, and skeletal muscles; increases HGH production	All animal protein sources*	Nuts, beans, brown rice
Lysine	Essential	Aids muscle growth; supports calcium absorption (which aids bone and muscle growth and fat burning); used to produce antibodies; supports hormones (HGH, testosterone, and insulin), enzymes, and collagen to repair damaged tissue	All animal protein sources*	Pistachios, pumpkin seeds, watermelon seeds, lentils, pinto beans, kidney beans, black beans
Methionine	Essential	Helps metabolize fat; improves digestion; promotes production of creatine monohydrate (for energy and muscle growth); helps eliminate toxins; protects the liver and brain; increases skin elasticity	All animal protein sources*	Sesame seeds, sunflower butter, Brazil nuts, seaweed, oats

(continued)

Amino Acid	Type	Benefits	Animal Sources	Plant Sources
Phenylalanine	Essential	With tyrosine, increases levels of norepinephrine and dopamine (which regulate mood); with glutamine, helps increase memory	All animal protein sources*	Avocado, almonds, nuts and seeds, quinoa, lentils, black beans, kidney beans, teff
Threonine	Essential	Necessary for collagen and elastin production; supports immune system; protects against fatty liver disease	All animal protein sources*	Pumpkin seeds, watermelon seeds, sunflower seeds, black beans, chickpeas, lentils
Tryptophan	Essential	Promotes production of vitamin B_3; in forms L-tryptophan and 5-hydroxytryptophan (5-HTP) helps form serotonin (a neurotransmitter that supports mood)	All animal protein sources*	Chia seeds, sesame seeds, sunflower seeds, flaxseeds, pistachios, buckwheat, beans
Valine	Essential Branched-chain	Promotes muscle growth and repair; provides an energy source for muscles	All animal protein sources*	Quinoa, millet, beans, lentils, teff, pumpkin seeds, pepitas, pistachios, mushrooms
Alanine	Nonessential	Increases muscle capacity; elevates carnosine, which supports muscle enzymes	Beef, lamb, chicken, turkey, pork, fish	Spinach, asparagus, beans, seeds, watercress
Arginine	Nonessential	Supports production of HGH; supports T-cell function (for immunity); precursor to nitric oxide, which regulates blood vessel flexibility (blood flow, blood pressure); assists detoxification	Chicken, turkey, pork	Nuts, seeds, rice, chocolate, chickpeas, spirulina, lentils
Asparagine	Nonessential	Supports the central nervous system; protects the liver; supports production of other amino acids in the body	Beef, chicken, turkey, fish, seafood, eggs	Asparagus, beans/legumes, nuts, seeds

Amino Acid	Type	Benefits	Animal Sources	Plant Sources
Aspartic acid	Nonessential	Supports health of central nervous system; supports functioning of DNA and RNA; aids production of antibodies and immunoglobin	Beef, lamb, chicken, turkey, eggs	Rice, amaranth, barley, millet, buckwheat
Cysteine	Nonessential	Supports function of T-cells for adaptive immunity; supports production of glutathione (our key antioxidant)	Chicken, turkey, pork, eggs	Broccoli, garlic, red pepper, onion
Glutamic acid	Nonessential	Serves as a chemical messenger in the brain that supports alertness, thinking, and mood; aids muscle recovery; supports carbohydrate metabolism	Fish, shrimp	Green tea, beans, oats, spirulina
Glutamine	Nonessential	Supports production of GABA (gamma-aminobutyric acid),† a key neurotransmitter that supports mental acuity, sleep, and mood; aids memory recall and concentration; regulates nitrogen levels and alkaline/acid balance; serves as a key building block of DNA and RNA; supports gut lining and gut health; supports liver detoxification; improves immune function	Meat, poultry	Broccoli, cabbage, asparagus, spirulina
Glycine	Nonessential	Contributes to protein synthesis; increases HGH; supports lean muscle mass; helps decrease inflammation and stabilize blood sugar levels; aids in mental performance	Collagen, bone broth, small amounts in other animal proteins	Spinach, kale, cauliflower, cabbage, pumpkin

(continued)

Amino Acid	Type	Benefits	Animal Sources	Plant Sources
Proline	Nonessential	Promotes cell regeneration, tissue repair, and collagen production; increases arterial elasticity; supports blood pressure	Collagen, bone broth, small amounts in other animal proteins	Asparagus, cabbage, mushrooms, spirulina, bamboo shoots
Serine	Nonessential	Promotes cell membrane health; supports DNA	Turkey, fish, eggs	Asparagus, kidney beans, spirulina
Tyrosine	Nonessential	Serves as a precursor to dopamine, our happy or reward hormone	Beef, lamb, chicken, turkey, fish, pork, eggs	Peanuts, pumpkin

* Note that not all animal-based protein powders contain all nine essential amino acids. For example, collagen protein powder doesn't contain tryptophan. Unfortunately, this type of information may not appear on the product label or nutrition facts. To determine whether a particular product has all nine essential amino acids, you may need to consult with the specific manufacturer or check their website.

† GABA can be found in beef, eggs, shrimp, fermented foods such as kefir and kombucha, and mushrooms.

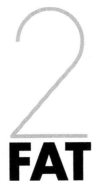

FAT

GOOD FOR BRAIN HEALTH AND MAKES YOU FULL, NOT FAT!

THE SECOND PILLAR OF the Fab Four is fat. A lot of my clients are afraid of eating fat. You might be, too, and it's not your fault. For decades, fat has been marketed as bad for us. It's an easy sell, and unfortunately it works. Take a stroll down the aisle of a typical grocery store, and you'll see foods labeled as "fat free" or "low fat." The message has been reinforced for years in commercials and other mass advertising. It's no help that a large data set that challenged the long-held view that saturated fat resulted in a higher incidence of heart attack and fatality wasn't published until over forty years after it was collected (this is the Minnesota Coronary Experiment). No wonder the idea has become so deeply ingrained. Putting aside the misinformation that is out there, I'll just stick to the science and say three things: (1) this way of thinking is based on old, outdated, and incomplete research; (2) it ignores *healthy* fats that exist in nature; and (3) the unhealthy, "bad" fats are actually man-made (these are trans fats and industrial seed and vegetable oils, which I discuss on page 82).

Eating healthy fat doesn't make you fat; it can actually support healthy weight loss efforts. Again, this goes back to blood sugar, satiety, and hunger hormones. As discussed in Blood Sugar 101, fat supports blood sugar balance. It doesn't break down into glucose, so it doesn't raise your blood sugar or cause the release of insulin. Fat helps slow digestion as a whole and lowers fasting insulin levels. It also causes the release of two satiety hormones, leptin and cholecystokinin (CCK), which help us feel full and satisfied. By having a neutral effect on blood sugar, slowing digestion, and suffusing the body with satiety hormones, fat helps us stay full in between meals and elongates our blood sugar curve. If your goal is weight loss or improved body composition, fat is very important.

BUT WHAT ABOUT ALL THE CALORIES?

Many of my clients are afraid to eat fat because it has more calories than other types of food. But not all calories are created equal, and a randomized 2018 clinical trial published in the *Journal of the American Medical Association* backs this up. The "DIETFITS" study had more than 600 participants replace added sugar and refined grains with whole foods—without worrying about counting calories or limiting portion sizes. Both groups of participants (low carb and low fat) lost a significant amount of weight. Quality whole foods will always trump quantity, and calorie counting is one of the ways many diets steer you wrong. Yet, just like the idea that fat is bad for us, the concept of needing to count calories and eat a low-calorie diet has become deeply and mistakenly ingrained. The latest research shows the negative health consequences that can result from calorie counting. (I am not talking about intermittently fasting.) Constantly restricting calories and chronic calorie deficits have been found to decrease metabolism and cause hormonal imbalances throughout the body, such as reduced active thyroid hormone function, the shutdown of sex hormone production, and the excessive release of cortisol (our stress hormone) by the adrenals. Chronically elevated cortisol levels may lead to both insulin resistance and leptin resistance.

The result of all these hormonal changes? Stalled weight loss, body fat retention, nutrient deficiencies, and other negative health effects. If you've been eating less and not losing weight, this could be what's plaguing you. Eating healthy fat keeps you out of the deficit zone (both in terms of energy levels and nutrients), which helps keep your metabolism strong and prevents hormonal imbalances. More important, healthy fat found in whole foods is good for you. It's a body-loving macronutrient. So don't count calories or fear healthy fat. You need them both.

Kimmy, age twenty-eight, a singer, was getting ready for a summer tour and wanted to look her best, so she decided to start counting calories. The first thing she cut back on was fat. What she didn't realize was that she had begun to re-place those calories with processed foods like popcorn and protein bars, and now her blood sugar curve was erratic. Inflammation ensued, and the nutrients needed to feed her cells and microbiome were scarce. The worst part was that her hunger (and mood) were now unpredictable. She was constantly left unprepared and looking for a stopgap. So I asked her to do something that sounded counterintui-tive to her: eat more whole food calories at every meal. She went back to healthy fats, stuck to the Fab Four, and lost seven pounds in a month. Even though she was eating more, she had changed the hormonal and inflammatory environment in her body, which unlocked the weight loss.

Fat is part of the Fab Four because it's the catalyst for vibrant, optimal health. It will truly help you thrive. Fat breaks down into fatty acids, which are essential to our overall health and play a crucial role in how the body functions. They enable hormone production, support brain health and cognitive ability, and help reduce the risk of disease. They support our immune system and metabolism, aid in cell development and cell signaling, and reduce inflammation. Fatty acids also allow us to absorb fat-soluble vitamins (such as vitamins A, D, E, and K) and phytochemi-cals (such as lutein, zeaxanthin, and beta-carotene). A lot of people have a vitamin

OTHER BENEFITS OF HEALTHY FAT

Healthy fats have also been linked with cardiovascular protection, improved body composition, easing of depression, cancer prevention, promotion of eye health, preservation of memory, decreased symptoms of ADD and ADHD, and reduced incidence of aggressive behavior. The benefits have even been so significant that at least one active study was ended prematurely. In a 2016 study comparing a high-fat Mediterranean diet with a traditional diet, the Mediterranean group reduced their risk of cardiovascular events (stroke and heart attack) so significantly that it was deemed unethical to allow the traditional group to continue. As you can see, fat affects many different aspects of our overall health and wellness.

D deficiency, and if you're not eating fat you're making it worse. Without healthy sources of fat and the fatty acids they contain, our bodies will function less optimally, and our long-term health will decline.

Fat is an integral part of the body on a cellular level. Our cell membranes are fat-based structures. Healthy fats keep these membranes fluid and flexible, while unhealthy fats cause them to be more rigid and inflexible. Fluid and flexible cell membranes allow the cells to communicate better. Cells are constantly signaling one another and transmitting vital information throughout the body, such as where to direct blood flow and how to adjust inflammation levels, nervous system impulses, respiratory system requirements, and flow of neurotransmitters like serotonin. By supporting cell signaling and communication, healthy fats help the body function more optimally. This is especially critical for the brain, which is mostly fatty tissue. A study out of UCLA showed that a high-fructose diet caused inflammation that actually reprogrammed certain genes responsible for cognitive functioning and metabolic control. For real! The only antidote was squelching the inflammation with DHA—an anti-inflammatory omega-3 fat. Conversely, unhealthy fats can weaken cell signaling and communication, creating rigidity and leading to less optimal functioning and other negative health consequences.

In my practice, I encourage my clients to regularly eat a mix of different healthy fats. *I generally advise them to eat at least 1 to 2 tablespoons of fat per meal, and I'm okay with more, too.* Fat is the second ingredient listed in every single Fab Four Smoothie recipe in this book and in *Body Love*. Many of my clients are initially hesitant to add fat to every meal, but time and again I've watched them do it and experience positive results. I can always tell when a client might be a "scaredy-fat." In our meeting, I discuss the need for fat and then a day or two later, I get a text that says something like, "½ an avocado, really???" My answer is always an all-caps YES. Gwen, age forty, a television producer, avoided all types of fat, fearing that even the healthy kind would lead to weight gain. But once we upped her intake, she felt full and satisfied after each meal and broke her bad habit of snacking on junk food while on set. She lost six pounds in her first month. Her skin had more glow and vibrancy, too.

Healthy fats aren't created in a lab. They're found in nature and come from the foods we eat. In this chapter, I list a number of body-loving foods that contain healthy fat. There are several types of healthy fat: monounsaturated fat, polyunsaturated fat, and saturated fat. One thing to note is that these foods contain multiple types of healthy fat, not just one. For example, on average, avocados contain approximately 70 percent monounsaturated fat, 17 percent polyunsaturated fat, and 8 percent saturated fat. I've mostly categorized foods by their predominant fat. In the chart on page 80, I list different cooking oils and include the average fat breakdown for each. The fat percentages listed in the chart generally apply to the whole food as well. I address cooking oils separately on page 75.

THE SALAD STUDIES

A little fat in your salad can go a long way. One study found that using fat in salad dressing significantly increased the absorption of carotenoids, which are healthy, fat-soluble phytochemicals like lutein, zeaxanthin, alpha-carotene, and beta-carotene. (Lutein and zeaxanthin protect the protein, fat, and DNA in the body. They also work together to fight free radicals and help recycle the body's strongest antioxidant—glutathione.) The study found that fat-free or reduced-fat salad dressings resulted in little or no absorption of these vital nutrients. In another study, one group of participants ate a salad of lettuce, carrot, spinach, and 2½ tablespoons of diced avocado. A second group ate the same salad but without the avocado. The group that ate avocado absorbed eight times more alpha-carotene and thirteen times more beta-carotene than the second group. The takeaway: by using healthy fats in your salad dressing or adding whole food fats to your salad, you can significantly increase nutrient absorption.

BODY-LOVING SOURCES OF MONOUNSATURATED FAT: Almonds, Cashews, Pecans, Macadamia Nuts, Brazil Nuts, Pistachios, and Butters Made from These Nuts; Avocado and Avocado Oil; Olives and Olive Oil; Macadamia Oil; and Algae Oil

Monounsaturated fats are heart-healthy, good for our brain, and full of antioxidants. The oils generally have a shelf life of six to twelve months and are good for salad dressings. For all of these foods, I prefer certified organic options.

Avocado is one of my favorite foods. It's nutritious, versatile, and a great whole food addition to virtually any Fab Four meal or smoothie. Nuts are another great option for healthy fat. As discussed in chapter 1: (1) choose raw or dry-roasted nuts (not roasted); (2) for packaged nuts, make sure there are only three ingredients maximum—the nut and possibly salt and maybe organic spices; and (3) steer clear of any added, refined, and processed sugars, man-made industrial seed and vegetable oils, and anything hydrogenated or partially hydrogenated. (I discuss these unhealthy "bad" fats on page 82.) These tips apply to nut butters as well. It's easy to grab your favorite brand of nut butter only to get home and find it has added bad oils or added sugar. Double-check the ingredients! It can be hard to resist your favorites and easy to justify buying them "one more time." But whether it's in nut butter, granola, sweeteners, or another food, a gram here and a gram there will eventually add up. Buy nuts in bulk, pull out what you need each week, and freeze the rest. This can extend their shelf life.

PEANUTS

Technically, peanuts are legumes, not nuts. Legumes are the seeds of plants in the legume family, which includes beans, peas, and lentils, as well. One common knock against legumes is that they contain antinutrients like phytic acid, which can disrupt digestion and nutrient absorption. In addition, peanuts are more susceptible to mold toxicity and are a common allergen. On the other hand, for kids, husbands, and the family dog, peanuts can be an efficient source of fat, protein, and fiber. Personally, I tend to choose almonds, cashews, pecans, walnuts, and their respective nut butters, but I don't mind my clients eating peanuts or peanut butter. If you buy peanuts or peanut butter, follow the same rules I've specified for nuts and nut butters.

Of note: one type of peanut that may be less susceptible to mold toxicity is the Valencia peanut, which is grown in more arid climates such as New Mexico and Texas. Also, if you're not allergic to peanuts, don't completely cut them out of your diet, because doing so may actually increase your chances of developing an allergy.

BODY-LOVING SOURCES OF POLYUNSATURATED FAT: Walnuts, Hemp Seeds and Hearts, Sunflower Seeds, Pumpkin Seeds, Pepitas, Watermelon Seeds, Sesame Seeds; Butters Made from These Seeds and Nuts; Wild Fish; Fish and Algae Oil Supplements

Walnuts and hemp hearts have 15 grams of fat per ounce, and hemp seeds have 12 grams of fat per ounce. Sunflower seeds, pumpkin seeds, pepitas, watermelon seeds, and sesame seeds average 5 grams of fat per ounce. As usual, seek out organic, raw, and sprouted options when possible.

Fish and algae are the best sources of EPA and DHA, the anti-inflammatory omega-3s that have been linked to numerous health benefits. A few fatty fish I like are wild salmon, sardines, herring, and mackerel (chub or Atlantic). If you're not a fan of eating fish, take fish or krill oil, which is essentially 100 percent healthy fat (see page 42). If you're a Plant-Based Devotee, getting EPA and DHA is critical, and you can get them both directly from algae oil. Nordic Naturals offers a vegan omega-3 from algae. Polyunsaturated fats are always good for eating as whole foods, but the oils generally have a shelf life of only two to six months. Always double-check how long you've had a given oil in the cabinet or pantry so you don't end up eating a rancid oil. As ever, seek out organic options.

KEY FATTY ACIDS DERIVED FROM POLYUNSATURATED FATS

A few highly beneficial fatty acids derived from polyunsaturated fats include:

- EPA (eicosapentaenoic acid), a long-chain omega-3 and powerful anti-inflammatory that reduces inflammation at the cellular level

- DHA (docosahexaenoic acid), a long-chain omega-3 that is vital for brain health, memory and cognition, and neural development

- ALA (alpha-linolenic acid), a short-chain omega-3 that supports cardiovascular health

- LA (linoleic acid), a short-chain omega-6 that has been linked with improved immunity, brain health, and cardiovascular health (I would prioritize eating LA from whole food sources. It can be inflammatory if eaten in excess from man-made industrial seed oils or oils that have gone bad.)

BODY-LOVING SOURCES OF SATURATED
FAT: Grass-Fed Ghee, Grass-Fed Butter,
Pasture-Raised Animal Fats (as Cooking Fats),
Coconut, Coconut Oil, MCT Oil, and MCT Powder

Saturated fats are good for cooking, and the oils generally have a shelf life of twelve to twenty-four months. I prefer to use organic, grass-fed, and pasture-raised products.

Ghee, or clarified butter, is 100 percent fat and is made by removing all of the milk solids (lactose, whey, and casein) from butter. The absence of these solids is what makes ghee healthier and an option for people with lactose intolerance. Ghee is also rich in conjugated linoleic acid (CLA), the only healthy, naturally occurring trans unsaturated fat. It contains vitamins A, E, and K_2, and has butyrate, which may help lower body fat percentage and decrease inflammation. Butter is also body-loving if it's grass-fed and pasture-raised. I cook with both ghee and butter, but I usually prefer using ghee. As for pasture-raised animal fats, I'm referring to cooking fats such as tallow, lard, schmaltz, and duck fat. I discuss these on page 78 in the section on oils.

MCT stands for *medium-chain triglycerides*. MCTs are a form of saturated fatty acid and one of my favorite body-loving fats. They help produce ketones, which serve as fat-based fuel for brains and bodies, and contain lauric acid, a potent antifungal. MCTs support our gut bacteria and gut microbiome and also have certain antioxidant-like benefits. Coconut and coconut oil are both good sources of MCTs, and MCT oil is a highly concentrated version, essentially 100 percent MCTs. More than half of my Fab Four Smoothie recipes incorporate MCT oil, coconut oil, or some form of coconut. In addition, coconut oil and MCT oil can both be blended into a hot beverage such as coffee, tea, matcha, or turmeric latte. (See the Girl on the Go plan, page 150, for recipes.) I use unflavored MCT oil, but flavors such as vanilla or mocha should be okay as long as there's no added sugar. MCT powder packets are convenient for flying or traveling. Some brands also add fiber to the

FAT IN YOUR COFFEE

You might have heard of Bulletproof Coffee, a meal replacement coffee drink created by Dave Asprey. It allows you to have a "fat fast" in the morning. Basically, you're blending MCTs (fat) into your coffee, which gives your body some fuel without spiking your blood sugar. I think it can be used occasionally as a tool, but the minute you start taking liberties with the recipe and adding sweeteners, you are defeating the purpose. And I wouldn't pair it with a full Fab Four breakfast or full Fab Four Smoothie. A few clients have done that every day and their weight has stagnated. If you do have it, consider it your breakfast. The official formula with Bulletproof products is on Dave Asprey's website, www.bulletproof.com. To do it yourself, blend 1 cup of coffee, 1 tablespoon of grass-fed ghee or butter, and 1 tablespoon of MCT oil or coconut oil in a blender.

powder, which is a plus. **Important: MCT oil has a low smoke point and therefore shouldn't be used for high-heat cooking, including sautéing, roasting, baking, or barbecuing. I discuss smoke points on page 79.**

For decades, we've been told saturated fat and cholesterol are the main causes of coronary heart disease and obesity. Yet this hypothesis was based on incomplete research and unpublished data. The Minnesota Coronary Experiment involved more than nine thousand participants. One group ate a diet higher in saturated fat and a second group ate a diet higher in corn oil, a man-made industrial seed oil. Even though the corn oil group's average cholesterol was lower, it had a higher incidence of heart attack and fatality. This challenged the long-held view that saturated fat resulted in a higher incidence of heart attack and fatality. However, this was not made public until over forty years after the data was collected. When you eat saturated fat, dietary cholesterol can only modestly increase, but it won't affect the ratio of good to bad cholesterol or increase the risk of heart disease. Note that the American Heart Association now refers to dietary cholesterol as a nutrient of no concern. Saturated fats can also help lower inflammation.

Here's how to incorporate healthy fats into your Fab Four lifestyle.

YOU SHOULD EAT A MIX OF HEALTHY FATS, NOT JUST ONE. Your body needs a mix of monounsaturated, polyunsaturated, and saturated fats. Even though the foods mentioned in the preceding pages contain all three types, one will usually predominate. For example, avocado contains mostly monounsaturated fat. If the only fat you ever eat is avocado, you'll always get some polyunsaturated and saturated fat, but long term you won't get enough. Can you still eat avocado every day? Yes, but you need to eat other fats as well, such as foods that are higher in polyunsaturated and saturated fat, in order to get a range of fat-soluble antioxidants and fatty acids.

Fats go in and out of style. Ghee and coconut oil became very popular when the paleo lifestyle took off. They're stable oils with good smoke points, making them options for cooking paleo meals. MCT oil surged in popularity with the rise of the ketogenic diet, and Bulletproof Coffee took off because of its efficiency in creating ketones in the body. Olive oil and olives are staples of the Mediterranean diet and come with heart and brain benefits. Whatever your personal preference, you still need to eat a mix of healthy fats. You don't need to obsess regarding eating all three types of healthy fat at every single meal. Instead, strive to eat a balanced mix over the course of a day or every couple days. (There's that Fab Four concept again—balance.) That might look like avocado in your smoothie, olive oil on your salad at lunch, and veggies roasted in ghee at dinner.

DON'T COUNT THE FAT IN YOUR ANIMAL PROTEIN AS YOUR 1 TO 2 TABLE-SPOONS (OR MORE) OF FAT. As discussed in chapter 1, animal protein can be a great source of healthy fat. Pasture-raised eggs and chicken, grass-fed beef, and wild fish are all good sources of the omega-3s EPA and DHA. In addition, grass-fed beef is a good source of conjugated linoleic acid (CLA), the only healthy, naturally occurring trans unsaturated fat. But you shouldn't count the fats in your animal protein as your 1 to 2 tablespoons (or more) of Fab Four fat. You should still use a separate fat source, such as your salad dressing, marinade, cooking oil, or a whole food such as avocado, nuts, or seeds.

On a similar note, as mentioned in chapter 1, if you're eating a plant-based meal and you use nuts or seeds as your protein, I would recommend using a different food from this chapter (and not the same nut or seed) as your fat.

YOU NEED TO EAT WHOLE FOOD FATS, NOT JUST OILS. Even though oils are a great source of healthy fat, you should strive to regularly eat a mix of whole food fats as well. One reason is that whole food fats are generally less oxidized than

THE RIGHT OMEGA-6 TO OMEGA-3 RATIO

To function optimally, our body needs a ratio of about 1:1 of omega-6 fats to omega-3 fats. Due in large part to the overconsumption of man-made industrial seed and vegetable oils (the unhealthy, "bad" fats, which are oxidized omega-6s), many Americans have ratios as high as 15:1 to 20:1, which is way out of balance. Studies have linked elevated omega-6 and deficient omega-3 levels with cardiovascular disease, stroke, autoimmune disorders, and other inflammatory diseases. To help rebalance the ratio, we need to: (1) eat or supplement with EPA and DHA, the omega-3s found in foods such as fish, nuts, and seeds; and (2) decrease our consumption of man-made oxidized omega-6 industrial seed and vegetable oils, such as safflower oil and sunflower oil.

oils. To oxidize means to chemically react with oxygen. Oxidation results in the release of harmful free radicals and other compounds. All food eventually oxidizes, but in whole foods, antioxidants and nutrients such as vitamin E naturally protect against oxidation. Oils are less protected and can oxidize more easily (see the discussion of oils' smoke points on page 79). You don't need to stop eating or cooking with oils, but you need to be aware of the potential for greater oxidation and consider ways to regularly incorporate a mix of whole food fats such as avocado, olives, nuts, and seeds. Indeed, this is why many Fab Four Smoothie recipes call for avocado, whole hemp seeds, and whole flaxseeds, not the oil versions.

Another reason to eat whole foods is they naturally contain more of the omega-3s EPA and DHA. Our bodies are not very efficient at producing these on their own. A few good sources are grass-fed beef, wild fish, and pasture-raised eggs and chicken (especially if the bird was fed flaxseeds—look for omega-3 on the carton).

BODY-LOVING GUIDANCE REGARDING OILS

Oils are a good source of healthy fat. However, it's important to know how to use them and when to incorporate them into a Fab Four meal. Some oils are good for cooking at high heat. Others are better for light cooking at low heat or for cold uses such as salad dressing. And some are best used occasionally and for cold purposes only. The chart on page 80 is divided into these categories and lists the smoke point and fat breakdown for each oil.

When deciding how and when to use an oil, there are a few factors to consider: smoke point, oxidation, and stability.

Smoke point is the temperature at which an oil begins to smoke. If you heat an oil above its smoke point, it will begin to oxidize and release harmful free radicals and other compounds that we don't want to eat or breathe. **Don't heat or cook with an oil above its smoke point. Stay at or below it. If you see smoke, turn down the heat on your stove or oven.** The more you heat an oil, the more oxidation will occur. The closer you get to the smoke point, the faster the oxidation rate will be.

Cooking isn't the only time when heat could be a factor; heat can be used in the processing or extraction of the oil from the whole food source. Ideally, you want oils that were processed with minimal heat (so as to limit or reduce oxidation) and without the use of chemicals. Opt for **extra virgin** oils, which are the least processed and heated; **virgin** is good, too. Also, look for **cold-pressed** on the label.

Exposure to light, air, and moisture will also cause an oil to oxidize. This means that oils can start to oxidize in transit to a store, on the shelf, or on your countertop at temperatures below their smoke point. Metal containers such as copper or iron may also cause oxidation. **Buy oils that come in dark glass bottles, tightly screw the lid down after each use, and store oils in a cool, dark place.**

Further, if you're cooking at high heat (450°F and above), it's important to use an oil that's stable, meaning it won't oxidize easily. In general, oils that are high in saturated fat are more stable and have higher smoke points. They're more resistant to heat and less reactive. Conversely, oils that are higher in unsaturated fat are usually less stable and tend to have lower smoke points. They're more sensitive to heat and more reactive.

These are not hard-and-fast rules, and not every oil follows them. But, in general, if you're cooking at high heat, oils with more saturated fat (ghee, butter, animal fats, coconut oil) are usually preferable to oils that have more unsaturated fat (olive oil).

Avocado oil is one of my favorite body-loving oils and a staple of my pantry. It has a very high smoke point of 520°F, but it's high in unsaturated fat (70 percent monounsaturated and 17 percent polyunsaturated, on average), which makes it less

HEALTHY OILS CHART

	Smoke Point*	Saturated Fat*	Monounsaturated Fat*	Polyunsaturated Fat*
High Heat				
Avocado Oil	520°F	8%	70%	17%
Algae Oil	485°F	4%	90%	2%
Ghee	450–485°F	65%	25%	5%
Pastured Tallow	400°F	49%	42%	4%
Pastured Duck Fat	375°F	33%	49%	12%
Pastured Lard	375°F	39%	45%	11%
Pastured Schmaltz	375°F	30%	45%	21%
Coconut Oil	350–365°F	87%	6%	2%
Grass-fed Butter	350°F	50%	23%	3%
Light Cooking and Cold Use				
Virgin Olive Oil	410°F	14%	74%	8%
Extra Virgin Avocado Oil	400°F	11%	70%	13%
Macadamia Oil	390°F	16%	83%	1%
Refined Olive Oil	390–470°F	14%	73%	11%
Extra Virgin Olive Oil (EVOO)	325–375°F	14%	73%	11%
Occasional and Cold Use Only				
Almond Oil	430°F	8%	70%	17%
Sesame Oil	350–410°F	14%	40%	42%
Hemp Seed Oil	330°F	10%	15%	75%
Walnut Oil	320°F	9%	23%	63%
Pumpkin Seed Oil	250°F	17%	20%	63%
Flaxseed Oil	225°F	9%	18%	73%

* The smoke points and fat percentages listed in the chart are approximate. The fat breakdown may not always add up to 100 percent due to the presence of certain other fatty acids in the food.

stable. So, I use it as an option for cooking at medium to medium-high heat (but not too high). It's great for cooking eggs because they cook fairly quick at medium heat. You can use it in marinades or drizzle it on your vegetables before baking or sautéing. It's also a great base for salad dressings. **Avocado oil** contains lutein, a fat-soluble carotenoid that has been linked to eye health. It also contains oleic acid, which has been found to help raise good cholesterol (HDL) and lower oxidized bad cholesterol.

Olive oil is another one of my favorite oils. I use **extra virgin olive oil (EVOO)**, which is minimally processed and heated. EVOO is so good for you I almost consider it drinkable. EVOO is full of monounsaturated fats and is very heart-healthy. I love using EVOO as a base for salad dressings. It has a smoke point range of 325 to 375°F, so if I use it for cooking, it's for low to medium heat only. I also love drizzling it on cooked proteins, raw chopped veggies with a pinch of salt, or a smashed avocado with a squeeze of lemon. If you find yourself hungry and scouring the pantry late at night, 1 to 2 tablespoons of a really good olive oil (or half an avocado) is the perfect way to curb sugary cravings, satisfy your hunger, and support fat burning when you sleep. *Virgin* olive oil has a smoke point of 410°F and *refined* olive oil has a smoke point range of 390 to 470°F; both can be used for higher-heat cooking.

Algae oil has a high smoke point of 485°F. However, like avocado oil, it's very high in unsaturated fat (90 percent monounsaturated, on average), which means it's less stable. I use it to cook at medium to medium-high heat (but not too high). Don't worry, algae oil doesn't make your food taste like algae or fish. It has a light, neutral taste that stays in the background. I like using it when I'm cooking fish.

Grass-fed ghee (clarified butter, discussed on page 75) is a staple in my refrigerator. It is 100 percent fat and has a high smoke point of 480°F. I use it in the pan when I cook my eggs in the morning, for sautéing vegetables, and as a side for my soup and crackers (my go-to gluten-free option is Jilz Crackerz). Grass-fed butter has a lower smoke point of 350°F. It should be used for cooking at lower heats.

Animal fats such as tallow, lard, schmaltz, and duck fat are high in saturated fat, which make them more stable options for cooking. They have smoke points ranging from 375 to 400°F. I don't recommend using fats from grain-fed, conventional feedlot animals; choose fats from pasture-raised animals only. Want to add a flavorful sear to your steak or crisp to your chicken? Use the fat of the animal you're cooking to get another layer of flavor.

Coconut oil is the highest in saturated fat (upward of 80 to 90 percent), with an average smoke point of between 350 and 365°F. You can't cook with it at high heat, but it's a stable option for low to medium heat. I use it to roast vegetables and make curries, and you can cook your eggs in it, too; just know that your food will taste a little like coconut. You can also blend it into a coffee (see page 76) or a tea (see page 142). As noted on page 75, coconut oil is high in beneficial MCTs.

Almond oil, **flaxseed oil**, **hemp seed oil**, **pumpkin seed oil**, **sesame oil**, and **walnut oil** are all high in polyunsaturated fat and shouldn't be used for cooking because they oxidize easily. For that reason, I would look for options that are cold-pressed, traditionally milled, or slow-pressed **without heat.** I would use them occasionally as part of a dressing or finishing oil.

WHAT OILS SHOULD YOU AVOID? Unhealthy, "bad" fats include artificial trans unsaturated fats (trans fats) and man-made industrial seed and vegetable oils. They result from the processing and overprocessing of foods. When the belief existed that saturated fat was bad for us (which research has shown to be inaccurate), processed food companies started using artificial trans fats and hydrogenated fats to give their foods longer shelf lives. Then, when research showed that these fats were harmful, many of these companies switched to man-made industrial seed and vegetable oils. The research shows that these are bad for us as well.

Artificial trans fats and man-made industrial seed and vegetable oils are bad for us for many reasons. Among other things:

- They cause cell membranes to become more rigid and inflexible, which weakens cell signaling and communication. As you may recall, cell membrane fluidity is critical for cell signaling and communication.
- They contain excessive amounts of oxidized omega-6 fatty acids, which throws our omega-6 to omega-3 ratio way out of balance. This leads to chronic inflam-

mation and has been linked to cardiovascular disease, stroke, and autoimmune disorders. (Our ancestors got their omega-6s from fresh, whole foods, which kept things in balance.)

- They're typically oxidized, which results in the release of harmful free radicals and other compounds. The small, hard seeds are processed at high heat often above their smoke point.
- They're often processed or extracted with chemicals, such as the neurotoxin hexane. Chemical processing can involve bleaching, use of toxic solvents, and deodorizing.
- They're inflammatory, bad for gut health, and may lead to increased risk of heart disease and cancer. They're also often made from genetically modified seeds and ingredients (GMOs).

You'll find artificial trans fats and man-made industrial seed and vegetable oils in processed foods such as chips, crackers, cookies, pastries, candy, hot dogs, and industrially raised animal products. They're in fried food, fast food, french fries, pizza, bread, pasta, condiments, margarine, and dairy. You'll even find them in "healthy" foods like protein bars, nuts, hummus, salad dressing, and foods labeled as "thin" or "skinny."

Avoid processed foods and fast food. Carefully read nutrition facts and ingredient lists. Avoid the following: peanut oil, cottonseed oil, grapeseed oil, canola oil, vegetable oil, safflower oil, sunflower oil, corn oil, soybean oil, palm oil, and anything hydrogenated or partially hydrogenated. If you see any of these man-made industrial seed and vegetable oils, steer clear. Remember, don't mistake whole seeds for any of these seed and vegetable oils. All of these oils sound natural, but they're not. If you're ever unsure about an oil, think about it this way: you want oils you could press out of the fruit or nut yourself. Oils from hard, small seeds tend to be processed with hexane (a toxic chemical) and oxidized because heat and/or chemicals will be needed to extract the oil.

Your favorite restaurant or takeout spot might be using these oils. Even though there's a risk, I think it's probably unrealistic to say you will never eat at or order from those spots again. A few tips to lower your load: (1) pull the skin from your chicken breast (because it can have a lot of bad oils on it), (2) dress steamed veggies with olive oil from the salad bar, and (3) stock your office fridge with #BWBKapproved dressings or your favorite olive oil. Use them when it's convenient. The stress of not enjoying a meal with friends can cause harm as well.

Avoid trans unsaturated fats. They will be clearly listed in the nutrition facts.

The only healthy, naturally occurring trans fat is conjugated linoleic acid (CLA), an anti-inflammatory antioxidant that can reduce the risk of heart disease and type 2 diabetes, increase insulin sensitivity, and support your metabolism. Good sources of CLA include grass-fed beef and grass-fed ghee. It is found in other grass-fed dairy products as well.

THE KETOGENIC DIET

The Fab Four lifestyle isn't a keto diet, which requires you to eat extremely low amounts of carbohydrates. However, when you follow the Fab Four, you might find yourself drifting in and out of a ketogenic state naturally based on your carbohydrate intake. That is exactly what I want for my clients. No counting or deprivation, yet still having the chance to occasionally and naturally benefit from the anti-inflammatory benefits of ketones.

If you're thinking of trying the keto diet, I would *strongly* recommend eating your carbohydrates from Fab Four sources (see chapters 3 and 4, on fiber and greens). Among other things, this will help support the health of your gut microbiome. Too often, devout ketotarians are cutting out fiber-rich vegetables due to carbohydrate content and replacing them with cream cheese. Vegetables should never be off the table!

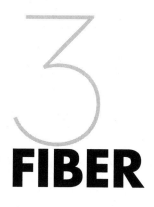

FIBER

FOR GUT HEALTH AND GLUCOSE CONTROL—AND IT HELPS YOU GO

THE THIRD PILLAR OF the Fab Four is fiber, and it's vital to overall health and wellness. When first I developed the light structure of the Fab Four, I specifically decided to include fiber because I found it was sorely lacking in many of my clients' diets. I wanted to make sure they would deliberately seek it out and not just get it on occasion or by accident. You need to eat fiber at every meal! The Fab Four is aimed at nurturing not only your cells, but the *bacterial* cells that live on and inside of you, because they directly affect your cells' health.

Fiber plays an essential role in the health of the gut microbiome, the ecosystem of bacteria and microorganisms that live in the small and large intestines. Fiber feeds so-called good or healthy gut bacteria, which in turn support a number of bodily functions. The benefits of eating fiber and nourishing our gut microbiome are felt and experienced all throughout our body. Among other things, healthy gut bacteria aid in digestion and nutrient absorption; produce butyrate, a short-chain fatty acid with anti-cancer and anti-inflammatory properties; provide protection from toxins, chemicals, and other harmful substances; support skin health and glow; bolster immune system function; and counteract the growth of disease-causing bad bacteria such as candida and yeast. Eating fiber also helps protect against "leaky gut," because the more fiber you eat, the more short-chain fatty acids you produce, such as butyrate. Butyrate strengthens the gut lining by fortifying the mucosal layer and nourishing intestinal cells.

Together with healthy gut bacteria, fiber helps to regulate bowel movements, improve digestion, and rid the body of waste. In addition, high-fiber foods are a key source of vitamins, minerals, and phytochemicals. Phytochemicals are crucial because they activate genetic pathways that stimulate the release of detoxifying and anti-inflammatory enzymes. (I discuss phytochemicals in more detail in chapter 4.)

Fiber also helps us live in balance. Again, this goes back to blood sugar, satiety, and hunger hormones. Fiber doesn't turn into blood sugar. Even though fiber is found in carbohydrates and listed under carbohydrates on nutrition facts, it isn't absorbed into the bloodstream and it doesn't break down into glucose. This is the basis for calculating **net carbohydrates**, which is simply **total carbohydrates minus fiber**. This roughly tells you how much of the carbohydrate content in a food will break down into glucose—because the fiber doesn't count. Many high-fiber foods also have less glucose to begin with.

In addition, fiber actually helps slow the absorption of glucose. Fiber is like an extra layer or shell around the molecules in food. We have to get through it first before we can access what's inside. This extra step adds time and slows the absorption of glucose. The result is a more gradual rise in blood sugar (not a steep spike) and a more measured release of less insulin (not a giant surge). The higher the fiber content, the lower the effect on blood sugar and insulin levels. Further, fiber regulates certain hunger hormones. It increases the production of peptide YY (PYY), a control hormone in our gastrointestinal tract that reduces appetite. It can lead to double the production of cholecystokinin (CCK), a satiety hormone that helps us feel full and satisfied. Fiber also physically stretches your stomach lining, which stops the release of the hunger hormone ghrelin. Ghrelin is released when our stomach is empty, and it tells us to eat until we're physically full.

Fiber is your friend for many reasons. It feeds your healthy gut bacteria, aids digestion, and keeps you regular. But it also helps balance your blood sugar and elongate your blood sugar curve. If your goal is weight loss or improved body composition, consistently eating fiber is very important.

It has been estimated that our hunter-gatherer ancestors consumed as much as 100 grams or more of fiber per day. Today, the average person eats only 13 to 15 grams per day. In my practice, I want my clients to get at least double that amount. *In general, I want their goal to be at least 10 grams of fiber per meal. Physically, I want fiber and greens combined to make up half of their plate, bowl, or dish.* A Fab Four Smoothie is a quick, easy way to get 10 to 15 grams of fiber, thanks to a few key seeds (like chia and flax) and raw powders (like acacia), as well as some of my most commonly recommended ingredients. In a regular Fab Four meal, the emphasis is usually on high-fiber, nonstarchy vegetables, but it can also be a team effort with leafy greens and other foods, which I discuss in this chapter and in the next. You gotta work for it, because this can actually be a challenge to do sometimes. You need to eat vegetables at every meal, add a side of vegetables at a restaurant, sneak them into your sauces or dips, and commit to thinking "vegetable forward."

There are three types of fiber: soluble, insoluble, and resistant starch. None of them are absorbed into the bloodstream.

Soluble fiber dissolves into a gel when eaten. Healthy gut bacteria then feed on the gel. This produces a number of healthy by-products we can absorb, strengthens the gut microbiome, and tends to slow digestion.

Insoluble fiber does not dissolve into a gel or other substance when eaten, and it does not feed healthy gut bacteria. Instead, insoluble fiber merely passes through the system. It helps move things along, tends to speed up digestion, and regulates bowel movements.

Resistant starches (also known as prebiotics) are starches that cannot be absorbed into the bloodstream. They're basically undigestible carbohydrates. Usually, starch is digested and absorbed as glucose. This isn't the case with resistant

PROBIOTICS

Probiotics are living bacteria that support gut health and enhance the proliferation of good bacteria. You can take probiotics in pill form as a supplement. Personally, I take them almost every day. The brand I take is Seed, and I prefer their probiotics because (1) they contain human-derived bacterial strains, which is most effective for our gut, as opposed to animal-derived strains; (2) they've been shown to survive through digestion, i.e., ending in the colon, which is where you want them to end up; and (3) they don't require refrigeration. To me, these are important factors to consider. If you're weighing different options, this information should either be listed on the bottle or in the product description online. Also, you'll see CFUs (colony forming units) listed on the label, which is simply a reference to quantity. My recommendation is to prioritize strain-specific CFU count over total CFU count. Different strains of bacteria support different bodily functions, so I would focus more on CFUs in the specific strain you want and less on total CFUs.

starches, which is good news from the standpoint of blood sugar. But more important, healthy gut bacteria love to feed on resistant starches. Again, this produces healthy gases and acids, supports the gut microbiome, and leads to various health benefits. (Technically speaking, resistant starches are a type of "fermentable" insoluble fiber, i.e., an insoluble fiber that can be eaten or broken down—fermented—by healthy gut bacteria.)

The importance of nourishing our healthy gut bacteria on a daily basis is critical. We used to think it took years to increase the quantity and diversity of gut bacteria. However, recent research from Stanford suggests there can be a large increase in bacterial quantity within just a few hours of eating a fiber-rich meal and, further, that diversity in bacterial strains (a good thing) can be seen in just a few months. What you eat today affects your gut microbiome more quickly than you think. In fact, not eating enough fiber may cause the permanent die-off of certain bacterial strains, which won't then be transferred to your child's microbiome. That's why it's important to consistently eat fiber. In addition to the benefits listed on page 86, feeding healthy gut bacteria increases the bioavailability of certain nutrients, including vitamins K and B_{12}, thiamine, and riboflavin.

Further, a person with a healthier gut microbiome may experience less of a blood sugar spike than a person with a weaker gut microbiome. Also, as noted in chapter 1, several studies have found that fiber and a healthy gut may help limit the production of trimethylamine N-oxide (TMAO), which has been linked to heart disease, diabetes, and colon cancer (see page 45). See *Body Love* for more detail on gut health, including probiotics.

The bacterial ecosystem in your small and large intestines accounts for the majority of the cells in your body. Nature is the best regulator. Eating whole foods wrapped in fiber will always be the best way to feed your gut microbiome, and avoiding processed foods will always help keep candida in check. The bottom line is that you want this ecosystem to thrive and flourish. Your health and wellness depend on a strong, robust, and resilient gut microbiome.

BAD INPUTS

Toxins, pesticides, chemicals, and other harmful substances, such as EDCs (see page 46), in the foods we eat wreak havoc on our gut microbiome. Antibiotics and birth control do as well. They destroy healthy gut bacteria, break down the gut lining and walls, and cause inflammation and disease (such as leaky gut syndrome). Further, sugar, alcohol, and overeating processed white carbohydrates all feed the bad bacteria in the gut (such as candida and yeast). An unhealthy gut microbiome can result from having too little good bacteria (quantity or diversity) or an overgrowth of bad bacteria. Some of the symptoms of an unhealthy balance of bad to good bacteria (dysbiosis) and thus an unhealthy gut microbiome may include excessive bloating, gas, cramping, constipation, diarrhea, abdominal pain and discomfort, and other irritable bowel syndrome symptoms. Even if you don't have these bowel or stomach-related symptoms, you might have other indicators of an underlying bacterial imbalance. For example, your gut has a direct effect on skin health, eczema, and certain types of dermatitis.

Of note: people with small intestinal bacterial overgrowth (SIBO) must adhere to a strict diet that severely limits their fiber intake, and they also must eliminate FODMAPs (a group of carbohydrates and sugar alcohols that cause bacterial growth). A breath test is used to test for SIBO, and antibiotics or herbal treatments are used to treat it. If you experience any of the symptoms mentioned above, consult with your physician. Food allergies, intolerances, and sensitivities may also contribute to gut issues.

BODY-LOVING SOURCES OF FIBER FOR A FAB FOUR SMOOTHIE: Chia Seeds, Flaxseeds, Acacia Fiber, and Psyllium Husk Powder

I generally prefer whole foods (like chia seeds and flaxseeds) or single-source powders (like acacia fiber and psyllium husk powder) over fiber blends. And, as always, I look for raw seeds and certified organic options when possible. NOW Foods has clean, certified organic options for all of these fiber sources.

Chia seeds pack an efficient punch. On average, 2 tablespoons contain 8 to 10 grams of fiber and 4 to 6 grams of protein. The fiber content is largely soluble. In addition to feeding healthy gut bacteria, it binds with old cholesterol and helps remove it from the body (which supports the body's natural process of recycling cholesterol). In general, soluble fiber can be better for people suffering from IBS because it absorbs water and is excreted more slowly during digestion. In addition to a Fab Four Smoothie, one of my favorite uses of chia seeds is in pudding. I whip up Fab Four Chia Seed Pudding (page 184) for breakfast when I'm not in a smoothie mood, or in the afternoon when I need a bridge snack. You can also check out Matcha Chia Seed Pudding (page 258).

One important thing to note is that eating dry chia seeds has been known to cause intestinal blockages. This is because the dry seeds absorb bodily fluid and can greatly expand in size. Hydrating chia seeds or blending them with liquid (such as in a Fab Four Smoothie) helps mitigate this risk and reduce internal expansion. I always hydrate or soak chia seeds in some manner before use. I wouldn't eat them dry.

Flaxseeds also contain both fiber and protein. On average, 2 tablespoons contain 4 to 5 grams of fiber and 3 to 4 grams of protein. Flaxseeds contain a good mix of soluble and insoluble fiber, so they feed gut bacteria and also help keep things moving. Acacia fiber is made from the gum or sap of the acacia tree and is a very rich source of soluble fiber. On average, 2 tablespoons contain 10 to 12 grams of soluble fiber. (To increase butyrate production, you can always add 1 tablespoon of acacia fiber to any Fab Four Smoothie. This would be on top of the fiber listed in the recipe.) Psyllium husk powder is made from the husks of the seeds from the *Plantago ovata* plant. On average, 2 tablespoons contain 6 to 8 grams of fiber.

Every single Fab Four Smoothie recipe also includes whole foods, many of which are good sources of fiber. For example, ¼ to ½ of an avocado contains 2.5 to 5 grams of fiber. In addition, leafy greens, nut butters, berries, herbs, and nonstarchy vegetables all add fiber as well. Together with your chia, flax, or acacia, getting up to 15 grams of fiber in your smoothie is easily attainable.

As for your protein powder, don't look to it as your source of fiber. It shouldn't be. Some protein powders might contain a small amount of fiber, which is fine, but remember—the most important thing about your protein powder is the protein. You don't need an excessively fortified supplement; you just need clean, high-quality protein. Get your fiber from the sources suggested here or from other whole food ingredients.

Occasionally, I add ½ to 1 cup of frozen cauliflower rice (see page 315) to my smoothie in order to add fiber and thickness, and make it colder. I also might add ¼ teaspoon of unmodified potato starch or plantain/green banana flour. These are potent sources of resistant starch, which our healthy gut bacteria love to feed on. But I only use them occasionally and keep it to a ¼ teaspoon max. A little goes a long way. They contain such high amounts of resistant starch that you might feel bloated and have discomfort if you overdo it (you'll essentially be overfeeding your gut bacteria). Caveat: if you have a nightshade allergy, unmodified potato starch may cause an allergic reaction.

For body-loving sources of fiber for a regular Fab Four meal, see the fiber and greens chart on pages 93–101.

The point of the Fab Four and body love is to allow you to find food freedom through light structure. In the preceding chapters, I've offered you a little more hands-on guidance regarding sourcing clean proteins and healthy fats. When it comes to fiber and greens, though, I really want you to feel empowered to choose the foods that are the right fit for you.

The chart on pages 93–101 is one big body-loving menu for you to choose from.

FERMENTED VEGETABLES

One way to help mix up your vegetable intake is to eat fermented vegetables. They're deliciously tart, palate cleansing, and full of fiber. In addition, fermentation increases the bioavailability of the nutrients present in the underlying vegetable, including iron (which is good for Plant-Based Devotees) and vitamin K. Fermented vegetables support glucose tolerance and insulin sensitivity and are a source of probiotics as well. Two of my favorite brands are Farmhouse Culture and Wildbrine.

It covers both fiber and greens because there is a lot of overlap between these two categories. There are so many delicious vegetables, leafy greens, herbs, and berries that are loaded with fiber and phytochemicals. When it comes to fiber and greens, variety is the spice of life, and mixing it up keeps things fresh. We all have our favorites, but I also want you to feel inspired to bring a new vegetable back from the farmers' market or grocery store. Read through the chart opposite and pick and choose as you see fit. Just keep the two general parameters in mind: **(1) Try to get at least 10 grams of fiber per meal; and (2) physically, try to have fiber and greens combined make up half of your plate, bowl, or dish.**

Eating a variety of foods from the chart will provide a mix of soluble fiber, insoluble fiber, and resistant starch. All the foods in the chart naturally contain a balance of soluble and insoluble fiber (which may include resistant starch). By eating a variety of these foods, nature will ensure that you receive a mixture of the different types of fiber. You don't need to obsessively seek out the different types. Again, the key is variety. I don't want you to limit yourself to one or two vegetables, and don't focus solely on one specific type of fiber. If you eat a mixture of the greens and vegetables in the chart, you'll support both your digestion and your healthy gut bacteria.

To hit the goal of 10 grams of fiber per meal, you can add the fiber content from all your food sources. The purpose of the goal is to make a conscious effort to add fiber to every meal. You can look to *all* the foods on your plate to help you do it. In addition to the vegetables, leafy greens, herbs, and berries listed in the chart, a few other body-loving sources of fiber include avocado, raw nuts and seeds, and nut butters.

In chapter 5, I cover my approach to certain starchy carbohydrates that contain fiber, including grains, potatoes, corn, beans/legumes, and high-glycemic fruit. In general, I count these foods but don't look to them as primary sources of fiber because of their effect on blood sugar and insulin levels. The starch is digested and absorbed as glucose, which causes the release of insulin and shuts down fat burning. I don't tell my clients they can never eat starchy carbohydrates—that would be a sad existence! I just ask them to focus on building their meals with the Fab Four. That should be plenty of food to keep them full and satisfied. If they want to add starchy carbohydrates, I just tell them to follow the body-loving guidelines and tools in chapter 5. Some people can eat more than that and still reach their goals. Ultimately, it depends on your unique body chemistry and how physically active you are.

Fiber and Greens	Fiber	Net	Body Love Benefit
Leafy Greens and Herbs			
Amaranth or Chinese spinach (1 cup)	< 0.5	1	Amaranth greens are easy to cook with a quick sauté and serve up vitamins C, B_6, and A.
Arugula (1 cup)	.5	1	A great alternative to cabbage, kale, cauliflower, and broccoli, this cruciferous vegetable is easier to digest. Rich in Kaempferol and quercetin and sirtuin-activating, it's a great leafy green to mix into any salad.
Basil (1 cup)	.5	1	This anti-inflammatory aromatic herb inhibits the release of pro-inflammatory cytokines and delivers the water-soluble flavonoids orientin and vicenin.
Beet greens (1 cup)	.5	1	A quick blanch removes oxalates and the bitter taste from this cruciferous vegetable; strain and blend into a smoothie, soup, or dressing.
Butter lettuce (1 cup)	.5	.5	A more nutrient-dense leaf for lettuce cup tacos, butter lettuce provides beta-carotene, lutein, and zeaxanthin.
Celery Leaf (1 cup)	< 1	< 1	Don't throw the leaves out; throw them in to your next smoothie for a dose of anti-inflammatory phenolic antioxidants.
Chicory (1 cup)	1.2	.2	Higher in fiber than most greens, chicory contains a healthy prebiotic fiber called inulin. Red chicory is sirtuin-activating. Chicory root fiber is occasionally used in processed food to increase the fiber content. It provides a subtle sweet taste. If you love the taste of coffee but want to ditch the caffeine, chicory coffee is an alternative.
Collard greens (1 cup)	3	2	The best sturdy wrap for your favorite warm or cold sandwich, collard greens are a cruciferous vegetable that is rich in vitamin K, vitamin A, fiber, manganese, and vitamin C.

(continued)

Fiber and Greens	Fiber	Net	Body Love Benefit
Endive (1 cup)	1.5	.5	A member of the chicory family, this fiber-rich green with a sturdy leaf is perfect for dipping into a thick hummus or heavy salmon or tuna salad.
Escarole (1 cup)	1	1	Another chicory family favorite, escarole is great chopped fresh in a salad, sautéed with garlic and lemon, or dropped into a white bean soup to wilt.
Garden cress (1 cup)	.5	2.5	Add a cup to your next salad! This isothiocyanate rich leafy green is a member of the cruciferous family and rich in beta-carotene, lutein, and zeaxanthin.
Iceberg (1 cup)	1	1	It isn't the most nutritious, but it's water-packed and offers up vitamin K so if it's all your kids will eat, offer it.
Kale (1 cup)	1	0	The sulforaphane found in cruciferous vegetables, like kale, increases enzymes that can deactivate free radicals and carcinogens. As a bonus, kale is also sirtuin-activating.
Lovage (1 cup)	<1	<1	Medicinal herb found in the Mediterranean that tastes like celery. Add this leaf to salad or soup. Lovage is loaded with anti-inflammatory flavonols like quercetin. It is also a sirtuin activator.
Mache (1 cup)	1	3	A European heirloom green that has a sweet and nutty taste, mâche is an excellent source of vitamin C and offers a gram of protein per serving.
Microgreens (1 cup)	<1	<1	Microgreens are the super-nutritious growth of a vegetable between sprout and plant. The tiny leaves offer close to ten times the phytochemical content and up to forty times the vitamin and mineral content of the full-grown plant.
Mustard greens (1 cup)	2	1	Mustard greens contain the phenolic antioxidant ferulic plus vitamins C and A; this trifecta helps protect skin from aging.
Parsley (1/4 cup)	.5	.5	Bitter herb linked to blood sugar shown to improve metabolic and liver function and regulate immune function in animal studies. Add this herb to your favorite Italian dish and throw the leftovers in your next smoothie.
Radicchio (1 cup)	0	2	Sometimes called red chicory, radicchio is a red leaf that can be mixed into salad like my Vegan Kale Caesar.
Romaine (1 cup)	1	.5	Hydrating and mineral-rich romaine provides calcium, phosphorous, magnesium, and potassium. Use it as taco shells or in your next salad.
Spring mix (1 cup)	1	1	Spring mix is a great way to get a mix of nutrients. Most mixed lettuces contain a blend of romaine, arugula, frisée, oak leaf lettuce, and radicchio.
Spinach (1 cup)	1	0	Spinach has a mild-tasting leafy green that is great for smoothies. Add a squeeze of lemon to cut the "green" taste. A spinach smoothie is full of phytonutrients, including lutein, kaempferol, nitrates, quercetin, and zeaxanthin and vitamins C, K, A, and folate. Organic frozen whole leaf spinach is a great option for smoothies too, no ice needed.

Fiber and Greens	Fiber	Net	Body Love Benefit
Swiss chard (1 cup)	1	1	Chard is a member of the Amaranthaceae family with spinach, but it's often compared to kale. Chard contains syringic acid, the flavonoid linked to lowering blood sugar levels. Chard is efficient at absorbing minerals from soil and rich in magnesium, iron, manganese, copper, potassium, calcium, phosphorus, and zinc.
Turnip greens (1 cup)	2	2	Turnip greens are anti-inflammatory and high in vitamins K, A, and C. Steam or sauté these leaves like spinach for the perfect green side.
Watercress (1 cup)	.2	.2	Watercress is a versatile leaf that can be added to soup, wraps, or salad. A member of the cruciferous family, this leaf contains the carotenoids lutein and zeaxanthin; vitamins K, A, and C; and more calcium than milk.
Nonstarchy Vegetables			
Artichoke (1 cup)	7	7	Fiber and folate full, artichokes are the perfect appetizer for any meal. You can purchase prepared artichokes to add to a salad or antipasto platter, or you can quickly sauté them. Buy water-packed chokes.
Asparagus (1 cup)	2.5	2.5	Asparagus contains inulin and resistant starch, two fermentable carbohydrates that feed probiotic bacteria. It also contains the amino acid asparagine, a natural diuretic that can help flush the body of excess sodium. Add asparagus to your plate the night before a photoshoot or if you're retaining water. Contains the phytochemicals beta-carotene, alpha-carotene, lutein, and zeaxanthin.
Beet (1 cup)	8	19	Beets, beet greens, and beet powder are high in inorganic nitrates that decrease blood pressure and support cardiovascular function through vasodilation, making beets a great carbohydrate to consume before or after your workout.
Beans (green, filet, wax, Italian, yard-long; 1 cup)	4	6	Technically a legume, green beans contain 2 grams of protein and 2 grams of fiber per cup to support satiety with a mild blood glucose response.
Bean sprouts (1 cup)	2	4	Bean sprouts can add fiber, vitamin C, and folate to your next wrap or salad along with a refreshing crunch.
Bok choy (1 cup)	0.7	0.8	A great source of selenium for thyroid health, bok choy is a cruciferous vegetable used most often in Asian cuisine.
Broccoli (1 cup)	1.8	2.9	Broccoli is a cruciferous family favorite rich in vitamin C, alpha-carotene, beta-carotene, lutein, and zeaxanthin. Due to its high respiration rate, it is important to buy this vegetable locally and eat it soon after purchase.
Broccoli rabe (rapini; 1 cup)	1	0	A turnip relative, broccoli rabe is quick to blanch or sauté for a weeknight side and a vegetable to add into the rotation if your family loves broccoli. The vitamins C and B, including folate, can help reduce homocysteine, an amino acid that is linked to heart disease when elevated.
Broccoli Romanesco (1 cup)	2.2	1.1	Packed with glucosinolate compounds, broccoli Romanesco is a cruciferous powerhouse with vitamins C, K, and folate.

(continued)

Fiber and Greens	Fiber	Net	Body Love Benefit
Broccoli sprouts (1 cup)	1	1	The richest source of sulphoraphane and an easy add to your salad or smoothie. Cruciferous family sprout.
Brussels sprouts (1 cup)	4	7	Shred Brussels sprouts through your food processor or peel off and roast leaves for a quickly prepared vegetable side.
Capers (1 cup)	0.4	0.1	Sirtuin-activating. Pairing capers with cooked protein decreases inflammatory by-products. Capers contain over thirteen phytochemicals, including quercetin, kaempferol, ginkgetin, isoginkgetin, sulfur-containing glucosinolates, and carotenoids.
Cabbage (green, Napa, savoy; 1 cup)	2	3	A salad and slaw staple, cabbage holds up even when it's covered in dressing for up to 48 hours, making it a great green to use for meal prep.
Cabbage, red (1 cup)	2	4	Swap in red cabbage for two times the vitamin C, ten times the vitamin A, and added cancer-fighting flavonoids called anthocyanins.
Carrots (1 cup)	3.6	8.4	I love baked carrot fries. Carrots offer skin-supporting beta-carotene, alpha-carotene, lutein, zeaxanthin, and the B vitamin Biotin.
Cauliflower (1 cup)	3	2	Frozen cauliflower rice can be blended into smoothies for a thicker consistency (like a banana but without the sugar) or sautéed for a quick weeknight bowl. This cruciferous veggie takes on the flavor of the dish and offers a dose of sulphoraphane.
Celery (1 cup)	1.5	1.5	Sirtuin-activating. Celery contains over thirty-five unique phytochemicals and the nonstarchy polysaccharides called Apiuman that support digestion. Fresh celery stalks are sturdy and snap when broken.
Cucumber, English (1 cup)	1	3	English cucumbers are a hydrating, crunchy cracker replacement. The skin is rich in vitamin C, silica, and caffeic acid, known to reduce skin inflammation and improve tone.
Cucumber, Persian (1 cup)	2	2	A small, thinner-skinned variety, the Persian cucumber is a refreshing addition to any smoothie.
Daikon (1 cup)	1.9	2.9	A white radish belonging to the cruciferous family. Daikon's root has a peppery bite perfect for pairing with dip, and its leaves can be added to salad. Daikon is the perfect start to any meal because it contains the enzymes amylase and esterase, which support digestion.
Eggplant (1 cup)	2.5	2.3	A part of the night shade family (Solanaceae), which includes peppers, potatoes, and tomatoes.
Garlic (1 cup)	<1	<1	A member of the Allium family, garlic is antimicrobial and supports the immune system to shorten the duration of colds. It provides vitamin C, vitamin B_6, and manganese, and research links it to an improved cholesterol ratio. See garlic prep tips on page 115.

Fiber and Greens	Fiber	Net	Body Love Benefit
Horseradish (1 cup)	< 1	< 1	Mustard, wasabi, and horseradish are cruciferous isothiocyanates that can be used as a condiment to spice up a dish and boost immunity. Horseradish specifically contains the glucosinolate sinigrin, which exhibits anti-cancer, antibacterial, antifungal, antioxidant, and anti-inflammatory pharmacological activities. If you enjoy creamy horse-radish, mix 1 tablespoon of minced horseradish root with 1 tablespoon of plain coconut yogurt or plain pastured Greek yogurt.
Jicama (1 cup)	1.8	1.5	Mandoline-sliced jicama is a fiber-full alternative to a lettuce cup for tacos with more crunch.
Kohlrabi (1 cup)	5	3	Kohlrabi is a cruciferous vegetable that provides more than your daily need of vitamin C and the cancer-fighting benefits of glucosinolates.
Leek (1 cup)	1.6	11	A great source of soluble fiber and the organic compound allicin, leeks can be enjoyed in a raw salad or replace onions in a soup.
Mushrooms (all types)	1	2.1	A great source of vitamin D, B vitamins, selenium, and potassium. A cup adds 2 grams of protein to your plate. Studies suggest shiitake and maitake mushrooms offer up the most potent phytochemical profile of the bunch.
Okra (1 cup)	3.2	4.2	Okra contains vitamins A and C and polyphenols, including flavonoids and isoquercetin. The gooey texture that is released when cooking okra is a healthy, soluble, gel-like fiber called mucilage. which is also found in chia, flax, agave, and aloe.
Onion (white, yellow, red; ½ cup)	1.4	7.5	Like other alliums, onions offer up vitamin C, B vitamins, and potassium. All onions have the anti-inflammatory quercetin, but the red variety also contains anthocyanins and is sirtuin-activating.
Onion, green (½ cup)	< .5	1.5	Green onions or scallions serve up the green vegetable vitamin profile of vitamins K, C, and A and folate, but for a garnish they are high in fiber.
Pea, sugar snap (1 cup)	2	4	Add this crunchy pea alternative to your next veggie platter to up the protein. Snap peas serve up 3 grams of protein and 3 grams of fiber per cup with a mild taste that is perfect for dipping.
Pepper (green, red, yellow, orange; 1 cup)	2	5	Technically a nightshade fruit, pepper is a bite of B_6 and lutein, quercetin, and luteolin. It's fun sliced into "boats" with a protein salad or stuffed and roasted for a weeknight dinner.
Pumpkin (1 cup)	7	12.5	A light starch alternative to potato with way more fiber and beta-carotene, the provitamin converted to vitamin A. Organic pumpkin puree is easy to source in a can or tetra pack. Add it to soups or baked goods to increase fiber and decrease acellular flours.
Radishes (1 cup)	3	3	When you bite into a radish, you get a jolt of spice from the isothiocyanates (present when you breakdown cruciferous vegetables) plus anthocyanins present in red vegetables.

(continued)

Fiber and Greens	Fiber	Net	Body Love Benefit
Rutabaga (1 cup)	3.2	8.8	Rutabaga is a more mild cruciferous root and a lower carbohydrate alternative for potato in your favorite recipe. Mash, cube, hasselback, or even eat this root raw in a slaw.
Shallots (½ cup)	2.6	10.9	Shallots have sulphur antioxidants that are antiviral and antifungal. Swap in shallots for white onions to increase the B_6 and mineral content of your meal.
Squash, acorn (1 cup)	9	20	Roast this high-fiber squash sliced or in halves. A squash half is about a 1 cup serving and can be used as a bowl to serve salad or soup.
Squash, butternut (1 cup)	6.6	15	Roasted butternut squash pairs well with warming spices like cinnamon, turmeric, and nutmeg.
Squash, Delicata (1 cup)	1.3	8	Squash provides vitamin C, magnesium, and carotenoid phytonutrients lutein and zeaxanthin.
Squash, spaghetti (1 cup)	2.2	7.8	A pressure cooker makes spaghetti squash noodles in under 10 minutes.
Squash, summer (1 cup)	1.6	3.3	Summer squash like zucchini is more readily available and easily prepared as zoodles to increase vitamins B_6, B_2, C, and folate.
Squash, zucchini (1 cup)	1.5	3.1	Avoid buying an overgrown zucchini. Look for a 6- to 8-inch-long dark green zucchini that is relatively thin but feels heavy for its size to guarantee the freshest fruit.
Tomato, processed (1 cup)	3.7	8.9	Prepared tomatoes (canned/tetra-packed, home-cooked, or sundried) provide the highest lycopene content and pairing them with a fat like olive oil increases the bioavailability of this fat-soluble phytochemical.
Tomato, fresh, (cherry, plum, vine-ripe; 1 cup)	2.8	8.2	Enjoying fresh tomatoes during the summer months can help provide sun protection. Studies suggest those who ingest lycopene before sun exposure had decreased intensity of skin reactions.
Tomato, heirloom varieties (1 cup)	2.2	4.6	My favorite tomatoes! "Heirloom" means the DNA of the tomatoes hasn't been manipulated. Opt for heirloom in any variety when available. Add a really good olive oil to your fresh tomato salad to increase lycopene absorption.
Turnips (1 cup)	3.1	4.6	A cruciferous family root, the turnip tastes like a carrot or potato depending on when it's picked. A medium-age turnip is a delicious potato replacement and a younger turnip can be enjoyed raw but avoid.
Water chestnuts (1/2 cup)	2	12	High in ferulic acid, gallocatechin gallate, and EGCG (epicatechin gallate), the longevity phytochemical in green tea these are a crunchy, fiber-rich addition to Asian cuisine.
Wasabi (1 tablespoon)	.5	3	Need a reason to make your sushi spicy? Wasabi is a cruciferous vegetable, high in levels of allyl isothiocyanate. Look out for knock-off wasabi made from horseradish or mustard.

Fiber and Greens	Fiber	Net	Body Love Benefit
Starchy Vegetables			
Corn (1 cup)	4	40	A grain, a vegetable, and a fruit, corn is starchy and sugary. Always buy organic to avoid pesticides.
Peas, green (1 cup)	7.2	15.4	A rich source of B vitamins, fiber, and protein (8 grams per cup), peas are an optional addition if you source certified organic.
Potato, sweet (1 cup)	8.4	44.2	Higher in vitamin A, sweet potato is a moderately starchy side and perfect for a post-workout meal.
Potato, white (1 cup)	4.8	43	At 5 grams of fiber and almost 4 grams of protein for a medium spud, the white potato offers half the net carbohydrates and twice the fiber of white rice.
Berries			
Açaí berry (½ cup)	6	1.4	Keep your açaí sugar-free. Freeze-dried powder or unsweetened frozen packets can be added to a smoothie with little blood sugar impact and three times the phytochemical content of blueberries.
Blackberry (½ cup)	3.8	3	Blackberries are a high-fiber berry with a strong flavor for smoothies or a sweet bite.
Blueberry (½ cup)	1.8	8.9	A phytochemical powerhouse full of anthocyanins and the flavanols quercetin and myricetin, sirtuin-activating blueberries are a Fab Four smoothie favorite that boost brain health and support blood sugar control. Buy frozen berries! Freezing blueberries actually improves the availability of anthocyanins found in the skin.
Boysenberry (½ cup)	3.8	3	Boysenberries are available July through August. Skip the syrup and buy up your boxes at the farmers' market instead.
Cranberry (1 cup)	3.6	8.4	Opt for fresh cranberries and avoid dried cranberries, which have added sugar. High in polyphenols and flavanols, cranberries also contain an oligosaccharide, which is active against UTIs.
Currant (½ cup)	3.8	4.8	The smaller and darker the berry, the higher the benefits. You can add currants to a salad or smoothie or eat them alone to support the immune system with vitamin C and increase anthocyanins.
Elderberry (½ cup)	5.1	8.3	Known for shortening the duration of cold and flu symptoms, elderberries are packed with vitamin C, phenolic acids, flavanols, and anthocyanins. Opt for sugar-free.
Goji berry (dried; ¼ cup)	2.9	14.7	High in vitamin C, goji berries are an occasional add to your smoothie bowl if you need a sweet treat. Keep your serving size to 1 tablespoon to keep sugar below 5 grams.
Raspberry (½ cup)	4	3.3	High in fiber, like blackberries, raspberries are a favorite for topping bowls, snacking, and tart smoothies.

(continued)

Fiber and Greens	Fiber	Net	Body Love Benefit
Other Fruit			
Apple (1 apple)	4	19	Granny Smith offer the most phytochemicals and animal research suggests the fiber supports a healthy microbiome. Red Delicious offer up anthocyanins and Honey Crisp offer a little more fiber at 5 grams per fruit.
Apricot (1 apricot)	.75	4	Rich in carotenoids, specifically pro-vitamin-A carotenoids like beta-carotene, apricots can be turned into retinol, an active form of vitamin A that is good for immunity as well as skin and eye health, by the liver or intestines.
Avocado (1/2 avocado)	6.5	2	My favorite food, avocados have been shown to improve cholesterol ration, decrease triglycerides, and be beneficial for metabolic health. Avocados deliver fiber.
Cantaloupe (1 cup)	1.4	11.7	It's a lower-fiber fruit, but it does contain 75 percent of your daily need for vitamin C and thirty times the beta-carotene content of oranges.
Cherries (½ cup)	1.6	9.1	Enjoy cherries occasionally fresh or frozen when they're in season. Tart cherries are best known for their ability to decrease muscle soreness and increase.
Coconut (½ cup)	14.6	10	A super-fat fruit. Coconut's MCTs support healthy brain function, reduce appetite, and increase fat burning while lauric acid kills off yeast. It's also high in fiber with a low net carbohydrate.
Grapes (½ cup)	.7	12.9	High in sugar (15g), grapes should be enjoyed only occasionally or earned in the gym. Red grape skins contain resveratrol, an anti-inflammatory phenol that increases insulin sensitivity in animal studies. Resveratrol is also found in wine and dark chocolate.
Grapefruit (½ medium)	2	11.6	Grapefruit has been linked to increased weight loss, decreased insulin, decreased appetite, and increased insulin sensitivity when eaten before meals, making it a good option to enjoy at your next breakfast buffet. Grapefruit is also loaded with beta-carotene, lycopene, and vitamin C.
Honeydew (½ cup)	.8	7.9	It can be tempting to buy precut melons, but your chances of bacterial contamination go up. Cut your own for the potassium, magnesium, and folate benefits.
Kiwi (1 fruit)	2.1	8	Eating the skin triples the fiber and protects the vitamin C present in the kiwi. Consistent consumption of kiwi shows that pectic polysaccharides and the dietary fiber present can increase probiotic bacteria in the gut, specifically lactobacilis and bifidobacterum.
Lemon (1 medium)	1.6	3.7	Add lemon juice to water in the morning to boost digestion. When you add a squeeze of lemon to spinach, the vitamin C present in lemon (and citrus) increases the absorption of non-heme iron in the spinach.

Fiber and Greens	Fiber	Net	Body Love Benefit
Mango (½ cup)	1.8	15.2	Along with polyphenolic compounds anthocyanins, catechins, quercetin, and kaempferol, mango contains a huge amount of magiferin, a potent phytochemical called a xanthone that is known to be more potent than vitamins C and E. Enjoy mango as a seasonal treat to ingest the benefits.
Orange (1 medium)	1.6	11.9	Oranges are rich in hesperidin and anthocyanins, but it doesn't mean you should drink OJ. Opt for the whole fruit seasonally or add a squeeze to flavor sparkling water.
Passionfruit (1 fruit)	1.9	2.3	Opt for the whole fruit as a snack instead of drinking the juice. If you have a latex allergy, you might have an allergy to the proteins present in passionfruit.
Peach (1 fruit)	2.3	11.7	A vitamin C–rich stone fruit, like plums, cherries, apricots, and almonds, peaches pair perfectly with iron-rich spinach salads.
Pineapple (1 cup)	1.2	9.6	Rich in phenolics, flavonoids, and vitamin C, this tropical fruit also contains bromelain, an enzyme that aids in healthy digestion. With 14 grams of sugar per cup, pineapple is the perfect holiday treat.
Plantain (½ cup)	1.3	22.3	A super-starchy fruit that is popular with paleo peeps, plantains can replace potatoes and give highly active individuals a good dose of glucose and potassium.
Plum (1 fruit)	1	6.1	Plums contain anti-inflammatory polyphenols and the ability to increase levels of adiponectin, a hormone that helps protect against metabolic syndrome. Prunes (dried plums) can relieve constipation, because they contain the alcohol sugar sorbitol and fiber.
Watermelon (1 cup cubed)	0.6	10.8	Mostly water and sugar (9 grams per cup) keep this fruit to a serving and use it as a hydrating pre-workout treat.

4
GREENS

NUTRIENT-DENSE, DETOXIFYING, AND HYDRATING

THE FOURTH PILLAR OF the Fab Four is greens, my body-loving term for both leafy greens (including herbs) and vegetables deep in color. When I first developed the light structure of the Fab Four, I noticed that many of my clients' meals were lacking in color. The monotone of beige, brown, and white was a sign of imbalance in their diet (too many processed, sugary, and starchy carbohydrates), which more than likely meant there was an imbalance in their blood sugar and gut microbiome. It also indicated a lack of nutrient density, phytochemicals, and water. Without leafy greens and colorful vegetables, you're missing out on many key nutrients and other health benefits.

Greens are a key source of phytochemicals, chemical compounds that activate genetic pathways and stimulate the release of antioxidants and enzymes to attack free radicals, help us detoxify, and fight inflammation. Certain phytochemicals can activate longevity and metabolism-enhancing genes as well. I discuss phytochemicals in more detail on pages 106–108.

In addition, greens are nutrient-dense and chock-full of vitamins and minerals, which help power all sorts of cellular processes and enhance overall vitality and beauty. They're an excellent source of fiber, which as discussed in chapter 3, aids in digestion and supports the gut microbiome. They also help keep us hydrated. Up to 20 percent of daily water intake comes from food, and water-packed vegetables are one of the main sources.

Greens nourish the body and elevate the nutritional content of every single meal. That's why they're part of the Fab Four, and why I always tell my clients to add color to their plate or smoothie. And not just the color green—the whole rainbow.

Greens also play a pivotal role in blood sugar balance, satiety, and hormonal balance. Leafy greens and colorful vegetables are carbohydrates, but they break down into smaller amounts of glucose than their processed, sugary, and starchy relatives. Coupled with the slowing presence of fiber, they don't raise your blood sugar as high, as fast, or much at all. Since there is less glucose in your bloodstream, your body doesn't dump a truckload of insulin into your bloodstream. And since your blood sugar is rising and falling more gently, your hunger is more predictable and manageable. Further, because of the fiber content, greens have the hormonal benefits listed on page 86 with respect to PYY, CCK, and ghrelin. They also increase the production of glucagon-like peptide-1 (GLP-1), which signals that you're full. The vitamins, minerals, and phytochemicals also support the metabolism on a cellular level. Deficiencies can negatively affect your metabolism.

Leafy greens and vegetables deep in color are some of the most body-loving foods you can eat. In my practice, I encourage my clients to add them to every meal and smoothie. *Physically, I want fiber and greens combined to make up half of your plate, bowl, or dish. Depending on the food, this will generally mean 2 to 4 cups (and sometimes more) of leafy greens and colorful vegetables.* Remember, the point is not to have you measuring your food at every meal. The point of the Fab Four is to give you light structure, so you can build a healthy, sustainable lifestyle that's right for you. The portion goals here and elsewhere in this book are intended to help guide your journey and give you a general sense of how to approach eating the Fab Four.

> TIP: Your hand can be a useful way to get an idea of portion goals. I often tell my clients that, for each meal, protein should be about the size and thickness of their palm (or a palm and a half), fat should be one to two thumbs, and fiber and greens should be two to four fists.

For body-loving sources of greens, see the fiber and greens chart on pages 93–101.

As I mentioned in the last chapter, there is a lot of overlap between fiber and greens, which is why I've grouped them together in the chart on pages 93–101. Use the chart like a menu and try to incorporate a variety of these foods into your weekly diet. It's easier than you think. Nearly all of my Fab Four Smoothie recipes call for something colorful, such as leafy greens (spinach, kale, microgreens), fresh herbs, or berries. Read the recipes in the plans in Part Two (and in *Body Love* if you want more inspiration) and don't be afraid to mix it up.

As for regular Fab Four meals, there's no shortage of creative ways to add more greens.

A recent study in neurology concluded that the consumption of approximately 1 serving per day of leafy green vegetables and foods rich in phylloquinone, lutein, nitrate, folate, α-tocopherol, and kaempferol resulted in a brain that performed on average eleven years younger and the slowing of the cognitive decline experienced with aging.

- Use clean swaps like squash or zucchini zoodles instead of regular flour noodles, or cauliflower rice instead of white or brown rice.
- Give your salad some added color or crunch with radishes, beets, carrots, red and orange peppers, cucumber, or celery.
- Branch out from broccoli, green beans, and asparagus (which are all amazing) and try something new like artichoke, eggplant, Brussels sprouts, bok choy, collard greens, or rutabaga.
- You can even elevate your meal with a simple topping: fresh cilantro on an omelet, minced green onion as a soup garnish, microgreens and watercress on a salad, or fresh herbs on your protein or in your marinade.

- Adding greens will also help you get more healthy fat into your diet, because of the fat-based cooking oils, dressings, and dips that often accompany them. This also helps increase the bioavailability of the phytochemicals present (see page 111).

Next, let's discuss one of the main benefits of consistently eating leafy greens and colorful vegetables: they're an excellent source of phytochemicals.

Phytochemicals are a specific type of chemical compound found in plants. They introduce a low-grade amount of oxidative stress to the body, which prompts a detoxifying or anti-inflammatory response. This is an example of *hormesis,* in which a small dose of something stressful can cause a beneficial or healthy result. Phytochemicals do this by interacting with the human genome to regulate gene expression. They activate specific genetic pathways in the cells and throughout the body. In turn, these genetic pathways up-regulate (stimulate) the production and release of detoxifying and anti-inflammatory enzymes. These enzymes are defenses, and regularly eating phytochemicals helps keep them strong and activated. It's like sending your cells to the gym. Over time, they become better at detoxifying, reducing inflammation, and dealing with oxidative stress.

We used to think that phytochemicals themselves were antioxidants and that they were directly responsible for eliminating free radicals, detoxifying, and reducing inflammation. However, in numerous studies over the past decade-plus, we've learned that phytochemicals are more like a biochemical wake-up call for our genes. It's our genes that then cause the production and release of antioxidants and enzymes that do the work. Phytochemicals activate some genes directly (such as sirtuin genes) and other genes indirectly by activating a gene regulator (such as NRF2).

NRF2 is one of the most important genetic pathways activated by phytochemicals. It's been referred to as a "master regulator" of detoxification and cell defense. You have about 25,000 genes total, and NRF2 regulates roughly 500 of them, or 2 percent. Imagine that each of your genes is controlled by a separate light switch—not a simple on-off toggle but rather a dimmer switch, so each gene can be turned up or down to a different level. NRF2 is responsible for roughly 500 dimmer switches and controls how much they get turned up or turned down. Or, said scientifically, NRF2 regulates and balances the "expression" of these 500 genes. Among them are survival genes that release antioxidants to eliminate free radicals, anti-inflammatory genes that release enzymes to fight inflammation, and antifibrosis genes that release enzymes to fight the formation of scar tissue. NRF2 also *deactivates* inflammatory genes.

What phytochemicals activate NRF2, and which foods are they found in? The phytochemicals include sulforaphane, catechins, curcumin, and resveratrol.

The most potent activator of NRF2 is *sulforaphane*, which is most prevalent in cruciferous vegetables such as broccoli, Brussels sprouts, cabbage, cauliflower, arugula, and kale. Sulforaphane belongs to a group of phytochemicals known as isothiocyanates, or ITCs (see Benefits of ITCs). Cruciferous vegetables contain compounds called glucosinolates and an enzyme called myrosinase. ITCs are produced when glucosinolates and myrosinase come into contact and chemically react with each other. Sulforaphane is produced when glucoraphanin (a specific glucosinolate) reacts with myrosinase. We help this reaction occur when we blend, chop, or chew vegetables. This breaks up the plant cells, and the damage allows glucoraphanin and myrosinase to mix.

BENEFITS OF ITCs

Isothiocyanates (ITCs) are powerful anticancer compounds. They have been found to detoxify and remove carcinogens, help kill cancer cells, and help prevent tumor growth. Specifically, ITCs deactivate phase 1 bio-transformation enzymes (carcinogens) and activate phase 2 detoxification enzymes (increase excretion). All the more reason to consistently eat greens. Also, the ITCs found in cruciferous vegetables help to reduce inflammatory chemicals, known as cytokines. Research shows that ITCs can lower common markers for inflammation seen on blood test results, including interlukin-6, by up to 20 percent, C-reactive protein by up to 16 percent,

(continued)

and tumor necrosis factor-alpha by up to 11 percent. These are specific markers that indicate inflammation in the body.

As noted on page 107, sulforaphane is an ITC. In addition to activating NRF_2, it helps reduce inflammation, assists in glucose regulation, increases glutathione levels (an antioxidant), and decreases cancer incidence.

Broccoli sprouts and cauliflower sprouts are particularly rich in glucoraphanin. To retain the most sulforaphane in cruciferous vegetables, steam them for 3 to 4 minutes. Cooking them for longer will deactivate myrosinase and result in less available sulforaphane. Only 20 percent of sulforaphane is bioavailable to begin with, so this is important to remember. You can also sprinkle broccoli sprouts or cauliflower sprouts over your cooked vegetables or add an external source of myrosinase to your cooked cruciferous vegetables. As it turns out, mustard seed contains myrosinase, so sprinkling your vegetables with mustard seed extract can increase the bioavailability of sulforaphane. Check out my Green Goddess dressing (see page 229) that contains mustard seed powder.

During a normal day, NRF2 is naturally activated every two hours or so. When you eat greens that contain sulforaphane, NRF2 is activated more often, approximately every hour. This is a significant increase—double the rate—and results in a more frequent release of antioxidants and beneficial enzymes. Again, this is good for your cells, like regularly sending them to the gym.

Further, phytochemicals don't stay in the system; our bodies actively neutralize them on a daily basis, which makes it important to eat leafy greens and vegetables every day. Balance and consistency are the keys. Overdoing it doesn't necessarily yield better results, so focus on consistency and low to moderate concentration. For example, EGCG (epigallocatechin gallate) is a phytochemical found in green tea. It's beneficial because it increases the production of glutathione, one of the most potent antioxidants. But EGCG works best at low to moderate levels. At high levels, glutathione production actually drops off. So, you don't need to drink eight cups of green tea or matcha per day. Just enjoy one cup per day consistently.

Here are several additional factors to consider when purchasing your greens:

CERTIFIED ORGANIC. For the reasons listed on page 33, I prefer certified organic produce. As always, it's a personal decision. If you want to buy certified organic, look for the "USDA Organic" label on the packaging.

TIP: Organic produce is typically more expensive than conventionally grown. To help reduce the cost, you can use the Environmental Working Group's annual "Dirty Dozen" and "Clean Fifteen" lists as resources to help decide what to buy organic versus conventionally grown (visit www.ewg.org for the most recent lists and other helpful information). The EWG uses data from the U.S. Department of Agriculture to analyze the amount of chemical pesticide residue on fruits and vegetables after being washed. The Dirty Dozen are crops that test positive for high levels of pesticides, which means they're good options to buy organic. The Clean Fifteen are crops that test for little or no trace of pesticides, which means they can be options to buy conventionally grown.

LOCALLY GROWN. To the extent possible, I try to source fresh produce from local farms and growers. One reason I do this is because locally grown produce is higher in nutrient value.

Plants start to lose nutrients from the moment they're picked as a result of a natural process called *respiration*. During respiration, plants break down and use their own stored nutrients to sustain themselves, which translates into fewer nutrients for you and me. All fruits and vegetables do this at different speeds, or cellular

SIRTUIN GENES

Sirtuin genes are a group of genes linked with longevity and metabolism. They help cells respond to different kinds of stress, and research indicates that increasing their activation may improve overall longevity. They're activated directly by certain phytochemicals (i.e., without the need for an intermediary/regulator such as NRF_2). We used to think that sirtuin genes were activated only during periods of fasting or strict caloric restriction, but now we know they're activated when we eat certain foods and aren't under a caloric restriction. In the chart on pages 93–101, I highlight which foods activate sirtuin genes.

respiration rates. The more distance and time your produce has to travel to get to you, the more nutrients it must use to stay alive. Further, shipping and transit can expose your produce to variations in temperature and rough handling that speed up the cellular respiration rate.

Locally grown produce has been recently picked from nearby locations. As a result, it generally contains higher nutrient values than produce shipped from the opposite side of the world. Foods with some of the most rapid cellular respiration rates include asparagus, broccoli, mushrooms, artichokes, Brussels sprouts, and green onions. Although refrigeration slows deterioration, you should try to eat these vegetables as soon as possible to maximize nutrient value. For example, one study found that vitamin C content in broccoli was undetectable just seven days after the pick date, even though when picked a single cup contains about 57 percent (on average) of our daily value.

> TIP: Buy local, store produce in the refrigerator, and try to eat vegetables with a rapid cellular respiration rate first. In the case of broccoli, if you can't find an organic local option, organic frozen broccoli is a good choice.

Buying locally grown produce has other benefits as well. It supports the community and reduces the environmental impact of transportation by using fewer natural resources and creating less pollution. Local produce also tends to be more seasonal.

Historically, specific crops were grown and harvested at the same time each year. Today, nearly every fruit and vegetable is available year-round, but before advances in agriculture and global supply chains, we generally ate what was grown seasonally in our geographic region. I try to incorporate what's in season as much as possible. One benefit is higher nutrient value (because seasonal produce is usually locally grown). It's also an easy way to spice up my shopping choices and add variety throughout the year. To find out what's in season, just ask the produce manager at your grocery store or visit your local farmers' market.

Shopping at a farmers' market every week is a great way to source fresh, local produce and get a sense for when different foods are produced in your area. Local farm cooperatives or associations are also good resources. At the grocery store or market, look for the country or state of origin on the label. It will give you a general sense of how far and long your produce traveled, and how close it is to its pick date. If you can't find local sources, flash frozen produce is also a great option. Most produce is flash frozen, but unfortunately there isn't a uniform labeling system to tell if it hasn't been.

GMOs. GMOs are genetically modified organisms. Modern science has given us the ability to genetically alter plants and engineer them for different purposes. This goes beyond crop and seed breeding, which has been around for centuries.

Today, many crop seeds are engineered to be resistant to pesticides and herbicides. This allows farmers to spray these chemicals without killing the crops. In the United States, more than 90 percent of the corn, soy, and cotton grown is genetically modified. Other foods that have been genetically modified include Arctic apples from Okanagan Specialty Fruits, Innate brand potatoes, AquaBounty's AquAdvantage salmon, certain dairy products, yellow squash, zucchini, papaya, alfalfa, sugar beets (sugar), and canola. The research on the health effects of GMOs is ongoing, and there isn't complete consensus yet. Whether you go non-GMO or not is a personal decision. For the time being, I'm taking a cautious approach and trying to source only non-GMO foods.

TIP: The Non-GMO Project is an organization that certifies products as non-GMO if the ingredients have less than 1 percent genetic modification. To know if you're buying a certified product, look for the Non-GMO Project label on packaging.

BIOAVAILABILITY. Bioavailability refers to the degree and rate at which a nutrient can be absorbed by your body. Nutrients that can be quickly and easily absorbed into the body are more bioavailable. Those that take longer or are more difficult to absorb are less bioavailable.

Bioavailability starts with the presence of nutrients in the first place, which depends on source quality, growing conditions, soil health, and time elapsed since the pick date. Unfortunately, recent research indicates there has been a nationwide decline in the nutrient content of our produce, which negatively impacts bioavailability. In a landmark study out of the University of Texas at Austin, an analysis of the nutritional data from forty-three different fruits and vegetables found "reliable declines" in the amount of vitamins and minerals over the past fifty years. Researchers have posited that the decline is the result of agriculture practices aimed at improving traits other than nutrition, such as size, growth rate, and pesticide resistance. Further, nutrient content in produce can vary greatly from region to region (or even farm to farm) due to specific growing conditions. One study found that soil health, exposure to sunlight, and water levels contributed to significant differences in iron, calcium, magnesium, and phosphorus content.

TIP: To help maximize nutrient content, incorporate microgreens and sprouts of vegetables such as broccoli, arugula, and cilantro into your diet. These small, week-old plants can serve up higher nutrient density than their full-grown counterparts—up to fourteen times as much.

Soil health is a key driver of nutrient content and thus bioavailability. This is one of the reasons behind the proposal of additional organic certifications that specifically take soil practices into account, such as Regenerative Organic Certified and the Real Organic Project mentioned on page 34. They aim to go beyond restricting the use of chemicals, and they incent growers to take additional measures to improve soil quality. Building and maintaining a healthy soil ecosystem depends on agricultural methods and techniques such as composting, aeration, root spacing, and reduced tilling. It also depends on the presence of microorganisms, other organisms, and the decomposition of organic matter.

TIP: If you buy produce from a farmers' market, ask the seller/grower about their food and farming practices. A few basic questions would be: Where was the food grown?

Who grew it? When was it picked? Is it certified organic? Were pesticides used? A few more probing questions: How do they control weeds (with chemicals or by hand)? Where do their seeds come from; are they heirloom (meaning used for generations and never modified)? How do they support healthy soil? You never know until you ask, and it could give you new or useful information to inform your purchasing decision. The goal is to help you find a seller/grower you feel comfortable going back to week after week.

Bioavailability also depends on the presence of so-called antinutrients, such as phytic acid or lectins, which can block the absorption of vitamins and minerals. Plants contain natural agents whose job is to prevent premature germination or growth. The problem is that in the process, they prevent access to vitamins and minerals. For example, phytic acid is an enzyme inhibitor that binds with zinc, iron, and calcium in the gastrointestinal tract, making these minerals inaccessible. Phytic acid is found in nuts, seeds, and beans/legumes.

One simple way to neutralize and eliminate phytic acid is to soak and/or sprout nuts, seeds, and beans/legumes before consumption. See page 51 to learn how.

Lectins are found in the skin or shell of plants, and are another natural protection against being eaten and digested. They're especially problematic for people whose gut health has been compromised by conditions such as leaky gut syndrome, Crohn's disease, celiac disease, and IBS. Lectins are highest in grains and beans/legumes. If you live a plant-based lifestyle and use grains and beans/legumes as a main source of protein, you'll need to pay special attention to this issue. To help reduce or neutralize lectins in beans/legumes, soak them or use a pressure cooker to cook them. Soaking also works for nuts and seeds. As for other fruits and vegetables, peeling and deseeding will help reduce or neutralize their lectins. Fermentation and pressure cooking also work. Lectins are something to be mindful of, but you shouldn't stop eating vegetables, nuts, or seeds. To me that's just ridiculous! If you're looking to have the largest impact, I would reduce or remove grains. If you're plant-based, use the simple methods here to help reduce or neutralize them. That said, I don't think you need to peel and deseed every single cucumber you eat, unless you want to.

Further, bioavailability depends on your unique biochemistry and your body's ability to break down and absorb food via digestive enzymes, hydrochloric acid, and healthy gut bacteria. To help the process along, chew your food completely. It sounds basic, but digestion starts in your mouth by physically breaking your food apart. Also, the enzyme amylase is present in your saliva and begins to break down carbohydrates and starches immediately. As food moves into your stomach, proteases and hydrochloric acid are released. Proteases are enzymes that help digest proteins. Hydrochloric acid helps inhibit bad bacteria and provides the acidic pH balance necessary for proteases to do their job. The pancreas releases additional enzymes into the stomach and small intestine, including lipase, which helps digest fat. By eating the Fab Four, you'll help support production of these enzymes and hydrochloric acid.

One of the reasons I developed the Fab Four Smoothie was to make digestion easier on your body. If you experience digestive issues, consult with your physician or functional medical doctor about being tested for low hydrochloric acid and/or supplementing with digestive enzymes or betaine hydrochloric acid.

Cooking vegetables can also affect bioavailability. On one hand, many vitamins can be lost during cooking, such as vitamins A, B_{12}, and C. On the other hand, some minerals and phytochemicals become more bioavailable with cooking, such as iron, calcium, and potassium.

TIP: Mix it up and eat both raw and cooked vegetables every day. One way to do this is to split your produce in half and prepare it both ways. For example, enjoy raw mushrooms and onions on a spinach salad for lunch, then sauté them for a savory side at dinnertime.

Pairing certain foods can affect the bioavailability of nutrients. Some combinations increase bioavailability, while others decrease it. Here are a few examples of specific food combinations:

• Turmeric: To increase the bioavailability of this anti-inflammatory spice and its phytochemical curcumin, pair it with healthy fat, black pepper, or tea.

- Sulforaphane: Pair cruciferous vegetables with mustard seed extract to increase sulforaphane absorption by an incredible 400 percent. (You can thank Dr. Rhonda Patrick for blazing the trail regarding the benefits of sulforaphane.)
- Red meat: To increase iron absorption, pair red meat with sources of vitamin C, including leafy greens, broccoli, or peppers. Iron absorption can be reduced by phytic acid, which is found in grains and beans/legumes, so perhaps avoid that pairing.
- Matcha: Matcha contains the phytochemical EGCG, which is a precursor to the antioxidant glutathione. To increase its bioavailability, add a squeeze of lemon to your matcha or green tea. Dairy milk will decrease its bioavailability.
- Healthy fats: As discussed in chapter 2, healthy fats help us absorb fat-soluble vitamins (such as vitamins A, D, E, and K) and phytochemicals (such as lutein, zeaxanthin, and beta-carotene) from vegetables. Boost the bioavailability of the nutrients in your salad by adding fats such as olive oil, avocado, or nuts.

Finally, here are a few other quick tips for increasing bioavailability:

- Garlic: Chop it ten to fifteen minutes before you need it. This releases an enzyme that increases the bioavailability of key nutrients, including organic sulfur compounds.
- Berries: Polyphenols are a type of phytochemical that can increase bioavailability when berries are frozen. Buy frozen berries at the market or buy fresh at the farmers' market and then freeze them.
- Shallots: They have more nutrient density than onions and are a great swap for many recipes.
- Dark chocolate: Try to source natural cocoa, and not Dutch-processed cocoa powder. Dutch processing removes polyphenols.

5
THE "NOT SO FAB" FOUR

YOUR OPTIONAL "PLUS-ONE"

THE PURPOSE OF THE Fab Four is to help you build balance on your plate, in your bloodstream, and ultimately in your life. It's light structure that prioritizes nutrient-dense, blood-sugar-balancing foods. When it comes to carbohydrates, the Fab Four emphasizes unprocessed whole foods that are rich in fiber, vitamins, minerals, phytochemicals, and water. These are your fiber and greens. It shifts the focus away from what I call the "Not So Fab" Four: processed, sugary, certain starchy, and liquid carbohydrates.

I chose the "Not So Fab" moniker, which is relatively mild, for a reason. It doesn't mean you can never, ever eat these foods. It just means they lack the full range of nutrients your body needs to function optimally and don't support optimal blood sugar balance. As a result, they shouldn't be the foundation of your meals or overall diet. Think of them as your "plus-one," an optional guest you can choose (or not choose) to invite to your plate party. The primary components of your meals should always be the Fab Four. Then, depending on your specific lifestyle or weight loss goals, you can decide if and when you want to invite your "plus-one."

In this chapter, I share my approach to these types of carbohydrates. I give you a few simple guidelines and practical tools that I call on and use every single day, both for myself and with my clients. My goal is to empower you to make body-loving choices, while still having the flexibility and freedom to enjoy life. Building a healthy, sustainable lifestyle isn't about deprivation or holding yourself to an impossible standard. I think it's unrealistic to say you'll never have another sushi roll made with white rice, fresh pasta if you're in Italy (or at Eataly), tortillas or chips on Taco Tuesday, corn on the cob at a summer barbecue, cake at a birthday party, glass of wine with friends, or cocktail on vacation. What is realistic is to prioritize the Fab Four and to use the Fab Four to bring yourself back into balance when you need to. When you commit to these simple ideas and turn them into action, your goals will always be within reach. You'll be nourishing your body and fostering a more positive relationship with food. And instead of beating yourself up about having an imbalanced meal or day, you'll be building self-confidence and resilience. That's the Fab Four lifestyle and body love in a nutshell.

Like everything else, my approach to processed, sugary, certain starchy, and liquid carbohydrates is driven by science and the biochemical effects these foods have on our body. Generally speaking, they have lower nutrient density and are either deficient in, or devoid of, many of the essential nutrients so vital to health. When you overeat these foods at every meal, you're missing out on the amino acids, fatty acids, fiber, vitamins, minerals, and phytochemicals that support your brain, organs, muscles, gut, skin, and cells. Instead, you're primarily getting one thing in excess: glucose.

As you'll recall from Blood Sugar 101, glucose or blood sugar is fuel for the cells. We use it to power all sorts of bodily functions, which is why our body keeps some available in our bloodstream at all times. The healthy range is between 70 mg/dl and 120 mg/dl. Carbohydrates break down into glucose and raise your blood sugar. In response, your body releases insulin, a storage hormone. Insulin takes excess glucose out of your bloodstream and stores it in the liver and muscles, then fat cells (after it has been converted into a triglyceride), thereby lowering your blood sugar and restoring balance. Overeating the "Not So Fab" Four at every single meal throws this process out of whack.

EXAMPLES OF THE "NOT SO FAB" FOUR

Here are several examples of the types of foods that fall into the "Not So Fab" category, most of which shouldn't be a surprise. Please note that this is not intended to be a comprehensive list. Also, keep in mind that depending on the ingredients, oils, and manner of preparation, some of these foods do have cleaner options (see the chart on page 125). That said, remember that even the cleaner options will raise your blood sugar and cause the release of insulin.

- **PROCESSED CARBOHYDRATES:** junk food, fast food, chips, and crackers.
- **SUGARY CARBOHYDRATES:** candy, cookies, pastries, and sweets.
- **CERTAIN STARCHY CARBOHYDRATES:** bread, pasta, grains, and corn.
- **LIQUID CARBOHYDRATES:** alcohol, soda, energy drinks, and mixers/fruit juice.

Processed, sugary, certain starchy, and liquid carbohydrates break down into larger amounts of glucose and therefore cause a more aggressive spike in blood sugar. As a result, your body has to release larger amounts of insulin. If your liver and muscles are already at capacity because you overate these foods at your previous meal (or because you don't regularly exercise), the excess glucose will (1) be converted into suboptimal free fatty acids (triglycerides) and stored as fat, and/or (2) linger in the bloodstream, resulting in elevated insulin levels (hyperinsulinemia), which increases the likelihood that other triglycerides, regardless of where they originate from (converted fructose, converted alcohol, dietary fat, or another source), will be stored as fat. Unlike your liver and muscles, your fat cells don't have a maximum capacity. Remember the car trunk analogy used in Blood

Sugar 101? Well, we can fill the trunk *and* hitch on a U-Haul with our food choices! Eating a large amount of the "Not So Fab" Four will cause excess insulin to linger in your bloodstream. When you have excess insulin in your bloodstream, your body won't burn fat. The presence of excess insulin shuts down fat burning because it's the chemical messenger that says, "Time to store." Finally, when your blood sugar starts to drop (or crash), your hunger hormones will kick in and trigger cravings for more carbohydrates, because they represent the fastest way to raise your blood sugar. If you act on the cravings, your body will release more insulin, and the spike-crash-crave cycle will start all over again.

If your goal is weight loss or improved body composition, this is why eating balanced meals consisting of the Fab Four can be so beneficial. It supports blood sugar homeostasis by encouraging you to eat fiber and greens first. Then, when it comes to other carbohydrates, it encourages you to eat them in the way nature intended: as whole foods wrapped in a fibrous cell (cellular carbohydrates). Your blood sugar won't aggressively spike or crash, your body releases less insulin, and your hunger hormones stay in balance. The result is an elongated blood sugar curve—you're full, fueled, and have balanced blood sugar for a longer period of time. This enables healthy weight loss. Remember, healthy weight loss happens in between meals and during sleep when your blood sugar is balanced and you don't have excess insulin in your bloodstream.

The bigger picture is the effect on your overall health, vitality, and longevity. Overeating the "Not So Fab" Four at every meal can pose real, long-term health risks. Not only are you missing out on all of the benefits of protein, fat, fiber, and greens (including the anti-inflammatory, detoxifying, and anticancer properties), but you're also potentially creating the conditions for disease and health issues to arise. Chronically elevated blood sugar can lead to diabetes and metabolic syndrome. Continuously high insulin levels can lead to insulin resistance and polycystic ovary syndrome (PCOS). Chronic inflammation can lead to cardiovascular disease, autoimmune disorders, and other conditions. Overeating these foods also feeds the bad bacteria in our gut (such as candida and yeast), which can lead to toxicity and increased inflammation throughout the body. In addition, these foods are often made with artificial trans unsaturated fats (trans fats) and man-made industrial seed and vegetable oils, which can be detrimental for the reasons listed on page 82 in chapter 2.

Regardless of your immediate goal, I want you to thrive and live a long, healthy life. I want you to build a sustainable lifestyle that promotes longevity, supports brain health, and helps reduce the risk of disease. It starts with prioritizing the Fab Four and eating balanced meals, and not overeating processed, sugary, certain starchy, and liquid carbohydrates at every meal.

So how should you approach these foods? In the following pages are a few simple, body-loving guidelines and tools I use every day, both in my own life and in my practice. How to approach carbohydrates is one of the most common questions people ask me. I hope this gives you a little more hands-on guidance and structure (if you want it), so you can determine what works best for you and your body. Remember, it's about elevating your food choices and prioritizing the Fab Four, which will balance your blood sugar and give your body a break from insulin.

Two quick notes before we dive in:

First, remember that these guidelines are only for carbohydrates in the "Not So Fab" category. They don't apply to fiber and greens!

Second, these recommendations are being made under the assumption that you're exercising daily or at least a few times per week, so that you're consistently dumping stored glucose from your muscles and making room for more.

HOW OFTEN SHOULD I EAT CARBOHYDRATES? It depends on your goal. If your goal is weight loss or improved body composition, once per day. If your goal is more about building a healthy lifestyle or optimizing your overall health, two (or occasionally three) times per day. Remember, these foods are an optional "plus-one." The priority should always be on the Fab Four.

For example, if you eat two pieces of gluten-free toast at breakfast, have a quinoa bowl at lunch, and eat sweet potato fries at dinner, you're essentially turning off fat burning all day long. Even though these are healthier carbohydrate options, they still raise your blood sugar and cause the release of insulin. Many of my clients have a specific weight loss goal, so dialing back carbohydrates to once per day is an easy way to give their body a break from repeated influxes of insulin and turn fat burning back on. Meanwhile, they're still eating Fab Four meals to keep them full, fueled, and balanced.

To be clear, I'm not telling you to stop eating carbohydrates completely. The Fab Four lifestyle isn't a no-carb diet. I never advise my clients to remove all carbohydrates. (See Low-Carb Purgatory.) Your body is more than capable of metabolizing them, including those in the "Not So Fab" category. I'm simply shifting your focus to make sure you get enough fiber and greens at every meal, which together with protein and fat are nutrient-dense, blood sugar–balancing, and give your body a break from excess insulin.

LOW-CARB PURGATORY

Some of my clients take it to the extreme, either by not eating any carbohydrates at all or by only ever eating greens that have the lowest possible carbohydrate content (i.e., spinach and asparagus on repeat). Not only is this overly restrictive, but it also puts you at risk of falling into what I call low-carb purgatory. If you're not actively pursuing a ketogenic state, going no-carb or extremely low-carb can result in low energy, poor recovery after workouts, and feeling depleted or exhausted. You're basically out of gas. As you'll recall from Blood Sugar 101, your body can run on two types of fuel: glucose from carbohydrates or fat-based fuel called ketones. If you don't have any glucose in your bloodstream or liver (or only a small amount) and you're not in ketosis, then you're stuck in a state of purgatory energy-wise. And you might binge your way out of it.

That's why I never advise my clients to remove all carbohydrates. I want them to stay fueled. You should feel confident making the choice to eat higher carbohydrate vegetables like sweet potato, carrots, and beets, as well as a "Not So Fab"

Four choice like a slice of pizza, a taco, or something sweet. If you prioritize the Fab Four, you give yourself the flexibility to live how you want and make choices, not cheats. Remember, even though you might have a goal, this is about building toward balance, not crash dieting.

HOW MUCH SHOULD I EAT? It depends on your goal and the type of carbohydrate you're eating. I cover two types below: cellular and acellular. Cellular carbohydrates are a cleaner, healthier option than acellular carbohydrates. I generally tell my clients to reserve acellular carbohydrates for a couple times per month or as an occasional add-on to a meal.

- If you're going to add carbohydrates to a meal and your goal is weight loss or improved body composition:
  - Cellular carbohydrates: 25 grams of net carbohydrates or less at that meal.
  - Acellular carbohydrates: 10 grams of net carbohydrates or less at that meal.
- If you're going to add carbohydrates to a meal and your goal is more about building a healthy lifestyle or optimizing your overall health:
  - Cellular carbohydrates: 50 grams of net carbohydrates or less at that meal.
  - Acellular carbohydrates: 15 to 20 grams of net carbohydrates or less at that meal.

Ideally, you also want the carbohydrate density of any given food to be 30 percent or less. Again, for the record, my intent is not to have you measuring your food at every meal. The point of the Fab Four is to give you light structure, so you can build a healthy, sustainable lifestyle that's right for you. These benchmarks and parameters are for those of you who want a little more hands-on guidance and structure to follow. And remember that these guidelines don't apply to fiber and greens!

Let's walk through net carbohydrates, carbohydrate density, and the difference between cellular and acellular carbohydrates.

Net carbohydrates is a rough measurement of how much of the carbohydrate

content in a food will break down into glucose or blood sugar. This goes back to fiber. As you will recall from chapter 3, even though fiber is listed under carbohydrates on the nutrition facts, it isn't absorbed into our bloodstream, and it doesn't break down into glucose or blood sugar. To calculate net carbohydrates, you simply subtract the fiber from the total carbohydrates.

Net carbohydrates = total carbohydrates minus fiber

Generally speaking, you should prioritize foods with lower net carbohydrate amounts. Lower net carbohydrate foods break down into less glucose and don't raise your blood sugar as high or as fast. As a result, your body releases less insulin. This helps keep your blood sugar and hunger hormones in balance, which supports healthy weight loss efforts. Plus, it likely means you're eating a higher fiber food source. As discussed in chapter 3, fiber is crucial for the health of the gut microbiome and aids in digestion. If you overeat higher net carbohydrate foods at every meal, you'll find yourself on the blood sugar roller coaster, be full of excess insulin, and miss out on the benefits of fiber.

Carbohydrate density is the percentage of a single serving that is carbohydrates. It helps answer the following question: how much of the food is carbohydrates? This generally tells us how the food will affect blood sugar and also gives an indication of its nutritional content. To calculate carbohydrate density, you divide net carbohydrates by the total number of grams in a single serving. The result is a decimal, which can also be expressed as a percentage.

Carbohydrate density = net carbohydrates divided by total grams in a single serving

CARBOHYDRATE CHART

Here is a sampling of the net carbohydrates and carbohydrate density for several body-loving carbohydrate options.

Food	Net Carbs	Grams/Serving	Carb Density
Seasnax seaweed crisps	0 grams	5 grams for 1 package	0%
Chopped broccoli	2 grams	91 grams per cup	2%
Flackers flaxseed crackers	1 gram	25 grams for 8 crackers	4%
NOW Foods macadamia nuts	2 grams	35 grams for ¼ cup	5%
Raspberries	7 grams	123 grams for 1 cup	6%
Cubed butternut squash	9 grams	100 grams for ½ cup	9%
Barely Bread grain-free bread	3 grams	26 grams per slice	12%
Trader Joe's gluten-free Norwegian crisp bread	3 grams	24 grams for 1 crisp	12%
Wild Friends Almond Macadamia Be Well Blend	4 grams	32 grams for 2 tablespoons	13%
Primal Kitchen macadamia nut bar	7 grams	49 grams for 1 bar	14%
Jilz Crackerz	5 grams	28 grams for 10 crackers	17%
Cubed sweet potato	23 grams	133 grams for 1 cup	17%
Bulletproof collagen protein bar	5 grams	21 grams for 1 bar	23%
GG Scandinavian Crispbread	2 grams	8 grams for 1 cracker	25%
Siete almond flour tortilla	14 grams	50 grams for 2 tortillas	28%

When you prioritize foods with lower carbohydrate density, carbohydrates account for a smaller proportion of each serving. As noted on page 123, a good benchmark to strive for is 30 percent or less. This is roughly the percentage found in many

If you constantly rely on dense carbohydrates, your brain and body will become accustomed to the constant supply of glucose. As a result, pulling back can make you feel sluggish, less energetic, and foggy. To ease the transition, gradually switch to lower net carbohydrate options with less carbohydrate density. For example, at breakfast, make a Fab Four Smoothie that has berries in the recipe for a week, then swap to a fruit-free recipe. At lunch, add ¼ cup of quinoa or ½ cup of roasted squash to your salad, instead of having a full grain bowl. If you typically eat an afternoon snack, ditch the cookie and opt for a small handful of raspberries and 1 tablespoon of almond butter. At dinnertime, focus on the fiber and greens, and if you feel the need for a starchier carbohydrate, opt for a sweet potato.

whole foods in nature, so eat vegetables without worry! Foods with lower carbohydrate density break down into less glucose, won't raise your blood sugar as high or as fast, and will release less insulin. In addition, it means the food contains a higher amount of fiber, which provides food for your gut microbiome.

THE DIFFERENCE BETWEEN CELLULAR AND ACELLULAR CARBOHYDRATES

Unprocessed whole foods contain cellular carbohydrates. All this means is that their carbohydrates are packaged inside of cells. The cells have an intact cell wall and contain fiber and water. Because they contain fiber, these foods generally contain lower net carbohydrates and have a lower carbohydrate density. They also contain more vitamins, minerals, and phytochemicals. Further, as you'll recall from chapter 3, fiber is like an extra layer or shell around the molecules in food. We have to get through it first before we can access what's inside. This extra step slows digestion and slows the absorption of glucose. Fiber also feeds healthy gut bacteria and helps prevent overfeeding bad gut bacteria. Overall, cellular carbohydrates are cleaner, healthier, and have less effect on your blood sugar than acellular carbohydrates.

If you add cellular carbohydrates to a meal, the goal should be 25 grams of net carbohydrates or less for weight loss, or 50 grams of net carbohydrates or less for general lifestyle. A few examples of starchy cellular carbohydrates include squash, quinoa, rice, black beans, sweet potato, parsnips, carrots, and cassava. A nonstarchy example is berries. As for corn and peas, I would eat them more occasionally. They tend to have higher carbohydrate density, and more than 90 percent of the corn in the United States is genetically modified (GMO).

Processed foods contain acellular carbohydrates—the carbohydrates are no longer packaged inside of intact cells. A few examples include flours, processed grains, and sugars, as well as all the foods made from these, such as cookies, cake, pizza, bread, and pasta. These foods have been milled, dehydrated, refined, or otherwise processed, which removes the cell wall and strips the cell of fiber, water, and other nutrients. What's left is just a concentrated version of one part of the original food. Because they no longer contain fiber, these foods generally contain higher net carbohydrates and have a higher carbohydrate density. You can guess what this will do to your blood sugar. The lack of fiber results in a quicker, higher spike. They break down into a sugary slurry, which enters the digestive chyme and is easier to absorb than fiber-wrapped molecules. If you read the list of ingredients on many processed foods, you'll also see they're often made with unhealthy fats—artificial trans fats and man-made industrial seed and vegetable oils.

As noted on page 123, I would reserve acellular carbohydrates for a couple times per month or as an occasional add-on to a meal. If you add them to a meal, the goal should be 10 grams of net carbohydrates or less for weight loss, or 15 to 20 grams of net carbohydrates or less for general lifestyle.

Overeating acellular carbohydrates at every meal may lead to several health risks and conditions. In a 2012 paper published in *Diabetes, Metabolic Syndrome and Obesity: Targets and Therapy,* Ian Spreadbury, a researcher in the Gastrointestinal Diseases Research Unit at Queen's University in Ontario, Canada, proposed that acellular carbohydrates might be responsible for the modern obesity epidemic. The author pointed to the fact that acellular carbohydrates expose gut bacteria to far greater amounts of glucose than ever before, which might result in an inflammatory microbial population. An overgrowth of this bad gut bacteria may cause production of bacterial endotoxins and intestinal permeability. In turn, if the intestinal permeability allows these endotoxins into the body, it could result in systemic inflammation. Inflammation caused by changes in the gut microbiota may cause damage to the hypothalamus and afferent vagus nerve endings, inducing leptin resistance. Leptin is a satiety hormone that tells us we're full and helps prevent overeating, and leptin resistance weakens the signal. Increased carbohydrate concentration could also lead to small intestinal bacterial overgrowth (SIBO) and gut dysbiosis, bacterial imbalances with side effects including gas, excessive bloating, IBS symptoms, and in severe cases, nutrient deficiencies.

This is why prioritizing cellular carbohydrates—whole foods with lower net carbohydrates, lower carbohydrate density, and more fiber—is crucial. They have a smaller effect on blood sugar, reduce the risk of endotoxin exposure and inflammation, and limit the overgrowth of bad gut bacteria. It's also why acellular carbohydrates are not everyday foods. Depending on your health, they might not even be every week foods. It doesn't mean you can never, ever eat these foods again. But it's important to understand how overeating acellular carbohydrates can disrupt satiety signals, undermine your self-control, and lead to an unhealthy gut.

Emma, age twenty-seven, a social media manager, came to me feeling out of control. During the week, she would eat zero carbohydrates. Then, when the weekend hit, that was all she ate. She would binge on late-night food like pizza, nachos, fries, and fro-yo, and indulge in cocktails and wine all the way up to Sunday night. She told me she felt like she had zero self-control and that on Monday she felt depressed. The first thing we did was bring back cellular carbs during the week. I asked her to find at least two meals per week post-workout to incorporate something like a cooked and cooled potato, quinoa, or fruit. By the second week, she felt less pressure to "be good" all week, and as a result found herself bingeing way less over the weekend. By the end of a month, she was making the choice to indulge in a few of her favorite things on the weekend without feeling out of control.

Also, even if a food is marketed as natural, gluten-free, or clean, you should still read the ingredients and nutrition facts. Every year, the largest food shows debut new "healthy" products that are just as processed as ever. Many are made with refined flours, loaded with sugar, and contain industrial seed and vegetable oils. Rice flour, quinoa flour, and arrowroot flour are still acellular, as is coconut sugar. Even though they're gluten-free and could be a healthier alternative, the effect on our bodies from the standpoint of blood sugar balance is essentially the same.

The takeaway: read the ingredients and nutrition facts, use the guidelines and tools in this chapter, and find the approach that works for you and your body. When in doubt, opt for organic, raw, and whole versions of foods. Here are some additional factors to take into account with respect to certain "Not So Fab" Four foods.

WHEAT:

- Dramatically spikes blood sugar levels and can contribute to diabetes, PCOS, heart disease, and cancer.
- Processed acellular wheat (flour) feeds candida and SIBO.
- Touted for being high in B vitamins, but during processing more than half of the vitamins B_1, B_2, B_3, and folic acid can be lost, as well as vitamin E, calcium, phosphorus, zinc, copper, iron, and fiber.
- Numerous research articles link it to autoimmune diseases, gut permeability, and inflammation.

CORN:

- More than 90 percent is genetically modified (GMO).
- Typically sprayed with chemical pesticides, such as glyphosate.

SUGAR:

- Studies indicate can be as addictive or more than narcotics.
- Full of empty calories that deplete the body of minerals, elevate glucose, and lead to exhaustion.
- Causes inflammation and can be a precursor to cancer.

DAIRY:

- Lactose, the sugar found in dairy, is a common allergen.
- May come with more than 60 growth hormones, and pasteurized dairy is hard to digest as it lacks lactase, an enzyme present in raw dairy.

- Raw dairy is digestible because enzymes are still present, increasing the bio-availability of calcium and protein.

The Fab Four is a light structure designed to help you put the most nutrient-dense, blood sugar–balancing foods on your plate. Protein, fat, fiber, and greens keep you vibrant, glowing, and fueled. They promote longevity and brain health, and help prevent disease. And they balance your blood sugar and give your body a break from excess insulin. The "Not So Fab" Four? Not so much.

PART TWO

THE BODY LOVE ARCHETYPES AND FAB FOUR PLANS

6
GIRL ON THE GO

FIND BALANCE WHEREVER LIFE TAKES YOU

ONCE WORK'S NOT SO crazy. Once I'm not traveling so much. Once the kids go back to school. Once the holidays are over. Once this project is off my plate. Once my in-laws or clients leave town. Once I'm not so exhausted. Once things finally settle down. Once I actually have time for me again. Once . . . upon a time.

Life can get so hectic that finding balance can feel like a fairy tale, or something you only see done on Instagram. How can I live a healthy lifestyle and reach my goals when I can barely catch my breath? At times it can feel daunting, but I'll tell you the same thing I tell all my Girl on the Go clients: start with one body-loving decision. Then make one more. Turn that hypothetical **once** into an actual twice. Because the truth of the matter is that **the small, everyday decisions you make in the here and now are what add up to balance.** One decision—your next—is all that matters. You don't need it to be a morning, a Monday, or a new month to start. I challenge you right now to make your next decision a healthy one.

When life is moving fast and you're constantly on the go and under stress, food quickly becomes a comforting reward. Many of my clients form an emotional bond with their sugary morning latte, their afternoon cookie from the office kitchen, their nightly glass of wine, or their favorite greasy takeout. These treats are a brief reprieve from the daily grind and they make us feel good . . . temporarily. The problem is that they add up as well. Eventually, these little daily derailments can take you so far offtrack that you feel out of control. That's when the wheels can really come off, and it's usually when my clients call me. What started as a busy couple of days turned into a three-week free-for-all and now they feel more anxiety, more pressure—and more overwhelmed.

We all want things to settle down so we can feel fully capable and committed to making healthier decisions. But life doesn't happen in a vacuum, and you can't sit around waiting for your calendar to clear. If yours looks anything like mine, it won't! And when you finally do manage a minute of calm, the temptation may be to let go entirely. I tell my Girl on the Go clients the same thing I tell myself: focus on the present moment. **Once you make one body-loving decision, you've dropped anchor and steadied the ship.** It stops the cycle of self-soothing that bleeds into the weekend and then next week. It's how you catch your breath. **Simple habits are what support a healthy lifestyle, and the Fab Four might be the simplest of all.** The plan in this chapter is full of actionable examples and easy ways to live the Fab Four lifestyle on the go. The temptation to overindulge and put off the changes you want is always there. But so is the Fab Four.

PLAN OVERVIEW

If you're a Girl on the Go, twenty-one days might take you twenty-one different places. Many of us perform a nonstop juggling act between work, family, travel, or all of the above (plus we have a social life). Then there are the days or weeks that pull us in twenty-one different directions mentally and emotionally. Wherever you go (or get pulled), this plan can work for you.

I've set up Week 1 as a travel week. Even if you don't travel that often, this is a great place to start and see the Fab Four in action. We all find ourselves in airports, hotels, and new cities from time to time, so the first week gives you some easy strategies to use in these environments. The travel week is also full of tips and tools that are just as useful at home, like what I keep handy in my purse, my advice on protein bars, surefire tips for ordering out, how to make a Fab Four Roadie using coffee, tea, or espresso drinks, and a body-loving reminder to ditch your phone, to sleep, and to find nature when you get home.

Weeks 2 and 3 bring you back home. These two weeks will show you just how easily the Fab Four can be incorporated into your everyday life—morning, noon, and night. There are delicious new Fab Four Smoothie recipes like Cinnamon Coconut (page 144), Green Ginger (page 161), Pecan Pie (page 177), and Happy Gut (page 181). There are a bunch of quick, easy, and tasty recipes that even the busiest Girls on the Go can make, like Wild Fish Boats (page 172), Chinese Chicken Lettuce Wraps (page 176), and Fab Four Chia Seed Pudding (page 184). In addition, you'll find suggestions for working out, tips for self-care, and a few easy ways to help manage stress. I also give you some tools and strategies for weekends away.

I want you to love your healthy lifestyle, so use this plan in the way that's best suited to you and your goals.

Travel Week

Air travel is taxing, both physically and mentally. It saps energy, challenges the immune system, and disrupts your sleep cycle. It can create stress and anxiety, test your patience, and make you puffy and bloated. Then there's the food. Many airport terminals and airlines have dramatically improved their offerings compared with a decade ago, but they're still not choices you can consistently rely on. The newsstand is usually bad news, and the biggest sellers are still junk food, candy, fast food, and alcohol—which are some of the biggest culprits in the "Not So Fab" Four category. All the hurrying, worrying, and waiting make you crave comfort food and perhaps something to take the edge off. That's why

FASTING ON YOUR FLIGHT

If done properly, intermittent fasting can be used as an occasional tool to aid weight loss efforts. Some of my clients like using their airport and flight time as an opportunity to intermittent fast. For example, if they have a morning flight, they fast at breakfast and then eat lunch as their first meal of the day once they reach their destination. Or if they have a midday or afternoon flight, they eat breakfast (or a Fab Four Smoothie), fast at lunch, and eat dinner at their destination. A few of my clients like a longer fasting period, too. If my clients want to fast while flying, I tell them to drink as much water as possible, sip on polyphenol-rich teas (such as black, green, or white tea), and limit their coffee intake to one or two cups maximum. I also tell them to consciously focus on taking full, deep breaths throughout the day. This sounds basic, but it's a calming practice for any situation and shifts focus away from the snacking and boozing that's probably going on around them. The point isn't to starve and deprive yourself, but to use a defined period of time to gain the benefits of intermittent fasting and then eat a full Fab Four meal that puts you right into balance. I discuss intermittent fasting on page 356.

airports can make McDonald's and a glass of chardonnay seem like a good combination. Here are a few simple strategies to tilt the situation back in your favor. When you're on the go, they can help turn any travel day—whether it's for a stressful work trip or a fun vacation—into just another body-loving day. That's the beauty of living in balance with the Fab Four.

FUEL UP WITH THE FAB FOUR BEFORE YOU GO. Heading to the airport on an empty stomach is just like grocery shopping on one: when you're hungry and surrounded by food, it can lead you to make decisions you otherwise wouldn't. The best way to counter the temptation is to fuel up and eat before you go.

- *Option 1*: Eat a full Fab Four meal at home or at your favorite healthy restaurant or market. Depending on your flight time, I would try to stick to your normal eating time for that meal and maintain normal eating hours throughout the entire day. For example, if I have an evening or red-eye flight, I stay fasted after dinner just like at home.

- *Option 2*: A Fab Four Smoothie is always a great option. If your flight is early in the morning, blend it up the night before and stick it in the fridge. The fiber can thicken overnight, so just add a little water or nut milk in the morning, shake a few times, and off you go. Then sip it in your car on the way to the airport. It saves time and money, shuts down hunger, and sets you up for the rest of the day.

- *Option 3*: If you're crunched on time, bring a Fab Four meal through security, then eat it in the terminal or even on your flight. Think of it as your Fab Four carry-on.
  - My favorite go-to is to build a wild salmon salad at Whole Foods or Erewhon Market. I also like putting together warm meals with grilled protein and sautéed vegetables. Build something that sounds good to you.
  - Another easy option is a rotisserie chicken salad. A rotisserie chicken is a fast, easy dinner option for Girls on the Go. If you have leftovers, make a simple salad to take with you the next day. Add a handful of greens, ¼ cup chickpeas, half an avocado, and sliced cucumber and bell pepper. A squeeze of lemon will keep the avocado from browning. Bring a mini container with your favorite dressing or a single-serving olive oil packet.

DON'T GO EMPTY-HANDED. In general, I don't recommend daily snacking because it can disrupt digestion and be detrimental to weight loss goals. But for a travel day, a Fab Four Snack Pack may help prevent bad decisions when anxiety, hunger, or boredom sets in. It can be a smart bridge tool and a better option than what's available at the newsstand or on the plane. Use a small soft cooler bag, travel container, or tin. If you have a long flight or layover that will overlap with your next meal time, I recommend taking a full Fab Four meal from home or from a healthy restaurant or market with you.

- **FAB FOUR SNACK PACK #1:** 2 hard-boiled eggs (protein), 1 bag raw nuts or nut butter (fat), and ½ to 1 cup chopped vegetables such as cucumber, celery, peppers, carrot, zucchini, or radish (fiber and greens). Recently, I had to get up at 4:15 A.M. for a work trip to New York. It was too early for me to have a Fab Four Smoothie, so I made this snack pack the night before, and it kept me fueled when I had the urge to graze once hunger hit.

TIP: Roughly 15 to 20 percent of our daily water intake comes from food. Water-packed vegetables like cucumber, celery, and peppers are great for travel days

LOCK IN A WORKOUT

I always lock in a workout before I fly. It calms my nerves and relieves some stress, and it feels good to sweat. It's a body-loving decision that can change your whole trip, because you're making the choice to treat your body well before you even leave. If you know things are going to be hectic on the day you fly, lock in your workout the day before. This will help you get a better night's sleep, too. My favorite workouts are Vinyasa yoga (I like an upbeat flow with music), Spin classes, and HIIT (high-intensity interval training). I love the Body by Simone app. This kick-ass app was developed by Simone De La Rue, who trains Jennifer Garner, Emmy Rossum, and others, and it offers all sorts of features—dance cardio, full-body strength exercises, and the option to live-stream classes (also, by the way, a food and nutrition plan written by yours truly). And don't underestimate the power of a power walk from one end of the terminal to the other. It's another way to get a thousand steps in. (See the client story on page 152.)

because they help hydrate you slowly without the immediate need for the restroom.

TIP: Splash a little olive oil and apple cider vinegar (ACV) on your vegetables when you pack them. ACV will give them a little bite and help curb cravings for salty airplane snacks.

- **FAB FOUR SNACK PACK #2:** 1 body-loving protein bar (opposite; protein), 1 packet MCT powder (fat), and ½ to 1 cup chopped vegetables (fiber and greens).

TIP: Stir the MCT powder into a tea or coffee for a warm, frothy fat-based beverage.

TIP: Make it easy on yourself. The night before traveling, stop at a grocery store that has a fresh salad bar. Load up a container with your vegetables and grab an empty dressing container to fill with your favorite dressing from home.

- **FAB FOUR SNACK PACK #3:** 1 bag raw nuts, seeds, or nut butter (protein), 1 avocado (fat), and ½ to 1 cup chopped vegetables (fiber and greens). Optional: ¼ cup blueberries.

TIP: If you're drinking a lot of almond milk each week, you're getting a steady dose of monounsaturated fat. To help mix up your fat intake, change up your nut choices. Walnuts are a great source of polyunsaturated fat, macadamia nuts offer more saturated fat, and cashews have a good ratio of all three. You can also make up your own bag with a blend of nuts.

PROTEIN BARS

Many protein bars could be renamed sugar bars (or carb bars). I look at a few factors when analyzing my options. First, I turn to the nutrition facts to figure out whether the bar is mostly protein, mostly fat, or mostly carbohydrates. To do this, I calculate the **net carbohydrates** in the bar (remember, **net carbohydrates = total carbohydrates minus fiber**). This roughly tells you how much of the carbohydrate content will break down into blood sugar. Then I compare this number with the protein and fat content in the bar. **Ideally, both the protein content and the fat content should each individually be greater than the net carbohydrates.** At the very least, one of them (preferably protein) should be greater than the net carbohydrates. That means the bar is either mostly protein or mostly fat. Otherwise, the bar is mostly carbohydrates (and probably has too much sugar). No thank you!

Ideal	Okay	No Thanks
Protein > Net Carbs	Protein > Net Carbs	Net Carbs > Protein
and	*or*	*and*
Fat > Net Carbs	Fat > Net Carbs	Net Carbs > Fat

Second, I look for good amounts of protein, fat, and fiber. **In general, I look for at least 10 grams of protein and around 5 grams of fat. Those are just minimums, and more is great. As for fiber, there should be enough to make net carbohydrates less than the protein and fat content.** Third, I look for minimal sugar. Nearly every bar on the market has some sugar in it, so **I try to look for options that have no more than 3 to 5 grams of sugar total.** Finally, I read the ingredients to make sure there aren't any man-made industrial seed oils (see page 83) and nothing hydrogenated or partially hydrogenated. Here are a few body-loving options I like, along with the types of protein in them:

- Primal Kitchen Bar (both collagen and egg-based options)
- Bulletproof (collagen)

(continued)

- Perfect Keto (collagen)
- Hemplete (vegan hemp protein)
- Julian Bakery (whey, egg, or vegan sunflower butter)

HYDRATE, HYDRATE, HYDRATE. Flying dehydrates us. Stay hydrated by sticking to H2O. The first thing I do when I get through airport security is head to the nearest filtered water fountain. Many airports now have filtered water fountains designed for refilling your water bottle. If you can't find one, Starbucks also has filtered water. I try not to buy plastic bottled water because BPA, phthalates, and other plastic additives have been linked to fertility and reproduction problems, blunted immune function, type 2 diabetes, cardiovascular disease, and obesity. I have a Fab Four Smoothie on the way to the airport in my stainless steel blender bottle. Then I put the empty bottle through security, give it a quick rinse on the other side, take out the blender ball, and use it as my water bottle. Depending on my flight time, my goal is to finish two bottles by the time I land at my destination. This usually saves between eight and ten dollars on plastic bottled water. (Plus, where do you buy that water? Usually at the newsstand, which is full of junk food and candy.) When you get to your destination, you can use your stainless steel blender bottle to make a Fab Four Smoothie. If you don't want to use the same bottle and don't mind carrying two bottles, a Hydro Flask, Corkcicle, or Yeti is a great way to stay hydrated on a flight.

> TIP: Sit in an aisle seat. It sounds silly, but I'm serious! If you run out of water, you can easily pop back to the galley to ask the flight team for more, and it's good to get up and move once or twice. Also, use an app or note in your phone to track how much water you've drunk that day. It helps reframe your focus.

I avoid soda (including diet), fruit juices, energy drinks, sugary coffee drinks, more than one cup of coffee, and especially alcohol when I'm flying. Alcohol is one of the biggest temptations at the terminal and on the plane. It's especially difficult to resist when you're traveling with friends or colleagues who like to drink when they fly. But alcohol dehydrates, sparks cravings for greasy food, causes bloating and puffiness, spikes blood sugar, and can give you headaches and hangovers. (It might even cause you to miss your flight.) If you're traveling for work or just on the go, don't drink at the airport or on your flight. Instead, make the body-loving decision to stay hydrated with water. Sparkling water works, too. My preference is Mountain Valley or Sound sparkling tea, which is tea-infused sparkling water. I love this brand because they have glass options and they don't use any artificial flavors, which can be made from ingredients that are actually inedible!

Staying hydrated sounds like common sense and the most basic piece of advice, but adopting this one change quickly adds up and results in a more balanced you the moment the plane touches down at your destination. Commit to making the healthier decision your new habit and save having a drink for a special travel occasion like a fun vacation, bachelorette party, weekender, or anniversary trip.

> **BYOT**
>
> If you find a clean, organic tea you love, bring a few bags with you on your trip. You can always ask the coffee shop or your flight attendant for a cup of hot water. White tea offers the biggest bang for your buck. It's low in caffeine, so it doesn't dehydrate you like coffee, and it's high in EGCG, a phytochemical that supports healthy blood pressure and blood vessels, which is especially helpful when flying. A calming hibiscus or chamomile tea is also a great way to settle yourself at the airport, so you don't head to the bar.

KEEP YOURSELF BUSY. Work never slows down for me. I don't have the time or luxury to take a break for the hours I spend at the airport and in the air. At any given time, I have a dozen client nutrition plans to write, scores of emails and texts to respond to, and deadlines to meet for my editors and partners. I like to keep working when I fly. For me, nothing makes the whole process go by faster. But a lot of my Girl on the Go clients end up doing the opposite, which I completely understand. We all need a mental breather sometimes, and a good movie or show to take our minds off things. The problem is that many of my clients develop bad habits around their plane relaxation time, like eating an entire bag of gummy bears and drinking three glasses of wine.

Marlene, age forty-five, is a successful financial executive who constantly travels for work. She often flies after long, exhausting days of meetings, so she developed a habit of indulging in several glasses (and sometimes a bottle) of wine between the airport and plane. "I don't know why I do it," she told me. After our meeting, I had a guess. She was a type A overachiever and had a million different things on her plate. In addition to a relentless work and travel schedule, she always had to be learning some new skill or bettering herself somehow—she was trying to teach herself a new language, studying art history like she was back in school, and forcing herself to work out every morning at 5 A.M. She was overscheduled, and the wine helped her unwind. The problem was that led to snacking, poor food choices, and weight gain. So I gave her permission to not achieve all the time. She needed a break from that part of her brain, so we decided reading a fun book was going to be her new habit at the airport. Like a lot of us, she hadn't had time to read a real book in a while, and she wanted to do it. Within days of her next work trip, she was hooked. She would become engrossed in her book, look forward to getting a chapter or two in before boarding, and in the process her airport drinking habit began to fade. In three weeks, she lost the five pounds she wanted to ditch before her birthday, too.

Do what works for you. It could be reading, answering a few work emails, crossing something off your to-do list, like a thank-you note, or even meditating. And if it's watching a movie or TV show, that's fine, too. Just commit to making body-loving choices along with it.

WHAT'S IN MY LUGGAGE? No matter where I'm going, my bag is always packed with items that will help support clean, body-loving decisions when I get to my destination. Here are some of my go-tos. Choose the ones that work for you and make them a must every time you travel, just like your toothbrush and toothpaste. (These are also examples of things I keep handy in my bag or car when I'm at home.)

- **DIY FAB FOUR SMOOTHIE PACKET:** You can premix the base of a Fab Four Smoothie and keep it in your purse for emergencies. Just scoop the following into a small travel container or tin: protein powder of choice containing 20 to

30 grams protein, 2 tablespoons fiber, and 1 tablespoon MCT powder. If you're in a pinch, it's great to have on hand.

- **SINGLE-SERVING PROTEIN POWDER PACKETS:** 1 packet per day of travel. Pick your favorite flavor or mix it up.
- **SINGLE-SERVING RAW NUT OR NUT BUTTER PACKETS:** 1 packet per day of travel. Some of my favorite nut and seed butters are from Wild Friends, with whom I partnered to create a new line of fun, delicious recipes.
- **SINGLE-SERVING OIL OR VINEGAR PACKETS:** 1 to 3 per trip. Use these as dressings to keep your salads healthy at a work conference, sports event, or back at the airport. A few favorites: Marconi Organic Extra Virgin Olive Oil, FBOMB Avocado Oil, and Vermont Village Apple Cider Vinegar Shots.
- **SINGLE-SERVING FISH POUCHES:** A "fish pouch" sounds a little fishy, but they're a great protein addition to any garden salad or a salad bar where the protein looks subpar. These have saved me at work conferences, corporate meetings, and the airport. A few options on Thrive Market and Amazon are Safe Catch, Wild Planet, and SeaBear. Cans work, too, but weigh more, are bulkier, and may contain BPA (look for BPA-free options).
- **SINGLE-SERVING COCONUT OIL, COCONUT BUTTER, OR MCT POWDER PACKETS:** 1 packet per day of travel. If you have an early morning during your trip or just want to take a break from eating after a big client dinner the night before, stir these into your tea or coffee to give yourself some fat-based fuel to start the day. Some MCT powders have fiber in them, which is a bonus.
- **DIY FIBER PACKETS:** Scoop 1 to 3 servings of chia seeds, flaxseeds, or acacia fiber into separate travel containers or tins. NOW Foods has great options for all three.
- **SINGLE-SERVING POWDERS:** Scoop 1 to 3 servings of greens powder into a travel container or tin. Use 1 tablespoon in your DIY smoothie. (Fresh leafy greens don't blend in a shaker bottle!) I like the Greens PhytoFoods powder from NOW Foods.
- **PROTEIN BARS:** 1 to 3 per trip. See page 131 for my tips on selecting a nutritious, body-loving option.

Day 1—Flight Day

BREAKFAST: Start the day with a blood sugar–balancing Fab Four Smoothie. It's a delicious way to fuel up, find balance, and nourish your body before takeoff. If you already have a favorite Fab Four Smoothie recipe, feel free to make your go-to. And if you want to start Day 1 with a different flavor, all four plans have other amazing options. (*Body Love* has more, too.)

BREAKFAST

CINNAMON COCONUT FAB FOUR SMOOTHIE

Try my new cinnamon coconut recipe; it tastes like healthy horchata. The fat in this recipe is a new one, too: sunflower butter, which is a seed butter and thus a great option for people with allergies to peanuts or tree nuts. It has a creamy, nutlike flavor and pairs well with everything.

Vanilla protein powder containing 20 to 30 grams protein
2 tablespoons sunflower butter
2 tablespoons flaxseeds
Handful of greens
1 tablespoon shredded coconut (unsweetened)
1 to 2 cups unsweetened coconut milk

Place all the ingredients in a high-speed blender and blend to your desired consistency.

LUNCH: Eat the Fab Four meal you brought with you or dip into your Fab Four Snack Pack. If you get antsy for more snacks, start with a hot tea, sip slowly, and reevaluate when you're finished. Odds are the craving will pass.

TIP: The hotel minibar is always tempting. If you don't want to stare at chips, cookies, and candy your whole stay, ask the front desk to remove the items from your room. Many hotels will happily oblige.

DINNER: You've been sitting all day, so get moving by walking to a restaurant around your hotel. Ask the front desk or concierge for a healthy recommendation, or do a quick search on your phone. Either way, pound the pavement a little. I can't tell you how many times I've happened upon a healthy market, yoga studio, or smoothie spot that becomes a go-to on my trip. Another option is to poke around your hotel and see what options it has. It's good to get your bearings and know what the hotel coffee shop, café, and restaurant have to offer. If all else fails, peruse the room service menu and find a healthy option.

SELF-CARE: Calm your body and support a good night's rest with a hot bath or shower about ninety minutes before bed. Your body temperature drops a few hours before bedtime to help induce sleep. Elevating your temperature with hot water can cause a steeper decline and support a deeper sleep. Also, wear ear plugs and an eye mask to create a quiet, dark environment. (*Body Love* has more good sleep-related tips.)

Day 2—Hotel Stay

MORNING MOVEMENT: Stop pressuring yourself to complete a traditional workout every single day you're on the road. A lot of my clients pack a bag full of workout clothes they never use. You don't need to go from zero to sixty; you just need to start a sustainable habit. Here's one: always work out on the second day of travel. Even if it's the only real workout you get, do it every trip. Treat it like your Monday workout at home. Consistency is the goal, and you can easily replicate this every time you travel. And you won't be flying clean clothes from state to state.

BREAKFAST: If it's a short trip or you didn't pack your smoothie stuff, head to a local breakfast spot, visit the hotel café, or maybe even order room service. Don't start your trip with a blood sugar spike (aka a bagel plus a bowl of fruit). Instead, go for a satiating egg breakfast such as a vegetable scramble, a spinach omelet, or eggs your way with a side of greens drizzled with olive oil. Add avocado to all three options.

> TIP: Tell your server to bring two glasses of water and leave the bread or toast in the kitchen.

LUNCH: Traveling for a conference or convention? Conference room cold cuts and convention food can be worse than the airport's. If I don't know what will be provided, I don't leave it to chance. One strategy is to order a salad the night before from room service. Ask them to make it to go, then save it in your mini fridge till the next day. A second strategy is to order your lunch from wherever you eat breakfast. A third option is to craft a Fab Four meal from the healthy market you found during your walk last night.

DINNER: Dinner out with co-workers or clients? No sweat. Here are a few pointers to help you make a clean, healthy choice.

- **AMERICAN:** Skip straight to the main courses or entrées and pick a protein meal that comes with a vegetable side. If the vegetable is starchy or creamy, peruse the menu for another clean, noncreamy vegetable option and ask to swap it.
- **ITALIAN:** If the bread basket always tempts you, consider ordering your own starter instead. Calm your hunger with a protein- or fat-based appetizer such as tuna tartare, fish or beef carpaccio, olives, or almonds. Italian restaurants usually have great pan-fried fish cooked with olive oil, lemon, capers, and a white wine reduction. That's my go-to, plus a fibrous vegetable like broccoli, eggplant, or zucchini.

- **INDIAN:** Vegetable or chicken curry (sans the starchy rice) is the way to go, because the coconut milk (healthy fat) will help keep you full. Ask if they use dairy, and if they do, opt for tandoori chicken.
- **MEXICAN:** Avoid eating tortilla chips by ordering a starter salad. You can enjoy the salsa and guacamole on your salad as the dressing without missing out on the flavor. For an entrée, fajitas with grilled protein and vegetables is a flavorful option. So is a large taco salad (without a shell).
- **MEDITERRANEAN:** There are a lot of good options, but I usually go for a protein skewer, cucumber salad, and hummus (I always swap vegetables for the pita bread).
- **SUSHI:** Opt for sashimi and a salad with ginger dressing, or if you don't like sushi, cooked fish and vegetables. If you want the rice, order one roll or two orders of sushi to help keep your overall rice consumption to one serving. White rice is gluten-free, but you don't want to end up eating two cups of it. (You'd be eating about 100 net carbohydrates, or the equivalent of about 7½ cups—about fourteen servings!—of butternut squash.) Also, consider a vegetable roll to add some fiber and greens.

TIP: Whether it's a conference mixer, team event, or client dinner, work travel often leads to a bar and the peer pressure to drink. Sometimes it's your boss or manager leading the charge. Part of adopting a healthy lifestyle is being confident in yourself and your decisions. We've all had people judge, guilt, or shame us for our choices, but we can't let that dictate what we do. You're reading *Body Love Every Day* for a reason. You have a deeper purpose—your "why"—that's motivating you. Remember it! Let that be your guide on nights like these, not what other people think or say to you. (For a few tips on alcohol, see Day 21, page 198.)

Day 3—Hotel Stay

MORNING MOVEMENT: Let's keep it simple today and just go for a brisk walk. Aim for at least twenty-five minutes. If there's a park, noteworthy street, or sight to see that's close by, make it part of your tour. If you want a little more burn, speed it up into a run. Make the finish line a smoothie shop.

> TIP: Want to move more when you're traveling? Pick one meal per day to walk to. It keeps you from feeling stagnant, and you end up banking way more steps than you otherwise would.

BREAKFAST: Last night's dinner might have you in the mood for something a little less heavy, so find your way to a smoothie shop. If your Google search isn't yielding great results, try a gym like Equinox or a market like Whole Foods. The key is to find a location that can offer you the Fab Four. Many smoothie shops use too little protein (sometimes as little as 8 grams), no fat, and large quantities of fruit. You don't need a whole apple, banana, or carton of strawberries in your smoothie; you need protein, fat, fiber, and greens! Even a smoothie labeled "green" can sneak in too much fruit. So ask to build your own or modify one on the menu by deleting the fruit and asking for more protein. A lot of "muscle builder" smoothies have good amounts of protein but not enough greens and fiber. In that case, ask for an extra serving of spinach or fiber powder.

LUNCH: If it's day two of the conference or convention, make it a BYOP (bring your own protein) day. If you packed a fish pouch and olive oil packet in your luggage, bring them to add to a garden salad. Another option is to buy a cooked chicken breast at the market and bring it with you.

> TIP: Does travel back you up? There are a number of reasons you might become constipated when you travel, including dehydration, lack of fiber, poor sleep, or lack of movement. I tell my clients to drink and refill their water bottle continuously. I also

recommend upping fiber intake with more leafy greens and vegetables every day. If you still can't go, magnesium may help. Try Natural Calm (available at most grocery stores) or another magnesium supplement.

BRIDGE SNACK: If you're running around on a busy day, you might need a protein or fat-based bridge snack to elongate your blood sugar curve. Two options are a handful of mixed raw nuts or a body-loving protein bar. Again, I don't recommend daily snacking. But I also don't want you ravenous going into dinner, because it can lead to deep-fried decisions and overeating. Use a bridge snack when you really need it.

DINNER: Steer your clients, co-workers, or friends to a healthy restaurant by taking care of the research and reservation. Two of my favorite resources are Eater and Thrillist because they highlight fun, healthy hotspots with innovative chefs. The Fab Four isn't about boring, bland food. Venture out and find somewhere that takes spices and flavor seriously. Always review the menu beforehand, and if you need some backup, check Yelp, TripAdvisor, or Foursquare.

Day 4—Hotel Stay

MORNING MOVEMENT: Roll out of bed and right into an app workout on your phone. It's quick, efficient, and over before you know it. There are a variety of twenty-five- to thirty-minute workouts you can stream and do in your hotel room. Whatever app you use, just make sure it's manageable, fun, and right for you.

BREAKFAST: Maybe your team is meeting downstairs bright and early, or you scheduled a last-minute coffee with a client. Whatever the case, you're really on the go this morning and don't have time to sit down for breakfast. The good news is that with your blender bottle, the supplies in your luggage, and a few key ingredients, you can turn a breakfast beverage into Fab Four fuel. Simply fill your blender bottle with the dry ingredients, then add the beverage on top. It's as easy as order, add, and shake.

- **FAB FOUR ICED COFFEE:** Order an iced cold-brew coffee. Pour over 1 packet chocolate collagen protein powder, 1 packet MCT powder, and 2 tablespoons acacia fiber.
- **FAB FOUR MATCHA:** Order an unsweetened iced green tea. Pour over 1 packet vanilla collagen protein powder, 1 packet MCT powder, 1 tablespoon acacia fiber, and 1 serving Matchaful Matcha.
- **FAB FOUR MOCHA LATTE:** Order an unsweetened iced almond milk latte. Pour over 1 packet chocolate whey protein powder, 1 packet MCT powder, and 1 tablespoon chia seeds. If the coffee shop doesn't have unsweetened almond milk, I might elect to go with an iced cold brew or regular coffee. Unfortunately, some places only have sweetened (sugary) almond milk. Whole Foods has unsweetened. (You can also make this recipe with unsweetened coconut milk or another nut or seed milk.)
- **FAB FOUR LEAN GREEN TEA:** Order an unsweetened iced green tea. Pour over 1 packet greens powder and 1 packet MCT powder.
- **FAB FOUR FAT COFFEE:** Order 1 cup regular coffee. Pour over 1 packet chocolate collagen protein powder and either 1 packet coconut oil or coconut butter.

All of these are considered Fab Four Roadies—easy ways to turn everyday beverages into modified versions of the Fab Four Smoothie. When you need a quick breakfast, bridge snack, or find yourself in a pinch, they can save you. It's also easy to keep the single-serving packets for your favorites in your purse, car, gym bag, or desk.

LUNCH: Nearly every grocery store has a salad bar. Building your own Fab Four salad takes no time at all. Here's a quick how-to:

- **GREENS:** Start with 2 to 4 cups of leafy greens like spinach, kale, or romaine base (or all three). Bonus points for adding a fresh herb or microgreens, too.
- **PROTEIN:** Add 4 ounces of chicken, steak, or salmon. Boost your protein with ¼ cup beans and 1 hard-boiled egg.

- **FAT:** Use a whole food fat like slivered nuts, seeds, avocado, or olives and then a fat-based dressing made with a healthy cooking oil like avocado or olive oil.
- **FIBER:** Choose 2 to 4 nonstarchy vegetables such as artichoke hearts, broccoli, Brussels sprouts, carrots, cauliflower, celery, cucumbers, peppers, or radishes.
- **OPTIONAL:** ¼ to ½ cup quinoa or ¼ cup berries or apple.

> **DON'T POUR DRY CHIA SEEDS ON YOUR SALAD**
>
> Chia seeds are a great source of fiber. But as noted on page 90, eating dry chia seeds has been known to cause intestinal blockages. Dry chia seeds absorb bodily fluids and can greatly expand in size. Always hydrate (via the blender) or soak chia seeds in some manner before use.

Check out the hashtag #fab4salad on Instagram. I love sharing my Fab Four salad creations to help you hit your needs!

TIP: You might have heard that there is more iron content in kale than in steak. The caveat is that plants contain a different type of iron than animal meat, so it's not quite apples to apples. In addition, the iron in plants (*nonheme* iron) is generally less bioavailable than the iron in animal meat (*heme* iron). To increase the bioavailability of the iron in your kale (and other greens), pair it with a source of vitamin C, such as a squeeze of lemon.

DINNER: Tomorrow you're flying home, and if you've made healthy choices all week long, you might be tempted to indulge at dinner and go out with a bang. To keep your body-loving momentum going, find a healthy way to have some fun. If you're craving a burger or tacos, get them lettuce wrapped. If you want something sweet, opt for dark chocolate and enjoy a piece or two. After a week of being out and about, maybe it's just a you night—order room service, kick your feet up, and dive back into the book you started on the plane. And if you want a drink, see Day 21 (page 198) for a few tips.

Day 5—Flight Day

MORNING MEDITATION: Home is on the horizon. If you wake up feeling stressed or anxious for your travel day, consider a simple meditation exercise to calm your nerves. Close your eyes and bring your attention to your breath. Focus on each breath, inhaling and exhaling slowly through your nose. Then start a body scan. Slowly work your way up from your toes to your head. Give each body part thirty to sixty seconds. Send a calm message to yourself on the inhales and release bodily tension on the exhales. If your thoughts begin to drift, simply reconnect with your breath.

TRAVEL TEMPTATION: You've had to be "on" for days. Meanwhile, your inbox has been filling up and your to-do list hasn't been touched. It all might hit you on the trip home, creating the temptation to blow off steam and self-soothe with fast food and alcohol. Abigail, age thirty-three, was constantly flying for work. She felt calm and in control on the road, but her Achilles' heel was always the way home. The stress finally caught up to her and she couldn't resist drinks, snacks, and fast food at the airport and on the plane. As with Marlene (page 142), I helped her create a new habit. I asked her to change into her workout clothes for the trip home. Then I told her to get to the airport thirty minutes earlier and walk the terminal after going through security. Did she drag her roller bag? Yep. And in the process she decompressed, locked in a few thousand steps, and ended up discovering the terminal's healthier options. She was already doing something body-loving (walking), and it led to more body-loving food decisions. Sometimes one decision *around* food has a huge impact on how you eat. Momentum works both ways. If there's a trigger that starts you in a "Not So Fab" direction, maybe something non-food-related can help you swing the mojo back in your favor.

BREAKFAST: I always encourage my clients to fuel up before flying. But if you feel like your body needs a little break or you want to try a morning fast, whisk up a coffee or tea with a few tablespoons of fat. The fat will give you fuel without releasing insulin. A handheld frother is easy to pack and travel with (mine is the size of a pen), and there are many fat-based creamers out there to choose from:

- Perfect Keto: MCT powder
- 4th & Heart: grass-fed ghee butter packets (Madagascar vanilla bean tastes great.)
- Trader Joe's or Artisana: organic virgin coconut oil packets
- Bulletproof: Instamix
- Know Brainer: casein- and lactose-free mocha creamer
- Laird Superfood: unsweetened superfood creamer
- Cave Fat Pack: vegan coconut powder creamer

TIP: If you have enough time, pop into a grocery store or market and build one of the Fab Four Snack Packs on pages 137–38. Sometimes cravings hit unexpectedly on the way home. Having something healthy on hand is a great way to neutralize them.

LUNCH: Go green. Pick the freshest, best-looking salad you can find, whether it's from a restaurant in your terminal, a grab-and-go counter, or Starbucks. Many airport dressings use unhealthy industrial seed oils, so use one of the oil and vinegar packets you brought with you. If the salad doesn't come with a clean protein, use one of the fish pouches you packed. Another option is to have a Fab Four Roadie (page 150) as your protein and fat, then to eat a garden salad as your fiber and greens.

DINNER: Temptation doesn't stop when the plane lands. After a long day of travel, takeout on the couch can sound like heaven. If you shop on a jet-lagged stomach, you might be tempted to buy a "Not So Fab" healthy snack or sweet. Your pantry and refrigerator might not be any help either. One simple strategy I use all the time is to hop on an app when I land or on my way home, and commit to ordering a healthy meal for takeout or delivery. You can use your self-made menu (see page 185). If you feel like something more indulgent, there are plenty of Fab Four Smoothies that can hit the spot: Cookies and Cream (page 163), Pecan Pie (page 177), Triple Chocolate Crunch

(Domestic Goddess plan, page 218), Sweet Spiced Carrot Cake (Plant-Based Devotee plan, page 284), or Salted Caramel from *Body Love*.

> TIP: I encourage my clients to eat as soon as possible after getting home. It gives them less time to fret over temptation and more time to digest their meal before bed, which will support a cleansing first night of sleep post-travel.

> TIP: Ditch your inbox, social media, or whatever else is on your screen and get in bed. Charge your phone across the room or, better yet, in another room entirely. The physical action of having to climb out of bed makes it harder to give in to the urge to check and refresh your feeds. After a long week of work travel, give your brain and eyes a breather. You'll sleep much better for it.

Day 6—Post-Travel Weekend Day

KEEP SLEEPING: Let yourself sleep in and wake up slowly today. Take your time during your morning routine and remind yourself it's the weekend. If you're an early riser, take your morning coffee or tea outside for the sunrise to help resync your circadian rhythm. Even if it's only for five minutes, shift down a gear.

LATE-MORNING MOVEMENT: We retain excess water and sodium when we fly, which can make us feel bloated and swollen the next day. To sweat it out, pick a workout class and go with a friend. Being around other people and feeding off their communal energy is a great way to bust through a travel hangover. If you pick a class you enjoy and go with a friend, there will be less anxiety about going and better odds you'll get it done. My favorite is a Vinyasa yoga class. Push yourself, but don't punish yourself. You don't need to atone for every food "sin" you might have committed that week. Have fun, sweat, and use it as a way to recharge with a friend at your side.

BRUNCH: Opt to make brunch at home. You can elevate your favorite classics at home with my Eggs Benedict (page 233) or Loaded Avocado Toast (page 271) from the Domestic Goddess plan.

FIND NATURE: If you've been on the road all week, you've probably spent a lot of time indoors, in planes or cars, or riding the subway. Recycled air, fluorescent light, endless hours of phone time, and traffic are all part of modern life, but we still have a physiological need for nature. Indeed, natural sunlight provides vitamin D. If you're a Girl on the Go, one way to slow yourself down and unwind is to find a bit of nature. Go for a walk or hike with your friends, plan a beach or lake day, or just take a blanket to your favorite park. Unplug for an hour or two and give yourself permission to just breathe and be. It will nourish a different side of you and connect you to something greater than yourself. We all need the balance, perspective, and rejuvenating energy that time in nature can provide.

MIDAFTERNOON SMOOTHIE: If you have a dinner out tonight, make a Fab Four Smoothie in the midafternoon. It will bridge you from brunch to dinner and place your blood sugar in balance, and you'll head to dinner less hungry.

DINNER: You're finally home, and your girls want you to go out. The good news is that your midafternoon smoothie already set you up to make a healthy decision, even if you end up at a "Not So Fab" restaurant. Pick a clean protein and pair it with a cruciferous vegetable option. If you really want something more carb-heavy or decadent, tell yourself it's a choice, not a cheat. Cheat meals or days imply that you're breaking some sort of rule or regimen. **Food freedom and body love mean accepting your decisions and knowing that you can always regain your balance at the next meal.**

INSPIRE THE CHANGE

A lot of my clients are people pleasers who want to make everyone happy. Often their agreeable dispositions can come at the expense of their own health and lifestyle goals. They let friends or family drag them to an unhealthy restaurant, end up sharing a bottle of wine on a random weeknight, or find themselves partaking in a flatbread appetizer or dessert they don't really want. Then the minute the meal is

(continued)

over, they feel bad about themselves and have the urge to rebound into a cleanse or be hyperrestrictive the next day. It can also make them start to resent their friends or family, especially those who seem to be genetically blessed and don't ever gain an inch or pound. (But remember, even if they don't, it doesn't mean their choices are good for their bodies. Anyone can develop diabetes, gut issues, and health problems as a result of their dietary choices.) You don't need to find new friends or family. You just need to have an honest conversation with them. It takes one conversation where you genuinely ask them to support your health and wellness efforts. If you don't, the unhealthy alpha will always get what he or she wants.

Jennie, age twenty-nine, had a fun group of foodie friends who went to dinner every week. It started to become an issue for her because she would let others order for the table, either for appetizers and dessert or sometimes the whole meal. She found herself eating things she didn't want to, which caused her to beat herself up afterward. She told me she wanted her friends to be happy and didn't want to deprive them of what they wanted or be "that girl." I gave her some homework and asked her to have a conversation with the friend who was the most vocal about choosing restaurants and ordering for the table. She was open and honest with her friend, reinforced that she wanted to eat cleaner and healthier, and expressed how the dinners were beginning to affect her emotionally. She felt like her opinion didn't matter and that their relationship was being strained as a result. She called me afterward. "We cried and had such a good moment. She never wants me to feel that way. She wants to support me and do it together. She said we don't need to drink to be friends, and we can even do health dates if I want." I followed up with her a few weeks later and she said their conversation was a game changer. My client had started choosing healthy restaurants for the group, and her friend had even started drinking Fab Four Smoothies, too.

When you eat out with healthy people, you make healthier decisions. Be that person for your friends and family. Inspire the change instead of letting them lead you down an unhealthy path. Be the one to bring everyone together and suggest a healthy restaurant or offer to host a healthy potluck.

Week 2: At Home

If you're constantly on the go, it can be a challenge to cook dinner at home. Many of my clients don't get home from work until 7 or 8 P.M. (or later) and are low on both time and energy. Some also just don't love cooking. But generally speaking, preparing your own dinner at home can be a cleaner, healthier, and cheaper option than eating out. You're the chef. That gives you control over your ingredients and how they're prepared. Plus, you learn so much. You learn about your food, its quality and nutritional content, and how it affects your body. You learn how to find balance and build and maintain healthy habits. And you learn how to use that positive momentum to healthily adapt and navigate through any menu, event, or situation you encounter out in the world. That's why I always encourage even my busiest, most on-the-go clients to make the effort to cook: it tunes you into your food, helps you build a healthy lifestyle, and the benefits travel with you.

I know some of you might be thinking, *Wait a minute—Kelly really wants me to cook and do meal prep? I'm way too busy.* I know it's a challenge; it is for me, too, especially as a mom who runs her own business. But there are just some things I want all my Girls on the Go to know how to do. Cooking a few simple homemade dishes is one of them. It helps elevate your everyday thinking, living, and eating. And if you shop smart, do some light prep work, and use a few key precooked ingredients, you can easily whip up a homemade (or semihomemade) Fab Four dinner in *fifteen minutes or less*. You don't need to become a Top Chef or try to beat Bobby Flay. For my Girls on the Go, it's about keeping things simple and being realistic. I'll show you some examples of how and give you a handful of easy recipes.

First, here are a few tips and ideas for quick, light prep on a Sunday.

WASH AND CHOP VEGETABLES. I do this right when I get home from the grocery store or farmers' market, so my vegetables are ready to be roasted, tossed into a salad, added to a Fab Four Smoothie, or eaten as a bridge snack during the week. It takes only five to ten minutes. OXO has a variety of GreenSaver containers that I

BACK TO *BODY LOVE*

If you end up enjoying your time in the kitchen and feel inspired to try other Fab Four recipes, check out my website or chapter 6 of *Body Love*. There are dozens of delicious recipes to choose from, along with more body-loving tips on prep and planning, including sample shopping lists, meal prep hacks, and many healthy swaps and substitutions.

use to store my vegetables in the refrigerator. Some come with an internal rinsing basket that stores directly in the container, and others come equipped with a charcoal filter to help keep the vegetables crisp and fresh. If you use a salad spinner to wash your lettuce and leafy greens, you can use it for refrigerator storage as well. Just pour out the bottom water, lay a paper towel over the washed lettuce, and place the lid back on. With this basic prep done, you can easily make a "fridge salad" anytime during the week.

MAKE A BULK SALAD DRESSING. Having a healthy, fat-based dressing on hand is an easy way to elevate your daily salad and increase nutrient absorption. One tasty option that takes less than five minutes to make is my Lemon Tahini. For other dressing options, see pages 229 and 259 and check out *Body Love*.

LEMON TAHINI DRESSING

½ cup tahini
½ cup filtered water
Juice of 1 lemon
3 garlic cloves, peeled
2 tablespoons extra virgin olive oil
Pink Himalayan salt

Combine the tahini, water, lemon juice, garlic, and oil in a blender and process until smooth. Taste and add salt as needed and pour into a glass container to store in the fridge.

COOK ONE OR MORE PROTEINS. You can do this in under 20 minutes. Even if you have time to cook only a single protein just for Monday night, you're setting yourself up for success.

- For boneless chicken, pork, or steak, season with salt and pepper, then cut into 1- to 2-inch pieces (or pound thin) and sauté on medium to high heat for 6 to 8 minutes, or until cooked through (chicken or pork) or done to your liking (steak). You can use these proteins for salads or other Fab Four dinners. Another option is my Easy Peasy Shredded Chicken (page 254).
- Sauté ground beef over medium-high for 10 to 15 minutes, or until the meat is browned and cooked through.
- You can roast a fish in 10 to 20 minutes. For a salmon fillet with no skin or skin on one side, preheat the oven to 450°F and bake uncovered for 4 to 6 minutes per ½ inch of thickness. For a dressed salmon (whole fish with the skin on), preheat the oven to 350°F and bake for 6 to 9 minutes per 8 ounces of fish.
- Sauté shrimp for 4 to 6 minutes (2 to 3 minutes per side), until opaque and cooked through.

> **PACKAGED DRESSINGS**
>
> I try to buy dressings with ingredients I would use to make a dressing at home. Your dressing shouldn't include added sugar, man-made industrial seed oils (see page 82), or any hydrogenated or partially hydrogenated ingredients. A few brands I like are Primal Kitchen and Bragg Organic.

If you don't have time to cook or do any prep, wild poached or canned salmon, sardines, and tuna are easy options for salads. My favorite brands are Safe Catch and Wild Planet, and I look for Alaska or sockeye salmon. One of my quick go-tos is a basic salmon salad: 1 (5- or 6-ounce) can salmon mixed with 2 tablespoons of Primal Kitchen mayonnaise. Also, bone broth can be heated up in minutes. Depending on the brand, 1 cup can provide between 6 and 12 grams of protein (see page 36 for a few I like).

USE A SLOW COOKER OR PRESSURE COOKER. These are great investments for Girls on the Go. They're an easy way to prepare quality protein without much time or fuss. All you have to do with a slow cooker is plug it in and set the time. As for pressure cooking, it significantly reduces cooking times. (See Italian Spaghetti Squash, page 173.) To make hard-boiled eggs in a pressure cooker, see page 168.

To make salsa chicken for tacos, place 2 to 4 boneless skinless chicken breasts in a pressure cooker, pour 1 jar of salsa over the chicken, cook for 20 minutes, then let the pressure release naturally. Or in a slow cooker, combine the same ingredients, then cook for 4 hours on High or 8 hours on Low.

DIY FROZEN SMOOTHIE CUPS. There are a number of frozen smoothie cups on the market. Unfortunately, many are loaded with added sugar or are low in protein, fat, and fiber. An easy Sunday prep move is to fill five travel cups or mugs with your favorite Fab Four Smoothie ingredients (except the nut milk). Take the cups to your office freezer on Monday, along with a container of unsweetened nut milk for the refrigerator and a small travel blender. During the week, pull out one of your cups, add the nut milk, and blend it up. In a snap you can have a real Fab Four Smoothie at the office. This is also a good move at home for moms or anyone with a hectic schedule. **Sometimes saving yourself as little as sixty seconds of prep time is what wins you the mental battle and helps you make a body-loving decision.**

The Fab Four Smoothie is your secret weapon. If you're always five minutes behind schedule, make it the night before so it's already done. If you always seem to run out of ingredients, prep the container ahead of time, so you're not disappointed in the morning when you discover you're out of something. If you're not hungry before you get to work, use the freezer cup technique.

Day 7—Light Prep Sunday

MORNING MOVEMENT: Let's start today with a brisk twenty-five- to thirty-minute walk, so you break a sweat and begin to counteract the Sunday Scaries before they hit you.

BREAKFAST

GREEN GINGER FAB FOUR SMOOTHIE

Try my new Green Ginger smoothie, which will help you hydrate and debloat if there was excess salt in your dinner out the night before.

Vanilla protein powder containing 20 to 30 grams protein
1 tablespoon MCT oil
2 tablespoons acacia fiber (I use NOW Foods)
¼ cup chopped cucumber
Juice of ½ lemon
1 teaspoon grated fresh ginger (or a fresh ginger turmeric shot)
1 to 2 cups filtered water or unsweetened almond milk

Place all the ingredients in a high-speed blender and blend to your desired consistency.

TIP: Acacia fiber is a soluble fiber that can help decrease elevated blood sugar and calm insulin. It helps support weight loss efforts by keeping you full and satisfied longer, and it increases butyrate production, which reduces inflammation in the gut.

LUNCH: Put that light prep to work and fix yourself a Fab Four salad with the fresh vegetables, Lemon Tahini Dressing (page 158), and one of the proteins you prepared for the week.

(continued)

SUNDAY SCARIES: The anxiety of going back to work on Monday can cause us to eat and drink emotionally on Sunday. If you can't get work off your mind or feel like you're procrastinating on something, spend fifteen minutes on the project or task that's making you feel anxious. The point is to take action and not let it continue to expand in your headspace. Another way to help shake off the scaries is to exercise. Whether it's another brisk twenty-five- to thirty-minute walk around the neighborhood or something more intense, working out is a positive way to diffuse that anxious energy. A third option is to do some of the light meal prep that I suggested on pages 157–59. Put yourself to work in a different way, use your hands, and chop up those vegetables. It will help make the healthy choice the easy choice all week long.

STUDY GUIDE: Studies have shown that exercise is linked with reduced anxiety and depression in clinical settings. One meta-analysis of more than ten thousand people found that physical activity decreased anxiety by more than 30 percent.

DINNER: Enjoy a light supplemental dinner by 5 P.M. today. Eating dinner on the earlier side will give you more time to digest before bed. If you've had a fun weekend, it will give you a longer fasting window and help you enter fat-burning mode while you sleep. Try my Vegetable and Cauliflower Rice Soup (page 304).

Day 8—Weekday

MORNING MOVEMENT: Sign up for a Spin class and power through any Monday stress. The dark lighting, pumping music, and positive instructors push me to break through the mental knots and anxious thoughts that form on Monday mornings.

TIP: What's the best time of day to work out? This is one of the most common questions clients ask me. Recent studies suggest that fasted morning workouts (i.e., without eating a preworkout meal) yield the best body composition results because your body uses more stored glucose for energy and has an opportunity to burn fat. If you work late, give first thing in the morning a try. But the A.M. isn't for everyone. If morning workouts interfere with your sleep or you find you're missing too many days, later might be better for you. The real key is to be consistent, so find the time(s) that suit you best, hold yourself accountable, and repeat.

FREEZER FUDGE

See page 214 in the Domestic Goddess plan for four scrumptious Freezer Fudge recipes: original, hazelnut, caramel candy, and praline. They're the perfect bite to pop in your mouth when your sweet tooth strikes—and super easy to make.

BREAKFAST

COOKIES AND CREAM FAB FOUR SMOOTHIE

You can thank Jennifer Garner for this scrumptious smoothie recipe. She took the Fab Four formula and created a delicious twist that tastes like cookies and cream.

Chocolate coconut Primal Kitchen Collagen Fuel powder containing 20 to 30 grams protein
1 tablespoon almond butter
1 tablespoon flaxseeds
Handful of fresh spinach
¼ cup frozen blueberries
1 to 2 cups unsweetened almond milk

Place all the ingredients in a high-speed blender and blend to your desired consistency.

LUNCH: Keep it simple with my Greek Chicken Salad (see the Domestic Goddess plan, page 259).

DINNER: Make it easy on yourself by using your slow cooker or pressure cooker today. To make salsa chicken for tacos, cook chicken in a pressure cooker or slow

(continued)

cooker as on page 159. Serve up a lettuce-wrapped taco bar with the following ingredients:

8 to 10 Bibb or iceberg lettuce leaves (or 2 Siete grain-free tortillas)
1 avocado, smashed
Tomatoes, diced
¼ cup salsa

BREATHWORK: Do you ever find yourself letting out big, long sighs during the day? If you're under a lot of stress, you may be taking rapid, fight-or-flight-type breaths. They trigger the release of cortisol (a stress hormone) and eventually lead to those big sighs. It's like you've been holding your breath . . . because you have been. One simple, daily practice that can help you slow down your breathing and reduce cortisol levels is called breathwork. For more details, see the Domestic Goddess plan, page 209.

Day 9—Weekday

BREAKFAST

SPA DAY FAB FOUR SMOOTHIE

Ease into the day with one of my most popular Fab Four Smoothie recipes from Body Love.

Vanilla protein powder containing 20 to 30 grams protein
¼ to ½ cup diced avocado
1 to 2 tablespoons chia seeds
Juice of ½ to 1 lemon
Fresh mint leaves
Handful of spinach
1 small Persian cucumber
1 to 2 cups unsweetened nut milk

Place all the ingredients in a high-speed blender and blend to your desired consistency.

TIP: If you want only half the lemon in your smoothie, squeeze the other half into a large pitcher of water. Drink it throughout the day to stay hydrated and help decrease inflammation.

LUNCH: Pack and bring a simple salad to work. Place 2 sliced hard-boiled eggs, avocado, cucumber, and tomatoes over a bed of greens and add Lemon Tahini Dressing (page 158).

DINNER

SHRIMP SCAMPI WITH ZOODLES

This dish is easy to prepare, no matter your cooking experience, and swapping zucchini zoodles for pasta noodles is a great, healthy way to add fiber and greens to your dinner. Zoodles are versatile and work well with many herbs, spices, and sauces. Italian and Asian dishes are two of my favorite ways to use them. Save the pasta noodles for fun occasions when freshly made pasta is on the menu—even gluten-free options are made from flours, aka acellular carbohydrates (see page 127).

Makes 2 servings

1 tablespoon ghee
4 garlic cloves, minced
10 to 12 large shrimp, tails on, cleaned, and deveined (you can buy them this way)
2 tablespoons chopped flat-leaf parsley
1 tablespoon dried oregano
Crushed red pepper flakes
2 tablespoons extra virgin olive oil
1 zucchini, zoodled (see Tip, page 166)
Coarse salt and freshly ground black pepper
Lemon wedges, for serving

(continued)

1. Heat the ghee in a large skillet over medium heat. Add the garlic and cook until soft but not browned, 1 to 2 minutes.

2. Add the shrimp, parsley, oregano, and a pinch of pepper flakes and cook, stirring frequently, until the shrimp are bright pink and opaque, 2 to 3 minutes per side.

3. Raise the heat to medium-high, add the olive oil and zoodles, and cook until the zoodles are hot. Remove from the heat and season with salt and pepper. Serve hot with a lemon wedge on the side.

TIP: You don't need a fancy zoodler with all sorts of parts. I use a handheld one, which costs about ten dollars and fits in your kitchen drawer. After rinsing the zucchini (or another vegetable), you can easily zoodle over a pan, pot, or cutting board.

TECH-FREE TUESDAY: When you have the power to stream, search, and scroll through an endless amount of digital content, that's what you end up doing . . . all the time. Tonight, try giving your eyes and attention span a break. Even if it's just for an hour, let all your screens stay dark. Don't worry—your favorite shows, websites, and apps will still be there when you pick up your phone or turn on the TV. See the Domestic Goddess plan, page 261.

Day 10—Weekday

MORNING MOVEMENT: Breathe, sweat, and clear your mind with an upbeat Vinyasa yoga class. In Vinyasa, you move from pose to pose with your breath. Yoga improves flexibility, enhances muscle tone, and builds core strength. Plus, the music gets you moving.

BREAKFAST

ORIGINAL GREEN FAB FOUR SMOOTHIE

Keep it simple with my original green smoothie from Body Love.

Vanilla protein powder containing 20 to 30 grams protein
¼ avocado (or 2 tablespoons coconut oil)
2 tablespoons chia seeds
Handful of spinach
1 to 2 cups unsweetened nut milk

Place all the ingredients in a high-speed blender and blend to your desired consistency.

LUNCH

EGG SALAD OVER ARUGULA WITH JILZ CRACKERZ

Sometimes I have only ten or fifteen minutes to eat lunch. One fast option I can whip up at times like that is this tasty egg salad. This is a perfect example of the type of meal prep and cooking I want you to know how to do, even if you're the busiest, least kitchen savvy Girl on the Go there is. The recipe is easy to follow, it takes only a few minutes, it tastes great, and it's incredibly healthy. Eggs are a good source of protein. Don't ditch the yolks—they're where the fat and B vitamins are, including choline, which is great for your central nervous system. Arugula helps you detoxify and reduces inflammation (see Tip, page 168). Even the gluten-free crackers give you a few extra grams of protein, fat, and fiber.

(continued)

Makes 1 to 2 servings

6 hard-boiled eggs (see How to Make Hard-Boiled Eggs)
¼ cup mayonnaise (I like Primal Kitchen)
1 teaspoon mustard (I like mine spicy, so I use Dijon)
1 teaspoon smoked paprika
¼ teaspoon pink Himalayan salt
¼ teaspoon freshly ground black pepper
3 cups arugula
1 teaspoon olive oil
1 tablespoon freshly squeezed lemon juice
8 to 10 Jilz Crackerz

In a small bowl, fork-smash the eggs. Mix in the mayonnaise, mustard, paprika, salt, and pepper. In a serving bowl, toss the arugula with the olive oil and lemon juice, then top with the egg salad. Enjoy with the crackers.

TIP: As a member of the cruciferous vegetable family (see chapter 4), arugula is an excellent source of *sulforaphane*, a phytochemical and a potent activator of NRF_2, which regulates the genes responsible for eliminating free radicals, detoxifying, and reducing inflammation. If you're at a salad bar, adding arugula is an easy way to help activate these cell defenses.

HOW TO MAKE HARD-BOILED EGGS

Place the eggs in a single layer in the bottom of a pot (don't stack them). Cover the eggs with 1 inch of cold water. Turn the heat to high, bring the water to a boil, then quickly turn off the heat (or remove the pot from the heat if you have a slow-to-cool electric stove) and cover the pot. Let the eggs sit for 11 to 12 minutes. Remove them from the pot and give them a quick dunk in cold water. Peel and serve, or refrigerate for later.

If you use a pressure cooker, your eggs can be done in half the time, and the shells will pop right off. Place the rack in the pressure cooker. Pour in 1 cup water and place the eggs in one layer on the rack (don't stack them). Close the lid and pressure cook on Low for 6 minutes. Once the time is up, quick release the lid and transfer the eggs to a bowl of cold water. Peel and serve, or refrigerate for later.

DINNER

STEAMED FISH AND VEGETABLES

Steaming is a quick, clean, and really easy way to prepare dinner. Steaming vegetables can increase the bioavailability of antioxidants and help eliminate certain compounds that block nutrient absorption. Need ideas for vegetables to use? Try bok choy, cauliflower, carrots, snap peas, green beans, asparagus, broccoli, and kale.

Makes 2 servings

2 (5-ounce) fish fillets, such as wild salmon or halibut
Vegetables of your choice
Kosher salt
Sauce of your choice: Curry in a Hurry Sauce or Lemon Butter Sauce (recipes follow), store-bought coconut aminos, vegan pesto, or olive oil with lemon juice

1. Pour 1 inch filtered water into a medium saucepan with a stovetop steamer or colander set above the water surface, cover the pan, and bring to a boil over medium heat.
2. Lay the fish and vegetables on the steamer rack (be sure they have plenty of room) and sprinkle with salt to taste. Steam, covered, for 4 to 8 minutes, or until the fish is done. (Another option is to use a pressure cooker: 3-minute cook time, rapid release.)
3. Drizzle the fish and vegetables with your sauce of choice.

CURRY IN A HURRY SAUCE

2 tablespoons extra virgin olive oil
3 garlic cloves, minced
1 teaspoon red pepper flakes
2 tablespoons red or green curry paste, or 2 tablespoons curry powder
1 tablespoon tamari

(continued)

1 tablespoon fish sauce (or coconut aminos, if you like it sweeter)
1 (13.5-ounce) can full-fat coconut milk
Lemon zest (optional)

1. In a medium saucepan over medium heat, add the olive oil. When it's hot, add the garlic and cook 1 to 2 minutes, until fragrant.
2. Add the pepper flakes, curry, tamari, and fish sauce (or coconut aminos) and whisk to combine. Add the coconut milk, whisk to incorporate, and bring to a low boil.
3. Remove the pan from the heat and add the lemon zest if desired. Store extra sauce in a jar in the refrigerator and rewarm it before using.

TIP: You can also make this sauce and simmer chicken or fish in it on the stovetop.

LEMON BUTTER SAUCE

¼ cup (4 tablespoons) ghee or butter
1 garlic clove, minced
1 tablespoon freshly squeezed lemon juice
1 tablespoon chicken bone broth
1 teaspoon dried parsley flakes
¼ teaspoon dried basil
¼ teaspoon paprika

In a small saucepan over medium heat, melt the ghee or butter. Add the remaining ingredients and cook, stirring, until hot. Pour the sauce over the cooked fish fillets.

TIP: You can also bake fish in the sauce at 350°F for 20 to 30 minutes, or until cooked through.

PRACTICE GRATITUDE: Take a moment to reflect on what you're thankful for in your life. Write it down, say it out loud, share it with someone. Do it every day. Practice it. Gratitude can give you perspective, bring a smile to your face, and shift your outlook on life in an instant. It has also been linked with improved health. In one study, participants who kept a journal most days of the week and wrote two or three things they were thankful for experienced reduced inflammation, improved biomarkers for heart disease, and better mood, sleep, and energy.

Day 11—Weekday

BREAKFAST

CHOCOLATE WALNUT FAB FOUR SMOOTHIE

Ever crave sugar first thing in the morning? Instead of a chocolate croissant, muffin, or coffee drink topped with whipped cream, use this rich, delectable smoothie to get yourself in balance.

Chocolate protein powder containing 20 to 30 grams protein
1 tablespoon walnuts
1 tablespoon flax meal
Handful of greens
1 to 2 cups unsweetened almond milk

Place all the ingredients in a high-speed blender and blend to your desired consistency.

LUNCH

WILD FISH BOATS

Five minutes to make lunch? No sweat. Go fish with these fish boats. Like my egg salad recipe (see page 167), this is a quick, easy, and delicious way to nourish your body with the Fab Four.

Makes 1 serving

1 (5-ounce) can wild salmon
2 tablespoons mayonnaise (I like Primal Kitchen)
6 to 8 romaine lettuce leaves
¼ to ½ avocado, diced
My Everything Bagel Seasoning (recipe follows), for sprinkling (optional)

Mix the salmon and mayonnaise in a small bowl. Spread it in the romaine lettuce "boats" and top with the avocado and a sprinkle of seasoning if desired.

MY EVERYTHING BAGEL SEASONING

One spice mix I love to sprinkle on top of Wild Fish Boats is Everything Bagel Seasoning from Gaby Dalkin of What's Gaby Cooking? *If I don't have any on hand, I sometimes whip up a quick riff on the recipe:*

¼ cup sesame seeds
¼ cup poppy seeds
3 tablespoons dried onion flakes
3 tablespoons dried garlic flakes
2 tablespoons coarse sea salt

Mix and store in a sealed container or seasoning jar.

BRIDGE SNACK: On days when you're planning a vegetarian or vegan dinner (spoiler alert: that's what's on the menu tonight), consider a protein-based bridge snack for the afternoon. For example, two hard-boiled eggs, grass-fed beef jerky, or a small handful of raw nuts.

DINNER

ITALIAN SPAGHETTI SQUASH

If you're a pasta lover, try this healthy spaghetti squash recipe for dinner. It's not only light, but it is also appropriate for vegans. If you want to add an animal protein, though, feel free. I like it with the Saucy Paleo Meatballs in Body Love.

Makes 1 to 2 servings

1 (2-pound) spaghetti squash
2 tablespoons olive oil
10 cherry tomatoes
4 cups fresh spinach
1 garlic clove, minced

1. Cut the squash crosswise, seed it, and pressure cook it for 7 minutes, rapid release. Once cooked, scrape the stringy squash flesh into a bowl.

2. In a medium skillet over medium-low heat, heat the olive oil. Add the squash, tomatoes, spinach, and garlic and cook, stirring often, until the dish is fragrant, the tomatoes are soft, and the spinach is wilted, 3 to 5 minutes.

TIP: Another option—though not as quick—is to bake the squash: Preheat the oven to 400°F. Place the halved and seeded squash on a baking sheet and bake for approximately 45 minutes.

LIE BACK AND RELAX . . . ON SPIKES: Acupressure mats have small plastic spikes that apply pressure to your back or feet. Lying down or standing on the mat at night can help calm your nervous system, relieve muscle tension, and ease aches and pains. There are a variety of affordable options on the market. Try it for between five and fifteen minutes and see how you feel. It's part of my nightly wind-down routine a couple times per week.

LIGHT PREP: If you have any leftover vegetables in the refrigerator, cook them for tomorrow's lunch. Coat a baking sheet with Primal Kitchen's avocado oil spray. Spread the vegetables evenly and give them another spray. Season with salt and roast them in the oven at 375°F for 25 to 30 minutes, flipping halfway through. When cool, store in a covered glass container in the refrigerator.

Day 12—Weekday

MORNING MOVEMENT: Wake up and work it. No excuses, no overthinking. Just thirty minutes of sweat.

BREAKFAST

SUPER GREEN MACHINE FAB FOUR SMOOTHIE

Reap the detoxifying benefits of broccoli sprouts and celery with my favorite new detox smoothie, the Super Green Machine. Broccoli sprouts help detoxify, reduce inflammation, and bolster cell defense (they contain the highest amount of sulforaphane). Celery contains coumarins, a group of phytochemicals that enhance white blood cell activity and help fight disease.

Vanilla protein powder containing 20 to 30 grams protein
1 tablespoon extra virgin olive oil
1 tablespoon chia seeds
Handful of greens (I like OrganicGirl Super Spinach or Super Greens)
1 to 2 tablespoons broccoli sprouts (preferably freshly sprouted; see Tip)
1½ cups fresh celery juice (recipe follows; see Tip)
Juice of ½ lemon

Place all the ingredients in a high-speed blender and blend to your desired consistency.

TIP: It's easy to grow your own organic broccoli sprouts. In a widemouthed sprouting jar, place 2 tablespoons of broccoli sprouting seeds (you can buy them online or at the grocery store) and cover with a few inches of filtered water. Screw on the lid and store in a dark location (a cabinet works great) at room temperature overnight. In the morning, drain the liquid and rinse with fresh water through the sprouting lid. Repeat this three or four times per day for two to three days. When the sprouts are an inch in length and dark green, replace the sprouting lid with a standard Mason jar lid and store in the refrigerator. The entire sprout is edible, so just pull out what you need; they should keep for up to one week in the refrigerator.

TIP: If you don't want to make celery juice, you can just use 2 cups filtered water and 1 cup roughly chopped celery. Be prepared for a few celery strings—the good news is that's roughly 2 grams of fiber you're getting.

HOMEMADE CELERY JUICE

Celery juice is too easy to make. Similar to homemade almond milk, you simply blend celery with water and then strain it through a nut bag.

1 head organic celery, including stalk and leaves
2 cups cold filtered water

Wash and chop the celery into 3-inch pieces. Blend the celery and water in a high-speed blender, then pour through a nut bag to strain. Store extra juice in the fridge for 1 to 2 days.

LUNCH: Take the roasted vegetables you cooked last night (see opposite) to work. If you have any leftover Lemon Tahini Dressing (page 158), take that, too. Then pick up a fresh prepared protein (chicken breast, grass-fed steak, wild salmon) at the market and enjoy it all together. If you didn't have time to cook your vegetables last night, no sweat. Just add fresh-cooked options from the market where you buy your protein.

DINNER

CHINESE CHICKEN LETTUCE WRAPS

Try this spin on lettuce wraps.

Makes 2 to 3 servings

1 tablespoon avocado oil
3 garlic cloves, minced
2 tablespoons minced fresh ginger
¼ cup chopped onion
1 pound ground pasture-raised chicken (or turkey)
3 tablespoons coconut aminos
¼ cup shredded carrots
½ cup shredded kale
1 cup chopped water chestnuts
Butter lettuce leaves, for serving
¼ cup chopped green onions
1 teaspoon sesame seeds
1 teaspoon sriracha (optional)

1. In a large skillet, heat the avocado oil over medium-low heat. Add the garlic, ginger, and onion and sauté until the onion is translucent, about 3 minutes.
2. Add the chicken and cook, breaking it up in the pan, until crumbled and lightly browned, 6 to 8 minutes. Feel free to drain off any excess oil.
3. Add the coconut aminos, carrots, kale, and water chestnuts and cook, stirring often, until the veggies soften, about 5 minutes. Serve the mixture in butter lettuce leaves and top with the green onions, sesame seeds, and sriracha if desired.

EVENING SELF-CARE: Take advantage of a night at home and jump in a Boosted Bath (see the Red-Carpet Ready plan, page 367).

Day 13—Weekend Day

BREAKFAST

PECAN PIE FAB FOUR SMOOTHIE

If your morning sweet tooth strikes again, try my Pecan Pie Fab Four Smoothie. The cinnamon adds a functional boost and is known to have blood sugar–balancing properties.

Vanilla protein powder containing 20 to 30 grams protein
2 tablespoons pecan butter or chopped pecans
1 tablespoon flax meal
½ teaspoon ground cinnamon (see Tip, page 239)
2 to 3 drops English toffee flavored Better Stevia liquid sweetener
1 to 2 cups unsweetened almond milk

Place all the ingredients in a high-speed blender and blend to your desired consistency.

GO GODDESS: If your schedule eases up and you're enjoying a slower Saturday, maybe it can be an opportunity to try cooking a recipe or two from the Domestic Goddess plan. Here are two options that don't take much time or prep.

LUNCH: Green Goddess Salad (page 229).

DINNER: Lettuce-Wrapped Pan-Fried Sliders and Roasted Root Fries (page 269).

Day 14—Weekend Day

BREAKFAST: Break your fast by cracking some eggs and making my Southwest Scramble (see the Domestic Goddess plan, page 239).

LUNCH: Get inspired by the season and create your own Fab Four Smoothie by using something from the farmers' market. Pick a seasonal fruit and create something fresh and different for yourself. Not feeling creative? Pick a recipe you haven't tried from this book or *Body Love*.

BE A TOURIST: Be a tourist in your own city. Pick a museum, venture to an up-and-coming part of town, see a sight you haven't seen, or take in a play or other type of performance. If you work in a creative capacity at your job, maybe it will give you the inspiration or invigoration you need. Maybe you'll learn something new or experience something fascinating about a different culture or time. Or maybe it will just give you a break from the four corners of your phone screen.

DINNER

MEXICAN CHICKEN VEGETABLE SOUP

Pick up a hot rotisserie chicken and some bone broth from the grocery store. You can use them to make this zesty soup. The fresh cilantro, lime, onion, and jalapeño give it that nice kick.

Makes 2 servings

1 tablespoon extra virgin olive oil
¼ cup diced onion
½ jalapeño, finely diced
1 garlic clove, finely minced
¼ cup chopped celery
½ cup chopped carrot

½ cup chopped zucchini
½ cup chopped summer squash
Pink Himalayan salt and freshly ground black pepper
2 cups shredded rotisserie chicken breast (or see Easy
    Peasy Shredded Chicken, page 254)
4 cups chicken bone broth
1 lime
Handful of cilantro, chopped

1. In a large saucepan over medium heat, heat the olive oil. Add half of the onion and jalapeño, and all of the garlic, celery, carrot, zucchini, and squash. Season with salt and pepper to taste. Cook, stirring often, until the onion is softened and the rest of the vegetables are tender, 6 to 8 minutes.

2. Add the chicken and bone broth and squeeze in the juice of half of the lime. Bring to a simmer. Serve hot and top with the remaining chopped onion and the cilantro; squeeze on a little juice from the remaining half lime, and add the remaining jalapeño for more kick.

> ## TO DRINK OR NOT TO DRINK
>
> There are some dinners, nights out, and other occasions when you're looking forward to a glass of wine or a cocktail. There are also times when you really don't want to drink, but end up doing it anyway. One way to keep yourself on track is to look at your calendar and mark the bigger occasions when you know you want to imbibe, like a birthday, dinner party, wedding, or date night. If you're going to drink, stick to those special times with family and friends, and leave the rest of your calendar alcohol-free.

TIP: Buying a hot rotisserie chicken is one of my favorite ways to cut down on cooking time. I opt for organic and pasture-raised chickens that are either unseasoned (naked) or minimally seasoned, without man-made industrial seed oils (see page 48), sugar, or other additives. You can pull off a breast and combine it with two handfuls of spinach, half an avocado, and a Primal Kitchen dressing to make a simple Fab Four salad in under 2 minutes.

ESSENTIAL OILS: Try using a calming oil in a diffuser tonight if you feel those Sunday Scaries creeping in. Essential oils are derived from plants and are used for various health and wellness purposes. My favorite way to use them is with a diffuser, which scents the air with a refreshing, calming aroma. You can also use essential oils topically or in other ways. Just be sure to read the instructions on the bottle carefully. Essential oils are powerful and highly concentrated. There is no shortage of brands out there to choose from to serve many different purposes, such as focus, calm, and sleep. Two blends I like from NOW Foods are Good Morning Sunshine and Cheer Up Buttercup. **Note: Certain essential oils are poisonous or toxic for animals. If you have pets, please check with your veterinarian before using essential oils in any fashion at home.**

Week 3: At Home

Let's keep the positive momentum going. You can always find balance and reach your goals with the Fab Four. The next seven days are full of more new recipes, helpful tips, and encouragement.

Day 15—Weekday

MORNING MOVEMENT: Choose a thirty- to sixty-minute workout that involves weight lifting, kettlebells, resistance, or strength training. A couple of class options include yoga with weights or a HIIT class (which combines aerobic and anaerobic exercise). Strength training helps tone, tighten, and build lean muscle mass. The point is to get an anaerobic workout that makes your muscles sore. This can help increase insulin sensitivity, lower blood sugar levels, and increase your metabolism.

BREAKFAST

HAPPY GUT FAB FOUR SMOOTHIE

Feed your healthy gut bacteria with this smoothie. Coconut yogurt comes with a dose of probiotics (live bacteria that support your gut microbiome) and a creamy, tangy flavor. GoldynGlow's Energy blend is a turmeric maca superfood that helps decrease inflammation and activates sirtuin genes, which have been linked to longevity and improved metabolism.

Vanilla protein powder containing 20 to 30 grams protein
1 tablespoon almond butter
1 tablespoon coconut yogurt
1 teaspoon GoldynGlow Energy blend
Handful of spinach
1 to 2 cups unsweetened almond milk

Place all the ingredients in a high-speed blender and blend to your desired consistency.

LUNCH

FLAKY TUNA AND TOASTED WALNUT SALAD

Not a huge fan of kale? Try baby kale. It's less bitter and easier to digest. It's perfect in this simple salad.

Makes 1 serving

2 tablespoons extra virgin olive oil
1 tablespoon champagne vinegar
4 (or more) cups baby kale
1 (5-ounce) can or 2 (3-ounce) pouches wild tuna, drained and fork flaked

(continued)

2 tablespoons toasted walnuts (see Tip)
Maldon salt or other big flaky salt

In a large bowl, whisk the olive oil and vinegar (see Tip). Add the kale, tuna, and walnuts and toss to coat them in the dressing. Finish with salt to taste.

TIP: Toasting nuts is an easy way to bring out more of their flavor. To do it, simply add a small handful to a frying pan and cook over medium-low heat for 2 to 3 minutes, stirring often, until browned and fragrant. Keep an eye on them as you toast—they burn fast.

TIP: Do you ever just drizzle olive oil and vinegar on your salad? Next time, drizzle them in the bottom of the bowl first, then whisk them together to emulsify (combine) for a more balanced flavor. Use a 2:1 ratio of oil to acid/vinegar. I like pairing olive oil with apple cider vinegar, lemon juice, or champagne vinegar. Looking to take it up a notch? Add a minced garlic clove to the dressing as well. It adds a nice bite and the phytochemical allicin (responsible for garlic's anti-inflammatory, anticancer, and immune-boosting properties).

DINNER

COCONUT CAULIFLOWER RICE WITH SWEET COCONUT CHICKEN AND BROCCOLI

With some precooked chicken from your own supply or a store-bought rotisserie chicken, it's quick to make this delicious dish with fiber-rich cauliflower rice, coconut chicken, and broccoli.

Makes 2 servings

2 cups broccoli florets
2 tablespoons coconut oil

2 tablespoons coconut milk (or coconut crème)

4 cups frozen or uncooked cauliflower rice (see page 315)

Meat from 1 rotisserie chicken (or 2 baked chicken breasts), shredded (or see Easy Peasy Shredded Chicken, page 254)

2 tablespoons melted ghee

¼ cup coconut aminos

2 tablespoons sesame seeds

2 tablespoons chopped chives

1. Heat 2 inches of water in a large saucepan to a simmer and quick-blanch the broccoli for 4 to 6 minutes, until fork tender (see Tip). Drain the broccoli and set it aside.

2. In the same pan, combine the coconut oil, coconut milk, and cauliflower rice. Stir-fry over medium heat until the cauliflower rice is done to your liking, 5 to 7 minutes. Add the broccoli and chicken to the pan and cook until warmed through, stirring as needed.

3. In a small bowl, mix the melted ghee, coconut aminos, and sesame seeds. Serve the cauliflower rice in bowls and dress it with the sauce. Garnish with the chives.

TIP: Blanching is a quick, easy way to prepare vegetables like broccoli, asparagus, cauliflower, and green beans. It's simply cooking the vegetables briefly in boiling water, then submerging them in ice water for several minutes. The technique works great for a crudité platter. Sometimes I do a "quick" blanch to cook vegetables for dinner. I just skip the step of submerging them in ice water and cook the vegetables just until fork tender. The cooking time will depend on the thickness of the vegetables, usually from 2 to 6 minutes (green beans and asparagus will cook faster than the broccoli in this recipe). Drain the water,

IT'S 2 P.M. . . . AND YOU HAVEN'T EATEN A THING

Some days it just happens. You're so busy at work that when you look up, it's 2 P.M. and you haven't eaten anything all day. Suddenly you find yourself staring at the vending machine in the office kitchen. If you ever have days like this, a small travel-size blender might be a worthwhile investment, so you can easily whip up a Fab Four Smoothie. NutriBullet has a few options for around fifty dollars. You can keep it at the office, along with the basics for a Fab Four Smoothie. Store protein powder, chia or flaxseeds, MCT oil, and a boxed unsweetened almond milk in a cabinet or in your desk. You can also throw a bag of frozen spinach in the office freezer. Unless you work with Popeye, I highly doubt it will be swiped! Now you have the ability to make a healthier decision than raiding the machine for chips, crackers, or cookies.

then use the vegetables as needed. (One option: place the vegetables back on the stove on low heat. Add salt and a light drizzle of extra virgin olive oil or avocado oil for flavor, and you're ready to serve.)

BREAKFAST PREP FOR TOMORROW

FAB FOUR CHIA SEED PUDDING

Chia seed pudding is a scrumptious way to start your day. Most chia seed puddings on the market have added sugar, though. Making it at home allows you to skip the sugar and fuel up on my protein-, fat-, and fiber-based version. Make it tonight so you can simply grab it from the refrigerator in the morning.

Makes 1 serving

¼ cup chia seeds
1½ cups unsweetened vanilla almond milk, plus more if needed
Vanilla protein powder containing 20 to 30 grams protein
1 tablespoon nut butter (I use almond or cashew)

1. Place the chia seeds in a mason jar (or other glass container with screw-on lid).
2. Place the almond milk, protein powder, and nut butter in a high-speed blender and blend, then pour the mixture over the chia seeds and screw the lid on tight. Shake well to mix.
3. Refrigerate for 20 minutes, then shake lightly again and taste. If the pudding is congealed but the chia seeds are still crunchy, add 2 more tablespoons almond milk, stir to incorporate, and return to the refrigerator until you're ready to eat. (You're more likely to need this added step if you use a plant-based protein powder.)

Day 16—Weekday

BREAKFAST: You already did the prep, so just grab your Fab Four Chia Seed Pudding and go. If you want to add a topping, try ¼ cup of blueberries or 1 tablespoon of your favorite nut butter.

LUNCH: If you have leftovers from last night (Coconut Cauliflower Rice with Sweet Coconut Chicken and Broccoli), dig in and supplement with anything you're missing. If you don't have leftovers, choose something from your self-made body-loving menu (see box below).

MAKE YOUR OWN MASTER MENU OF BODY-LOVING OPTIONS

This is one of my favorite tips from *Body Love* and bears repeating for my Girls on the Go. It may seem basic, but making your own menu is an extremely effective way to guide yourself to healthier decisions. All you have to do is take a few minutes and make a master menu of the clean, healthy dishes available from your favorite restaurants, takeout spots, and grocery stores with a hot bar. Then, the next time you're going out or ordering in, let the menu steer you in a healthy direction. If you have a long menu of clean options in front of you, you'll be less likely to act on emotional cravings at the end (or in the middle) of a stressful day. It's also a great tool if you find yourself being easily swayed toward an unhealthy decision by your significant other, kids, friends, co-workers, or food-delivery apps. Yes, I said your apps! At the end of a stressful day, they can make ordering an unhealthy dinner all too easy.

One way to elevate this concept a step further is to plan out your entire week of takeout dinners from your menu. *In my world, this still counts as meal prep!* If you have a family, let them know where you'll be ordering from for each night of

(continued)

> the week and just collect their orders for each restaurant. It can work for lunches, too. You'll build a healthy habit of eating the cleanest thing on the menu at the locations in your neighborhood without even trying. Over time, these decisions are what add up to a lifestyle. And remember, this doesn't mean you can never, ever have pizza or pasta from your favorite Italian place. It just puts a few bumpers on your bowling lane.

DINNER: Choose a healthy takeout option from your self-made menu. See page 185.

TIP: A few small purchases at the grocery store can easily elevate takeout from restaurants that might not be super healthy. Buy a head of butter lettuce, in case the Mexican restaurant or burger spot doesn't lettuce wrap their tacos or burgers. Stock salad dressings and condiments made with clean oils. Primal Kitchen has some delicious options. If you're going to dip into ranch, why settle for the sugary, industrial oil option that many restaurants carry? Keep a loaf of high-fiber gluten-free bread in the freezer so you can swap it for sandwich bread, buns, or rolls. Avocado pretty much goes with everything and is an easy way to add healthy fat and fiber to any meal. Siete chips and tortillas are clean, gluten-free swaps on Taco Tuesday. And sliced celery, carrots, and peppers are a great stunt double for French fries for kids. Okay, they might see through that one. . . . Roasted carrot and parsnip fries should do the trick . . . fingers crossed.

ROLL IT OUT: One body-loving routine I do several times per week is foam rolling. It's quick, easy, and feels phenomenal. Foam rolling can help improve fascia health, lymphatic drainage, and alignment. Fasciae are the connective tissues that wrap and protect the muscles, organs, and nerves. See the Domestic Goddess plan, page 251.

Day 17—Weekday

MORNING MOVEMENT: Let's balance Monday's strength/weight training with a cardio workout this morning. Pick your favorite app, go for a brisk thirty-minute power walk or two- to three-mile run, or use the elliptical machine at the gym.

BREAKFAST: Let's take the training wheels off. Without referencing a recipe or the formula, build a Fab Four Smoothie using your favorite protein, fat, fiber, and greens. I want you to become comfortable with the formula and with not always having a recipe in front of you. Also, understanding the components helps you decide what to order if you're out at a smoothie bar or restaurant.

LUNCH: Missing eggs? If you're having a Fab Four Smoothie most mornings, treat yourself to breakfast for lunch. Eggs are nutritious and warm, and can be a welcome change from your typical salad. Pick a café that serves breakfast after noon, or if you're at home, make eggs your way.

SIMPLE EGGS AND GREENS

One simple, satisfying option.

Makes 1 serving

3 eggs
1 tablespoon ghee or avocado oil
2 handfuls of spinach
½ avocado, diced
Pink Himalayan salt
Your favorite hot sauce

1. Fry the eggs in the ghee in a large skillet over medium heat. Remove the eggs to a plate. *(continued)*

2. Add the spinach to the pan and stir over the heat until wilted, about 2 minutes. Plate with the eggs. Top with the avocado, a sprinkle of salt, and hot sauce.

THE BE WELL BY KELLY PODCAST: It's here! I cover so much ground and have a blast doing it. Pick an episode and give it a listen on your way home from work today.

DINNER

SAUSAGE AND PEPPER SKILLET

Time can be one of the biggest deterrents to cooking. Buying precooked proteins is one of the easiest ways to make a weeknight meal in a flash. My Sausage and Pepper Skillet takes less than 10 minutes.

Makes 2 servings

6 ounces precooked sausage, chopped (I like Applegate Organics brand)
1 tablespoon avocado oil
1 cup diced bell pepper (any color)
½ cup diced yellow onion
1 zucchini, diced
2 garlic cloves, minced
2 tablespoons bone broth or water
2 cups shredded or baby kale
Pink Himalayan salt and freshly ground black pepper
Red pepper flakes

1. In a skillet over medium heat, combine the sausage, avocado oil, bell pepper, onion, zucchini, and garlic. Cook, stirring occasionally, until the onion pieces are translucent, the vegetables are fork tender, and the sausage is lightly browned, 6 to 8 minutes.

2. Add the bone broth and kale, and stir until the kale is wilted and the skillet is deglazed (the brown bits lift from the bottom). When the liquid has evaporated, transfer the mixture to a plate and sprinkle with salt, black pepper, and red pepper flakes to taste.

Day 18—Weekday

BREAKFAST

DARK CHOCOLATE OLIVE OIL SEA SALT FAB FOUR SMOOTHIE

Mix up the fat in your smoothie with this elegant recipe. Extra virgin olive oil is a great source of monounsaturated fat and is one of the most brain-healthy foods out there. It also contains oleocanthal, a compound that helps reduce inflammation throughout the body. This smoothie is a dual threat: it can satisfy that morning sweet tooth or be the perfect thing to curl up with when your hubby digs into a bowl of ice cream at night.

Chocolate protein powder containing 20 to 30 grams protein
2 tablespoons extra virgin olive oil
1 tablespoon chia or flaxseeds
½ teaspoon coarse sea salt
½ teaspoon cacao nibs
Handful of spinach
1 to 2 cups unsweetened almond milk

Place all the ingredients in a high-speed blender and blend to your desired consistency.

TIP: There might be a day or two when you don't have greens in your refrigerator or freezer. It's okay. Just because you're missing that component doesn't mean you have to miss out on protein, fat, and fiber. My advice is to lock in those nutrients and still have your smoothie. (Same goes for any meal.) Then, go a little extra green at lunch with a super green salad.

LUNCH: Head to a grocery store that has a salad bar and make yourself that super salad. Start with a base of romaine, add a handful of spinach or arugula, and if there are microgreens available, add those as well. Add ½ avocado for fat and fiber. Other green vegetables you can use as toppings could be cucumber, green bell pepper, and an herb that sounds good to you. Add your choice of protein and an approved body-loving dressing.

TIP: Most salad bars won't have avocado available because it browns quickly, so you might have to buy a whole avocado in the produce area. If you use half for your salad at lunch, save the half with a pit for a healthy bridge snack. Lightly dampen a paper towel or napkin and wrap the pitted half, then throw it in your work refrigerator. This will help keep the avocado from turning brown for about a day. If hunger strikes while you're at your desk, grab a spoon, sprinkle the avocado with salt, and enjoy.

DINNER: If you're feeling up for it, try cooking a more adventurous recipe from the Domestic Goddess plan. See if you can step out of your comfort zone and try something new.

CONSIDER JOINING A TEAM: Did you play a team sport in high school or college? A lot of my clients miss their days playing soccer, softball, volleyball, basketball, or whatever their sport was. One way to mix up your exercise routine is to join a recreational league or coed team. Not that you need another thing on your calendar, but it's a healthy way to work out, stay social, process stress, and tap back into your competitive spirit. Do a little research tonight and see if there's a season starting up soon.

Day 19—Weekday

JUST MOVE: Movement is a mind-set. See if you can shift into gear by walking somewhere today. A few simple ideas: take the stairs when you have the opportunity, walk to lunch instead of ordering it to a conference room or your desk, tackle an errand or two on foot, or walk to a coffee shop for the afternoon if you work from home.

BREAKFAST

CINNAMON PROTEIN PANCAKES

Whip up these pancakes for a sweet start to your Friday.

Makes 1 serving

Vanilla protein powder containing 20 to 30 grams protein
1 egg (or 2 egg whites, if your protein powder doesn't mask the yolk flavor)
¼ cup unsweetened almond milk
¼ teaspoon ground cinnamon
1 teaspoon coconut oil
1 teaspoon unsalted butter (optional; I like Kerrygold)
1 tablespoon monk fruit syrup or pure maple syrup (optional)

1. In a bowl, whisk the protein powder, egg, almond milk, and cinnamon, forming a batter.
2. Melt the coconut oil in a large skillet and pour the batter onto the griddle, using approximately ¼ cup for each pancake. Brown the pancakes on both sides, turning them after small bubbles appear on the top, 1 to 2 minutes per side.

IT'S OKAY TO SAY NO ONCE IN A WHILE

If you're like me, you say yes to almost everything. But sometimes you just gotta say no and thank yourself for it. Indulge in a little JOMO (joy of missing out) and take a night off just for yourself. Soak in a hot bath, give yourself a facial or mask, open a book for a chapter, journal for twenty minutes, or dive into a show you've been wanting to watch. And if FOMO strikes, remember you can always surprise your friends and meet them out.

3. Serve warm with butter (if using) and drizzle with monk fruit syrup (if using, make sure it's a single ingredient, with no high-fructose corn syrup or other added sugar).

LUNCH: Shrimp Louie Salad (see the Domestic Goddess plan, page 206).

DINNER

HERBY ITALIAN CHICKEN

It's tempting to order takeout on a Friday night, but this recipe is full of flavor and ready in less than 15 minutes.

Makes 2 servings

2 (6- to 8-ounce) boneless, skinless chicken breasts, butterflied
2 garlic cloves, minced
2 teaspoons dried oregano
2 teaspoons thyme
2 tablespoons minced fresh Italian parsley
2 tablespoons lemon juice
¼ cup extra virgin olive oil
1 teaspoon pink Himalayan salt
2 tablespoons minced fresh basil
2 tomatoes, chopped
6 cups arugula

1. Place the chicken breasts between two pieces of parchment paper. Using a meat tenderizer, pound the breasts until they are about ¼ inch thick.

2. In a large bowl, combine the garlic, oregano, thyme, parsley, 1 tablespoon of the lemon juice, 1 tablespoon of the olive oil, and the salt. Using tongs, add the chicken breasts to the bowl and mix to coat. (Optional: let the coated chicken breasts marinate in the refrigerator for 20 minutes.)

3. In a large skillet, heat 1 tablespoon of the olive oil over medium-high heat. Pan-fry the chicken breasts until cooked through, 3 to 4 minutes per side.

4. In a large salad bowl, add the remaining olive oil and lemon juice and the basil. Add the tomatoes and arugula and toss to coat.

5. Plate each chicken breast with half of the salad mixture.

Day 20—Weekend Day

BREAKFAST: A frittata may sound like something a fancy chef would make, but it's easier than you think. My Farmers' Market Frittata is a great recipe to try; see the Domestic Goddess plan, page 210.

GET INVOLVED: Find a way to volunteer your time or do something positive for your community today. Get involved and give back in a way that's meaningful to you. Even an hour makes an impact. When you're constantly on the go, it's easy to become consumed with what's happening in your world. But we're all part of a larger community. Do something today to nurture, heal, or help the world beyond your own. Someone or something out there needs your spark.

LUNCH: If you found yourself out last night, detox and hydrate with the Super Green Machine Fab Four Smoothie from page 174.

AFTERNOON MOVEMENT: Here are a few ideas for some light weekend movement. The goal is to get outside and not turn into an all-day couch potato: (1) go for a thirty-minute walk; (2) find a bit of nature and go for a hike; or (3) be a tourist in your own city, visit a museum, or explore an unfamiliar neighborhood—those steps will add up fast.

DINNER: What's faster than takeout and just as comforting? Tonight's dinner!

DINNER

COWBOY SKILLET

This spiced-up skillet dish takes less than 15 minutes to make and is a warm, satisfying meal that hearkens back to Hamburger Helper. This is a great recipe if you're looking to put any leftover vegetables in your refrigerator to use. I like to add shredded or finely diced broccoli, asparagus, zucchini, or carrots.

Makes 4 servings

1 pound ground beef
1 tablespoon smoked paprika
1 tablespoon chili powder
1 tablespoon unsweetened organic ketchup
½ tablespoon garlic salt
1 (12-ounce) bag frozen organic cauliflower rice (see page 315)
1 to 2 cups shredded or finely diced vegetables (optional)
8 cups fresh spinach
2 tablespoons nutritional yeast (optional)

1. Place the beef in a large skillet and cook over medium-high heat until browned and cooked through, 7 to 10 minutes, breaking it into smaller pieces with a wooden spoon as it cooks. Add the paprika, chili powder, ketchup, garlic salt, cauliflower rice, and vegetables (if using) to the meat in the skillet. Stir to combine and cook until heated through, 3 to 4 minutes. Add the spinach and cook until lightly wilted, 1 to 2 minutes.
2. For a cheesy flavor, sprinkle the nutritional yeast on top (if using) and serve.

Weekend Away

Weekends away are supposed to be a time to relax, have fun, and recharge. But I can't tell you how many of my clients have anxiety surrounding their next girls' trip, couple's retreat, or three-day weekend. I remember feeling that way, too. For those who've adopted the Fab Four lifestyle, it can be a time when their positive momentum gets stalled or when they're on the receiving end of judgy comments from their friends. For new clients, it can be a time of uncertainty or feeling like one bad decision means their only option is to let go in the moment and start over on Monday. But no matter what the weekend throws at you, be it nachos, s'mores, tequila, or peer pressure, the Fab Four is always there for you. As I said at the beginning of this chapter, one decision—your next—is all that matters. Focus on having fun, accept that you might not have as much control as you do at home, and use the tips and sample day below to help make your next decision a body-loving one. And if it isn't, don't dwell on it. Just turn your attention to the one after that.

PACK PREPARED. Give yourself the ability to elevate everyday situations (and rescue yourself from cravings) by packing items that will help support clean, body-loving choices. See the list starting on page 142 for examples of things I bring with me on trips. These small items can make a big impact if you're on a bachelorette trip where the rental house is filled with junk food, or a sports weekender with your sorority sisters or boyfriend/husband when you're eating at bars and stadiums. If you've been living the Fab Four lifestyle for a while, going back to imbalanced meals can make you feel less satiated, and you might experience strong carbohydrate cravings again. Packing your blender bottle and a few key ingredients can give you the ability to nip hormonal hunger in the bud. For example, you can quickly make any of the Fab Four Roadies that start on page 150.

TELL YOUR HOST OR PLANNER IF YOU'RE CELIAC OR GLUTEN-FREE. If you have special dietary needs, give the host or planner a heads-up. If they're preordering lunches, they can order you a gluten-free sandwich, an individual pizza, or a salad from the pizza place, or at least let you know if you need to plan ahead for restaurants without acceptable options.

LOVE IT ON THE LAST DAY. When you're on vacation or traveling for fun, enjoying a location-specific dessert, treat, or "Not So Fab" Four meal can be a highlight of the trip. If you're gone for a week or longer, the risk is that it can turn into a daily habit, which can lead to a week or longer of imbalance. One way I coach my clients to stay on track is to "love it on the last day." Save that dessert, treat, or meal for your last day in that particular location and tell yourself, "If I still want it on the last day, I will love it." It doesn't necessarily have to be the last day of your entire trip, and it can even be spur of the moment. The point is to choose when you're going to indulge and then enjoy it, sans guilt. Saving it for the last day at each location is just a way to help you stay focused on making healthy decisions until that point. This works great when you're on a multicity tour in Europe, and is equally helpful for shorter weekends away closer to home.

A LITTLE RESEARCH GOES A LONG WAY. Take a few minutes online and make a list of healthy restaurants where you'll be traveling. We can all wing it, but part of building a healthy lifestyle is making nutrition part of your travel thought process, which starts before you leave. Even if you end up eating only a single healthy meal at one of the restaurants you found, it's a success. Get as excited about trying that one place as you do about indulging in local sweets. Plus, you might discover different neighborhoods or sights to see while you're researching.

Day 21—Weekend Away

BREAKFAST: Breakfast on a girls' trip is typically one of three things: a continental breakfast with sugary pastries, fruit, granola, and yogurt; a late brunch to which you arrive starving; or a piecemeal homemade breakfast at your rental house. If the continental offerings aren't ideal, lean on a few protein- or fat-based items you packed, such as the protein in a Fab Four Roadie or a fat-based creamer for your coffee or tea. If you know your girlfriends might lag and brunch won't happen till noon, eat a protein bar after your coffee (see the list starting on page 139 for my go-tos). It's better to arrive fueled than famished, so you're not tempted by French toast and pancakes. If the group cooks up eggs at your house, but you've been consistently having Fab Four Smoothies back at home, the meal might leave you wanting more. Aim to eat three eggs to get the protein and fat you're used to, add any vegetables available, or supplement with one of the other items on pages 142–143.

> ### THE HEALTHY HERMIT NO MORE
>
> Some people feel the need to close off from the world and stay at home in order to make healthy decisions. Using the light structure of the Fab Four means you don't have to. You can live your life, see your friends, and always elevate your next meal or food choice. I hope the tips, tools, and recipes in this chapter empower you and help you drop anchor on a healthier lifestyle.

TIP: Here's a slimmed-down list of what to bring: 2 protein bars; 2 protein powder packets; 2 fat-based creamer packets (MCT powder or coconut oil); and 2 raw nut packs.

LUNCH: One of the best orders you can make for lunch is a large salad. I know it's a simple suggestion, but during a weekend that might expose you to more carbohydrates than normal, it's important to lock in some fiber and greens. This nets you at least one meal that feeds your healthy gut bacteria. Try to opt for a more fibrous lettuce, such as kale or cabbage, add avocado, and ask for a side of olive oil.

TIP: If you're going to be drinking over the weekend, it's important to be cognizant of your sugar intake, specifically fructose. Just like alcohol, fructose is metabolized in the liver. If you're going to drink more than normal, you can give your liver a bit of a break by avoiding things like fruit juice mixers, simple syrup, and agave in your drinks, and cookies, candy, and other sweet junk food.

DINNER: Instead of trying to soak up alcohol with starchy carbohydrates, focus on eating a high-protein, high-fat dinner such as wild salmon, a lettuce-wrapped grass-fed burger, or a baked chicken dish. A protein- and fat-based dinner will take longer to digest. If you're drinking alcohol at dinner or afterward, the alcohol will also take longer to digest. In addition, while it is in your stomach, the enzyme ADH (alcohol dehydrogenase) can break down up to 20 percent of the alcohol, which reduces the load on your liver and makes you less tipsy.

TIP: If you're going to drink hard alcohol, do it responsibly and in moderation. Stick to clear alcohol (such as vodka or tequila blanco) and clear mixers (like water or soda water). I always add a lemon or lime wedge. Avoid sugary or juice-based mixers, as they will tax your liver and spike your blood sugar. You want to continuously hydrate and also take a multivitamin because the alcohol will deplete your body of vitamins A, B_1, B_2, B_6, C, D, E, and K.

7

DOMESTIC GODDESS

BUILD YOUR HEALTHY DREAM HOUSE

WE ALL HAVE DREAMS and aspirations. One of mine is to build a healthy home for my family. Home is where the heart is, and it's also where clean eating, healthy habits, and body love begin. It might sound quaint or old-fashioned, but I can't wait to buy a house, put down roots, and live life to the fullest with those I love most. (As a bonus, I'd also really love what my aunt Cindy built in her backyard: a sprawling garden full of fresh herbs and vegetables to inspire her cooking, and a coop with two hens laying eggs every day!)

Whether you live in the city or the suburbs, you're a mom of toddlers or teenagers (or not a mom at all), or you're just starting out like me, I want to help you build your healthy dream house. The good news is that you don't need a big kitchen, fancy appliances, a home garden, your own hens, or even a house to do it. With the Fab Four as your foundation, you can create a healthy lifestyle that's right for you and your family and be the Domestic Goddess you want to be.

For me, it starts in the kitchen. It's one of my happy places. I'm not the world's greatest chef by any stretch, but I love cooking. It connects me to my food and where my ingredients come from. One of the simplest ways to apply the Fab Four to your home life is to source high-quality ingredients for your pantry and refrigerator. Part One gave you some practical advice for how to do this, and the plan in this chapter will build on that advice.

I also don't like eating bland food, and cooking helps me spice it up. After all, a sustainable lifestyle you actually want to live has to be flavorful. In the following pages, I share a bunch of delicious new Fab Four recipes and give you some tips on how to elevate a few classic comfort foods. Also, the Girl on the Go plan has a bunch of amazing (and easy) recipes you can make in a flash, and the Plant-Based Devotee plan is full of tasty vegetarian and vegan dishes that can help expand your culinary horizons. (And if you need even more inspiration, you can always revisit *Body Love*.)

Cooking helps you eat clean, balance your blood sugar, and stay fueled throughout the day. Whether it's one meal per day, all three, or just prep for later in the week, cooking will help you integrate the Fab Four into your daily life. And this extends out into the world. **If you're balanced and fueled at home, you'll make healthier choices when you're out and about.** Being a Domestic Goddess doesn't mean you have to cook like a Food Network star or bake every day. It just means using cooking and the kitchen as tools to support your healthy lifestyle and help you reach your goals.

If you have kids, your home base will have a lifelong effect on how they eat, drink, and exercise. It also shapes the way they think about food, nutrition, and their own health. **When you live the Fab Four lifestyle, the message you send and the example you set is one of nourishment.** The Fab Four emphasizes eating complete meals consisting of whole, nutrient-dense foods. It's an approach that supports blood sugar balance, longevity, and overall health. It's not about deprivation, dieting, or perfection. When you live a healthy lifestyle for yourself, it trickles down to the rest of your family. If one of your "mom goals" is to adapt or implement the Fab Four for your family, I hope the recipes, tools, and ideas in this chapter (and the rest of the book) help you do it.

But what about those other goals—*your* goals? I work with so many women (both with and without children) who yearn to reconnect with themselves and make their health goals a priority again. I've also had clients who feel selfish or guilty once they finally do. Even if the whole world seems to depend on you (and in your family or at your job it actually might), one of the healthiest things you can do is take the time to nourish and nurture yourself. That's a form of body love we sometimes forget. *Body love isn't solely about accepting your shape or figure (although that's a huge part of it); it's also about prioritizing your health and giving your body the nourishment and love it deserves.* If you feel like you've lost touch with yourself, I hope this sparks a reconnection. Even if it's been a few years, you're only one decision away from reconnecting with who you are and what you want. Whether it's a new relationship with food, a weight goal, or a healthier overall lifestyle, the plan in this chapter can help you get there. Each day is rooted in the Fab Four and will help you slow down and find your footing.

A few final words of encouragement to all the mothers out there. There's nothing easy about raising a family or running a household. Being a Domestic Goddess isn't a vacation from life. (Having my own little one has taught me that lesson pretty quickly.) It's no less draining or stressful than working an office job. Just like me, many of you have career goals and ambitions to balance. So don't hold yourself to an impossible standard. Being a Domestic Goddess doesn't mean you have to become Martha Stewart. It doesn't mean having everything under control, hosting elegant dinner parties every weekend, or raising kids who make themselves Fab Four Smoothies. It means doing your best, valuing yourself, and building confidence one healthy decision at a time. There's a balanced, brave, and beautiful woman inside every one of us, and she deserves body love.

PLAN OVERVIEW

Whether you're already an established Domestic Goddess like my aunt Cindy, or an aspiring one like me, I hope this plan gives you a fresh outlook and new inspiration. All three weeks have you home cooking some amazing Fab Four meals and smoothies that prioritize clean, nutrient-dense ingredients. Each week has tips for evening self-care, ways to approach working out, and ideas for applying the Fab Four to your family's needs.

The Fab Four meal recipes are mostly home-cooked from scratch, which can make them a little more time-intensive, but all the more enjoyable and satisfying as a result. For many women who cook for their families, food is love, which sometimes can mean a lot of flour, sugar, and bad oils get used. The recipes in this plan show you new ways to show your love and do it in a cleaner, healthier way. Food is medicine, too!

As for the Fab Four Smoothies, they still take mere minutes. The recipes in this plan are out of this world and cover a flavor profile just as big. For example: Chocolate Almond Butter Crunch (page 216), Green Goddess (page 213), Turmeric Almond Bliss (page 237), Detox Winter Mint (page 240), Anti-Inflammatory Vanilla Spice (page 246), Sun Butter and Jelly Swirl (page 261), Creamy Mocha (page 264), and Sweet and Savory Basil (page 266).

EVERYDAY ELEVATION

If the kitchen is your happy place, then sourcing ingredients, meal prep and planning, and cooking might already be well-honed skills. But as with nearly everything in life, there are still ways to elevate your game every day.

- You might be a master chef, but you can always learn something new. I would encourage you to browse through the Girl on the Go and Plant-Based Devotee plans to discover new ways to augment your healthy lifestyle. There are tips for

Sunday prep, healthy hacks to use during the week, and a bunch of delicious Fab Four recipes. And if you're in a funk or need a little motivation, the Red-Carpet Ready and Inner Perfectionist chapters can give it to you.

- In some of the recipes in this plan (and the others), you might see a new or unfamiliar ingredient. Everything I included is there because it's what I cook with. (I'm not trying to send you on a wild goose chase!) Even if you only use something occasionally, such as Dr. Cowan's Threefold Blend Powder (see page 273), here's how I would think about it—you're elevating your game by having these items in your pantry. Another example is salt. I keep Real Salt (see page 275) in my pantry because it's an unrefined mineral salt from an ancient, uncontaminated salt deposit in Redmond, Utah, and contains an abundant variety of trace minerals.

- Part One went in-depth on my approach to sourcing protein, fat, fiber, and greens. For instance, I explained why I prefer grass-fed and grass-finished beef from a health and nutrition perspective, then gave you a few options to source it (see page 37). Take a look through those chapters and see if there's a way you can update a few things on your shopping list with cleaner, more nutrient-dense options.

Day 1—Weekday

BREAKFAST: If you have kids, a smoothie bowl is a great way to sneak more greens into their diet, especially if you tweak it (see Tip, page 204) and go with a fun flavor like Triple Chocolate Crunch (page 218) or Cookies and Cream (see the Girl on the Go plan, page 163). You can even sub in avocado as the fat for greater benefit and thickness. Nut and seed toppings add a fun crunch—as well as fat and fiber—to every bite.

BACK TO *BODY LOVE*

For more recipes, sample shopping lists, meal prep hacks, and healthy swaps and substitutions, you can revisit *Body Love*. It also includes recipes for a bunch of sauces, dressings, and dips, such as Pistachio Mint Pesto, Cilantro Pesto, Chimichurri Sauce, Lemon Aioli, Roasted Garlic Cashew Cream Sauce, Fab Four Vinaigrette, Dill Ranch Dressing, Lemon Vinaigrette, Homemade Hummus, and Avocado Hummus.

BREAKFAST

GREEN FAB FOUR SMOOTHIE BOWL

This morning let's start with a lean, green bowl.

Vanilla protein powder containing 20 to 30 grams protein
¼ avocado
1 tablespoon chia seeds
1 cup frozen spinach
1 to 1½ cups unsweetened almond milk or Homemade Plant-Based Milk (recipe follows)
Dry topping options: 1 tablespoon hemp hearts, slivered almonds, goji berries, or cacao nibs
Fruit topping options: ¼ cup blueberries, blackberries, strawberries, or in-season sliced fruit

Place the protein powder, avocado, chia, spinach, and almond milk in a high-speed blender and blend to your desired consistency. Pour into a bowl and top with a dry topping and/or a fruit topping.

TIP: With a few simple tweaks, you can make any Fab Four Smoothie into a smoothie bowl. Begin by choosing your favorite recipe. To help thicken the smoothie base so you can eat it with a spoon, reduce the nut milk to 1 to 1½ cups and use frozen vegetables instead of fresh. For an extra-thick and cold bowl, consider adding ¼ cup of frozen cauliflower rice. If you want to use nut and seed toppings, reduce the fat and fiber in your recipe to 1 tablespoon each (for avocado, use only a quarter, rather than a half). Save your fruit for the top, too.

HOMEMADE PLANT-BASED MILKS

On page 54, I gave you some pointers for choosing a plant-based milk for your Fab Four Smoothie. You can also make your own at home. This recipe works for almonds, cashews, hazelnuts, pecans, macadamia nuts, flaxseeds, hemp hearts, and gluten-free oats.

Makes 5 to 6 cups/servings

1 cup raw, unsalted nuts, seeds, or oats
8 cups filtered water, room temperature

1. Place the nuts, seeds, or oats in a glass jar or bowl. Add 4 cups filtered water and cover with a mesh lid or cloth. Let soak overnight. In the morning, drain and discard the soaking water and thoroughly rinse the food. (Optional: for the creamiest almond milk, peel the skins off the almonds after soaking. To do so, pinch each almond between your fingers to loosen the skin and then gently peel.)

2. In a high-speed blender, blend the nuts, seeds, or oats with the remaining filtered water until the mixture reaches a creamy consistency, with no visible sign of whole nuts, seeds, or oats, 4 to 5 minutes.

3. Using a nut milk bag, strain the blended nut mixture into a glass pitcher (one that has a lid). (Optional: you should be able to skip this step for cashews, flaxseeds, and hemp hearts. Due to their softness, they should blend completely.)

4. Store the milk (lid on) in the refrigerator for up to 3 days.

STREAM A MORNING WORKOUT: You don't need to leave home to get your workout in. Some of my most successful clients do all their exercise at home. This week let's commit to three thirty-minute at-home workouts on Monday, Wednesday, and Friday. Whatever app (or other method) you use, just make sure it's manageable, fun, and right for you.

LUNCH

SHRIMP LOUIE SALAD

*Cooking your own shrimp is an easy way to expand your culinary repertoire and try some-
thing new, like this salad. You get the benefit of a fresh, wild, and clean protein in under
ten minutes. I've planned it so you make a dozen and save half in the refrigerator. They're
great for a quick salad (you'll also have extra dressing) or bridge snack later in the week.
(And if you're also going to be a Girl or Mom on the Go today, you can always make this
recipe with precooked shrimp.)*

Makes 1 serving

SHRIMP
½ onion
2 garlic cloves, peeled
2 celery stalks
1 bay leaf
1 dozen large shrimp, cleaned and deveined, tails removed

CHIVE VINAIGRETTE
Juice of ½ lemon
1 teaspoon Dijon mustard
¼ cup chopped or snipped fresh chives
⅓ cup extra virgin olive oil
Pink Himalayan salt and freshly ground black pepper

SALAD
2 baby romaine hearts
½ small avocado, diced
2 radishes, thinly sliced

1. To prepare the shrimp, pour 4 cups of filtered water into a medium saucepan. Add the onion, garlic, celery, and bay leaf and bring to a boil for 5 minutes. Remove the pan from the heat and drop in the shrimp. Return to heat and cook for 3 minutes, stirring occasionally, until the shrimp are pink and curled. Drain the shrimp and discard the aromatics. Rinse and cool them to room temperature.

2. To make the chive vinaigrette, in a small bowl, whisk the lemon juice and Dijon, then add the chives. While whisking, pour in the olive oil in a slow stream. Add a pinch each of salt and pepper.

3. To assemble the salad, layer the romaine, avocado, and radishes on a serving plate. Top with 6 of the shrimp and drizzle with 2 tablespoons of the vinaigrette.

4. The remaining 6 shrimp will keep, covered, in the refrigerator for up to 3 days. Transfer the leftover dressing to a jar with a lid and store it in the refrigerator for use later in the week.

TIP: Having themed dinner nights can help you mix up your proteins and flavors throughout the week. It's also an easy way to plan ahead for your family and develop your own version of light structure. I like having Meatless Monday once or twice per month to incorporate a plant-based dinner. Taco Tuesday is an automatic in my household, but I mix it up with chicken tacos one week, steak the next, and fish or shrimp after that. We often default to chicken and vegetables, so seeking out wild fish on Wild Wednesdays ensures we get brain-healthy omega-3 fats every week. Come up with a few days of your own that you and your family can look forward to (such as Birdsday Thursday, Grass-Fed Friday, or Souper Sunday). We all thrive on a little light structure.

DINNER

ITALIAN BUTTER BEAN BAKE

Speaking of Meatless Monday, let's give it a go tonight. This dish is a comforting alternative to pasta or lasagna. Butter beans are a high-fiber, lower carbohydrate alternative to flour-based pasta and bread products. Serve up the bake with your favorite mixed green salad.

Makes 4 servings

2 tablespoons extra virgin olive oil
2 garlic cloves, minced
½ cup chopped white onion
2 (15-ounce) cans organic butter beans, drained and rinsed
2 cups marinara sauce (I like Rao's or Thrive Market brands)
½ cup pesto
1 cup shredded mozzarella cheese (vegan option: Parmela Creamery mozzarella-style shreds; see Tip)

1. Rinse and drain the beans. In a large skillet over medium-high heat, heat the olive oil, then add the garlic and onion. Sauté, stirring continuously, until the onion is translucent and the garlic is aromatic, about 3 minutes. Add the beans and cook, stirring, until they are heated through and the flavors are mingled, 3 to 5 minutes.
2. Preheat the broiler or preheat the oven to 375°F.
3. Transfer the beans to a 9-inch square baking dish and cover with the marinara. Place spoon-size dollops of pesto on top and sprinkle with the cheese.
4. Bake for 5 minutes, until the cheese is melted.

TIP: If beans aren't great for your digestion or you want an animal protein instead, ground turkey can be used in place of the butter beans (just be sure to cook it thoroughly when you add it to the onion mixture). Also, to add fiber to either version, sauté diced zucchini and summer squash along with the protein (beans or turkey).

TIP: Be careful with nut-based cheese spreads. Many are full of bad oils, refined flours, soy, emulsifiers, and gums. I like Parmela Creamery because they use limited ingredients.

MOODY MONDAY: We've all had a case of the Mondays. One way to process those emotions and the residual stress of the day without resorting to a glass of wine is to try breathwork. My friend and instructor Ashley Neese's new book, *How to Breathe: 25 Simple Practices for Calm, Joy, and Resilience,* is a perfect place to start. Breathwork uses specific breathing techniques and exercises to calm your nervous system. You set an intention, connect with your breath, and then move through different breathing patterns. For me, the effect was dramatic. I felt a great swell of emotion rise to the surface, followed by a total release of all the stress and anxiety I was holding on to. It was like meditation and therapy combined. Breathwork can relieve stress and anxiety, help you process your thoughts and emotions, and clear blockages and stuck energy.

SNEAKY GREENS

I'm a new mom (relatively speaking), so I won't pretend to know all the crafty mom tricks to sneak vegetables and greens into meals for kids. But I do have a few ideas:

- Add finely grated zucchini, carrot, or summer squash to pasta or meat sauce.
- Blend fresh spinach into pesto or broccoli soup.
- Add cauliflower rice (see page 315) to macaroni and cheese, mashed potatoes, or potato salad.
- Bulk up burgers, meat loaf, or meatballs with finely grated mushrooms.
- Whip up a Fab Four Smoothie Bowl (see Tip, page 204) with a fun flavor like Chocolate Almond Butter Crunch (page 216) or Blueberry Muffin (from *Body Love*).

Day 2—Weekday

BREAKFAST

FARMERS' MARKET FRITTATA

A few fresh vegetable buys at the farmers' market or grocery store can turn a standard egg breakfast into this delicious frittata.

Makes 4 to 6 servings (if your kids are little)

10 eggs
½ teaspoon pink Himalayan salt
¼ teaspoon freshly ground black pepper
1 tablespoon avocado oil
4 garlic cloves, minced
1 cup sliced shiitake mushrooms (see Tip)
1 cup roughly chopped broccoli rabe
3 cups baby spinach
Basil, cut into chiffonade

1. Preheat the oven to 350°F.
2. In a medium bowl, lightly whisk the eggs. Season with salt and pepper and set aside.
3. In a large cast-iron frying pan over medium heat, heat the avocado oil, then add the garlic, mushrooms, and broccoli rabe. Sauté for 3 to 5 minutes, until softened, stirring occasionally. Remove the pan from the heat, add the spinach, and stir to wilt.
4. Spread the sautéed vegetables evenly over the surface of the pan and pour the eggs on top. Bake for 20 minutes, until the frittata is puffy and the center is firm. Serve warm with the basil chiffonade on top.

TIP: Shiitake mushrooms are a good source of vitamin D and lentinan, an immunity-boosting polysaccharide that has anticancer properties and heals chromosomal damage. They have greater nutrient density than white button mushrooms, which is why I use them in the frittata. Another nutrient-dense option is oyster mushrooms, a good source of the amino acid ergothioneine, which supports skin health by protecting the mitochondrial membrane and helping the skin use oxygen more efficiently. This can aid with wrinkles and sun damage.

LUNCH

SPICY SALMON NORI BURRITO

Try my spicy salmon nori-wrapped burrito (as seen in Body Love*).*

Makes 2 servings

¼ cup mayonnaise (I like Primal Kitchen)
1 to 2 tablespoons sriracha (I like Organicville's gluten-free Sky Valley)
1 (6-ounce) can or 2 (3-ounce) pouches wild salmon, drained (or cooked salmon fillet, flaked)
2 sheets full-size dried nori wrap
1 cup cooked quinoa or brown rice, room temperature (optional)
1 cup mixed greens
1 tablespoon extra virgin olive oil
1½ teaspoons lite seasoned rice vinegar
1 avocado, thinly sliced
½ cup peeled, thinly sliced cucumber
½ cup shredded carrot
1 tablespoon sesame seeds
¼ cup coconut aminos

1. Preheat the oven to 350°F. Line a baking sheet with parchment paper.
2. In a medium bowl, combine the mayonnaise and sriracha. Add the salmon and mix gently with a fork.

(continued)

211

3. Place two nori sheets on the prepared baking sheet and top each with ½ cup of quinoa (if using) and half the salmon salad. Warm the wraps in the oven for 3 to 5 minutes, until the nori is malleable.

4. In a medium bowl, dress the greens with the olive oil and vinegar. Toss to coat.

5. Layer the avocado, cucumber, carrot, and mixed greens on top of the salmon salad. Roll each into a burrito (the ends of the nori tucked in) and cut them in half. Garnish with the sesame seeds and serve with coconut aminos for dipping.

DINNER

MARISA'S CARNITAS KALE SALAD

This tasty slow cooker recipe comes directly from my sister-in-law's kitchen.

Makes 6 servings

CARNITAS

1 (2-pound) pork roast (or use 2 pounds chicken breast)

1 tablespoon pink Himalayan salt

1½ teaspoons freshly ground black pepper

1½ teaspoons ground cumin

1½ teaspoons smoked paprika

1½ teaspoons chili powder

1½ teaspoons garlic powder

1½ teaspoons onion powder

1½ teaspoons dried oregano

1 cup chicken broth or water

2 bay leaves

½ white or yellow onion, sliced

2 tablespoons avocado oil

CILANTRO-PEPITA DRESSING

1 (7-ounce) can diced green chiles

3 tablespoons pepitas

2 garlic cloves, peeled

3 tablespoons cotija cheese (optional; avoid if dairy-free)

1 teaspoon freshly ground black pepper

½ teaspoon pink Himalayan salt

2 tablespoons freshly squeezed lime juice

⅓ cup avocado oil or olive oil

1 tablespoon red wine vinegar

Leaves from ½ bunch fresh cilantro (no stems)

¼ cup cold filtered water

QUICK PICKLED ONIONS

1 cup filtered water

½ cup apple cider vinegar

1 tablespoon coconut sugar

1½ teaspoons pink Himalayan salt

1 red onion, thinly sliced

SALAD

8 to 10 cups chopped, stemmed kale (or romaine)

2 avocados, pitted, peeled, and diced

½ cup roasted pepitas

½ cup crumbled cotija cheese (optional)

1. To make the carnitas, season the pork roast with the salt, pepper, cumin, smoked paprika, chili powder, garlic powder, onion powder, and oregano. Set it in a large skillet over medium-high heat and sear it until brown on all sides.

2. Place in a slow cooker (fat side up) with the chicken broth, bay leaves, and onion. Cook on Low for 8 hours, until it's completely tender and shreds easily with a fork. Remove the pork from the slow cooker and shred on a cutting board. If you like the pork juicier, use a large spoon and dress the pork with drippings from the slow cooker, to your desired amount.

(continued)

3. Meanwhile, make the cilantro-pepita dressing: Place all the ingredients in a high-speed blender and blend until the consistency is similar to pesto.

4. When the pork has finished slow-cooking, heat the avocado oil in a large skillet on high heat. Add the pork and pan-fry to give it a crispy carnitas texture.

5. To make the pickled onions, in a medium bowl, whisk the water, vinegar, sugar, and salt together until the salt and sugar dissolve. Place the onion in a mason jar and pour the vinegar mixture on top. Secure the lid and let the jar rest at room temperature for 1 hour.

6. To assemble the salad, in a large serving bowl, toss the chopped kale and dressing. Top with the carnitas, avocados, pickled onions, pepitas, and, if desired, cotija cheese.

TIP: Speaking of my sister-in-law, see the Teacher Training box on Day 8, page 238. Marisa was a branding and marketing executive who thrived on leading her team through complex campaigns. When she took time off to raise her two boys, one of the ways she was able to tap back into that leadership role was to become a Pilates instructor. She had fallen in love with Pilates postpartum and wanted to teach her newfound passion to others. It also helped her carve out time for herself and her body—which rocks!

FREEZER FUDGE

If your sweet tooth strikes, this fudge is a clean dessert option. This recipe makes enough to fill a standard ice cube tray, but you can double it if your trays are larger (or you want to fill two). Then, on nights when you're craving a bite of something sweet, pop a cube in your mouth. (Just try to keep it to one cube per night.) This is my original recipe from Body Love, *along with three scrumptious new flavors.*

Makes 12 to 14 bite-size servings

ORIGINAL

1 cup coconut oil
¼ cup organic unsweetened cocoa powder
8 to 10 drops liquid stevia
¼ to ½ cup almond butter (optional)
Pinch of Maldon sea salt or pink Himalayan salt (optional)

HAZELNUT

1 cup coconut oil
¼ cup organic unsweetened cocoa powder
8 to 10 drops liquid stevia
¼ to ½ cup hazelnut butter

CARAMEL CANDY

1 cup coconut oil
8 to 10 drops liquid Caramel Stevia
¼ to ½ cup cashew butter
½ teaspoon ground cinnamon (see Tip, page 247)
¼ teaspoon pure vanilla extract

PRALINE

1 cup extra virgin olive oil
8 to 10 drops liquid Caramel Stevia
½ cup tahini
¼ cup chopped pecans
Pinch of Maldon sea salt or pink Himalayan salt (optional)

1. To make the original, hazelnut, or caramel candy, melt the coconut oil for approximately 30 seconds over low heat. For all flavors, place the oil in a medium glass bowl.

2. Add all the other ingredients to the bowl, except the salt, if using, and whisk to combine. Divide the mixture evenly in an ice cube tray (do not fill all the way to the top). Sprinkle with salt, if called for and desired.

3. Freeze for 30 minutes, or until solid, then turn them out of the tray. Store the fudge bites in an airtight container in the freezer.

Day 3—Weekday

FASTED MORNING WORKOUT: Lock in your second at-home workout of the week. If you need to set your alarm thirty minutes earlier to make sure you have the time, do it. If your Day 1 workout was more cardio focused, choose a workout that includes resistance or weight training. Resistance and weight training can help build lean muscle mass, tone your figure, and increase strength. (The scientific reason: it has been found to increase IGF1 gene expression with an increased protein synthesis after two to four hours.)

BREAKFAST

CHOCOLATE ALMOND BUTTER CRUNCH FAB FOUR SMOOTHIE

The subtle crunch in this decadent-seeming smoothie comes from the cacao nibs. They don't completely blend in. If you want a full crunch, sprinkle on an extra teaspoon of nibs as a topping.

Chocolate protein powder containing 20 to 30 grams protein
1 tablespoon almond butter
1 tablespoon chia seeds
1 teaspoon cacao nibs, plus 1 teaspoon for topping if desired
Handful of spinach
1 to 2 cups unsweetened almond milk

Place all the ingredients in a high-speed blender and blend to your desired consistency. Top with extra cacao nibs if desired.

BREAKFAST: Not in the mood for chocolate this morning? Try a vanilla recipe from the Girl on the Go plan, such as Cinnamon Coconut (page 144), Super Green Machine (page 174), or Happy Gut (page 181).

LUNCH: One of the simplest hacks to incorporate on a weekly basis is to make one or two extra servings of a given dinner and then enjoy the leftovers for lunch the next day. Today, let's put any leftover carnitas over a mixed green salad or in lettuce cups. If you don't have any, build a Fab Four salad with your choice of protein.

DINNER: Steamed Fish and Vegetables (the Girl on the Go plan, page 169). Flip back to the fiber and greens chart that starts on pages 93–101 and pick a new vegetable for tonight's dinner, one you haven't had in a while or tried before.

GIVE YOUR FEET SOME LOVE: An easy form of self-care is to use a spiky foot massage ball to stimulate the nerve endings on the bottoms of your feet. You can find a variety of options online for under ten dollars; they're about the size of a tennis ball or baseball (either of which can be used if you don't want to purchase one, though I personally like the stimulation provided by the spikes). This can relieve tension and help you relax. Place the ball under the sole of your foot. Pressing down, roll it over the heel, arch, and ball of your foot, one foot at a time for five minutes per foot. You can do this while sitting down or, for more pressure, standing up (just make sure you're near a wall or something to hold on to for balance). Another simple (and spiky) self-care option is to lie back on an acupressure mat; see the Girl on the Go plan, page 173.

Day 4—Weekday

BREAKFAST

TRIPLE CHOCOLATE CRUNCH FAB FOUR SMOOTHIE

If you love chocolate, you'll love this new Fab Four Smoothie recipe: intense chocolate flavor, plus the lively crunch contributed by the cacao nibs.

Chocolate protein powder containing 20 to 30 grams protein
¼ avocado
2 tablespoons chia seeds
1 cup frozen spinach (or two large handfuls of fresh spinach)
1 tablespoon cacao nibs
1 teaspoon raw cacao powder
1 to 2 cups unsweetened almond or coconut milk

Place all the ingredients in a high-speed blender and blend to your desired consistency. Or, if preferred, blend in 2 teaspoons of the cacao nibs and use the remainder as a topping.

TIP: To add a functional boost, add ½ teaspoon of He Shou Wu, a plant extract from the buckwheat family known to have immunity and stress-reducing benefits.

LUNCH

BLT WRAPS

Bulk up your next BLT and balance your hunger hormones with egg and avocado. Half an avocado adds 5 grams of fiber and two pasture-raised eggs add 12 grams of protein. A simple swap that can add more detoxifying and anti-inflammatory phytochemicals is to use baby plum tomatoes instead of regular beefsteak tomatoes. Usually I like my BLT without bread, but if I have a gluten-free option in the refrigerator or freezer, I might toast up a piece. Two options I like are the unBun from Keto Buns (high in fiber and only 3 or 5 net carbohydrates, depending on the type of bun) and Bread SRSLY (great-tasting sourdough made in the traditional way with a starter that helps break down the grains for easier digestion).

Makes 4 lettuce-wrapped BLTs

4 organic, pasture-raised bacon slices
8 romaine leaves
¼ cup baby plum tomatoes
½ avocado, peeled, pitted, and sliced
2 hard-boiled eggs, sliced (see page 168)
2 tablespoons mayonnaise (I like Primal Kitchen)

1. Cook the bacon to your desired crispness.
2. Layer 2 romaine leaves with bacon, tomato, avocado, egg, and mayonnaise. Fold or wrap the romaine and enjoy.

DINNER

CHICKEN PICCATA AND ASPARAGUS

Chicken piccata might already be a family favorite, but you can easily elevate the dish by using gluten-free flour supplemented with a bit of unmodified potato starch. As discussed in chapter 3 (see page 91), unmodified potato starch is a source of resistant starch, which feeds healthy gut bacteria. One caveat: because it's so potent, it may cause bloating and discomfort if you eat too much. I would keep to ¼ to ½ teaspoon per person, as in this dish. Also, if you have a nightshade allergy and must avoid potato, just swap in additional coconut flour for the potato starch.

Makes 4 servings

4 chicken breasts, butterflied and pounded thin
Pink Himalayan salt and freshly ground black pepper
2 teaspoons unmodified potato starch
2 tablespoons coconut flour
3 tablespoons ghee
1 cup low-sodium chicken stock
1 tablespoon extra virgin olive oil
$^1/_3$ cup freshly squeezed lemon juice
Handful of capers, rinsed
12 asparagus stalks, trimmed
2 garlic cloves, minced
1 tablespoon unsalted butter (optional)
Lemon zest, for garnish

1. Season the chicken with salt and pepper. In a small bowl, combine the starch with the flour. Dust all sides of the chicken breasts with a very light layer of the mixture.
2. In a large skillet over medium-high heat, melt the ghee. Pan-fry the chicken for 3 to 4 minutes per side, then transfer it to a plate.
3. Remove the skillet from the heat and add the stock, olive oil, lemon juice, and

capers. Whisk to deglaze the brown bits from the bottom of the skillet, return the chicken to the skillet, and simmer on medium heat for 5 minutes. Transfer the chicken to a clean plate (it wasn't fully cooked earlier) or to serving plates.

4. Add the asparagus and garlic to the skillet and cook for about 5 minutes, until tender, turning often. Transfer the asparagus to a bowl or to the serving plates, alongside the chicken.

5. Add the butter to the skillet and whisk to deglaze the pan and thicken a little if desired. Serve the butter sauce poured over the chicken and asparagus. Garnish with lemon zest.

ADULT COLORING: Coloring might be the simplest form of art therapy. It's a creative way to chill out and can help you unwind, relieving some of that stress or anxiety you might be feeling. Buy an adult coloring book and give it a try tonight. Or if you have kids, fill in a page or two of one of their coloring books. (Maybe leave them a loving or silly note, too, as a little surprise for later.)

Day 5—Weekday

MORNING MOVEMENT: Seize the morning and get your third at-home workout of the week done and dusted before breakfast.

BREAKFAST

GREEN GODDESS FAB FOUR SMOOTHIE

Continue the positive momentum by going a little extra green with this smoothie. That added serving of greens powder boosts the vitamins and minerals even more.

Vanilla collagen protein powder containing 20 to 30 grams protein
¼ avocado

(continued)

2 tablespoons chia seeds
1 cup frozen spinach (or 2 large handfuls of fresh spinach)
1 to 2 cups unsweetened almond or coconut milk
1 tablespoon greens powder (I like NOW Foods Green Phytofoods)
Juice of ½ lemon

Place all the ingredients in a high-speed blender and blend to your desired consistency.

LUNCH

TUNA PATTIES

These quick and easy tuna patties are warm and satisfying. Pair them with a small mixed green salad or crudités for a complete healthful lunch.

Makes 1 serving

TUNA PATTIES
1 (5-ounce) can or 2 (3-ounce) pouches light tuna, drained (I use Safe Catch or Wild Planet)
1 teaspoon mayonnaise (I like Primal Kitchen)
1 teaspoon Dijon mustard
1 teaspoon freshly squeezed lemon juice
1 teaspoon lemon zest
1 teaspoon minced chives
1 teaspoon chopped fresh parsley
Pink Himalayan salt and freshly ground black pepper
1 egg, lightly whisked
1 tablespoon coconut flour, or ¼ teaspoon unmodified potato starch
2 tablespoons avocado oil

TARTAR SAUCE
1 teaspoon mayonnaise (I like Primal Kitchen)
½ teaspoon capers
½ teaspoon dill relish

1. In a medium bowl, use a fork to mix the tuna, mayonnaise, mustard, lemon juice, lemon zest, chives, parsley, and salt and pepper to taste. Add the egg and coconut flour and mix to incorporate. Mold the mixture into 3 or 4 equal-size patties.

2. In a large frying pan over medium heat, heat the avocado oil.

3. Meanwhile, to make the tartar sauce, mix the tartar sauce ingredients in a small bowl.

4. When the frying pan is good and hot, fry the tuna patties for 2 to 3 minutes per side, until crispy. Enjoy with the tartar sauce.

DINNER: One of the core concepts of my nutritional philosophy is to elevate your everyday food choices. Healthy swaps, whole foods, and clean, nutrient-dense ingredients are all great ways to do this. Sometimes it's about elevating the things *around* your main entrée. At the end of a long week, not everyone in your family (including yourself) may want a piece of wild salmon; something more comforting might be calling your name.

DINNER

OVEN-BAKED RIBS

My husband loves barbecue, especially ribs. The ribs themselves can easily be prepared to suit the Fab Four. And luckily, there are also ways to elevate some of the classic side dishes—see the recipes that follow. That way he's happy and I'm happy. And for the record, you can source cleaner ribs, too—from companies like US Wellness Meats, ButcherBox, or Thrive Market.

Makes 2 servings

1 tablespoon garlic powder
1 tablespoon onion powder
1 tablespoon chili powder
1 tablespoon smoked paprika
1 teaspoon cayenne pepper, or to taste
2 teaspoons pink Himalayan salt
1 rack (about 1½ pounds) baby back ribs
3 to 4 tablespoons barbecue sauce (see Tip)

1. Preheat the oven to 275°F and line a baking sheet with parchment paper. In a small bowl, mix all the dry spices and seasonings.
2. Dry off the ribs and peel off the membrane. Rub both sides of the ribs with the dry mixture. Place the ribs on the prepared pan and bake for 3 hours.
3. Glaze the ribs with the barbecue sauce and bake for 5 minutes longer, or use the barbecue sauce for dipping. (Optional: to add a light char, broil for 5 minutes.)

TIP: Ideally, you want to look for a barbecue sauce that contains less than 4 grams of sugar per serving. Primal Kitchen has two awesome flavors that fit the bill, Classic and Golden BBQ Sauces.

DINNER

FERMENTED COLESLAW

Coleslaw is a barbecue staple. My recipe elevates it by using cleaner ingredients and also by adding caraway kraut. Sauerkraut is fermented cabbage—it adds a nice tang and feeds your healthy gut bacteria in the process—and caraway seed is rich in vitamins and minerals.

Makes 2 servings

¼ cup mayonnaise (I like Primal Kitchen)
3 tablespoons extra virgin olive oil
1 tablespoon apple cider vinegar
1 tablespoon freshly squeezed lemon juice
½ teaspoon pink Himalayan salt
2 cups shredded green cabbage
1 cup shredded red cabbage
½ cup shredded carrot
¼ cup Farmhouse Culture caraway kraut (or other sauerkraut along with a pinch of
   caraway seeds)

In a large bowl, whisk the mayonnaise, oil, vinegar, lemon juice, and salt. Add the cabbage, carrot, and kraut and mix well. Refrigerate for at least 1 hour and serve cold.

TIP: One thing that can contribute to watery coleslaw is excess moisture from the cabbage. You can salt the cabbage first to help pull out the moisture. Place the shredded cabbage in a bowl, sprinkle with 1 to 2 tablespoons of salt, and toss to coat. Transfer to a salad spinner and refrigerate for 1 to 2 hours, to allow the cabbage to soften. Thoroughly rinse the cabbage under cold water (to remove the salt) and spin to dry.

DINNER

CAULIFLOWER POTATO SALAD

Adding cauliflower is a great way to elevate your potato salad. Cauliflower is a great source of sulforaphane, a phytochemical that activates detoxification, reduces inflammation, and supports cell defense.

Makes 6 servings

1 pound small white potatoes
2 tablespoons plus 2 teaspoons pink Himalayan salt
3 cups cauliflower florets
1 cup mayonnaise (I like Primal Kitchen)
1 tablespoon extra virgin olive oil
2 tablespoons Dijon mustard
2 tablespoons whole-grain mustard
½ cup chopped fresh dill
2 teaspoons freshly ground black pepper
½ cup chopped celery
½ cup chopped red onion

1. Place the potatoes and the 2 tablespoons of salt in a large pot of filtered water. Bring the water to a boil over high heat, lower to a simmer, and cook for 10 minutes, or until fork tender. Using a slotted spoon, transfer the potatoes to a colander (keep the water simmering in the pot) and cover them with a clean, dry kitchen towel to steam for 15 minutes.

2. Place the cauliflower in the pot and simmer for 2 to 4 minutes, or until crisp-tender. Drain the cauliflower and rinse with cold water to stop the cooking. Set aside.

3. In a small bowl, whisk the mayonnaise, oil, mustards, dill, 1 teaspoon of the salt, and 1 teaspoon of the pepper.

4. When the potatoes are cool enough to handle, cut them into quarters. Place the potatoes and cauliflower in a large bowl and add the dressing, celery, red onion, and remaining 1 teaspoon each salt and pepper. Toss to coat.

5. Refrigerate for 1 to 2 hours to cool the potatoes and amp up the flavor. To elevate the nutrition even further, refrigerate overnight (see Cooling Potatoes [and Rice]).

FRIDAY NIGHT LIGHTS: If you have kids in high school, you might find yourself at a game or match on Friday night. To avoid the temptation to choose candy, popcorn, or nachos at the concession stand, use one of these tools from the Girl on the Go plan:

- Fuel up before you go (page 136).
- Take a Fab Four Snack Pack or body-loving protein bar (page 137).
- Whip up a Fab Four Roadie (page 150).
- Use a fat-based creamer for a coffee or tea (page 76).

These tools can help for any other event or outing where concession food might tempt you, such as movies, concerts, fairs, weekend tournaments, or professional sports games.

COOLING POTATOES (AND RICE)

The two-step process of cooking and then cooling potatoes creates resistant starch. The same applies to rice. Resistant starches (also known as prebiotics) are starches that cannot be absorbed into the bloodstream. They're essentially undigestible carbohydrates, and healthy gut bacteria love to feed on them. In turn, this produces short-chain fatty acids that support the gut microbiome and lead to various health benefits. For example, it produces butyrate, an anti-inflammatory short-chain fatty acid that increases the health of your intestinal cells and helps to prevent barrier permeability (known as "leaky gut"). Making potatoes or rice the day before and letting them cool overnight in the refrigerator can result in up to three times (for potatoes) or two and a half times (for rice) the amount of resistant starch. Consuming cooked and cooled potatoes and rice can also lower your blood sugar response as compared with eating potatoes that haven't been cooled.

Day 6—Weekend Day

BREAKFAST

LOW-SUGAR AÇAI BOWL

Many açai bowls are loaded with added sugar, sometimes up to 60 grams or more. My version uses unsweetened açai or freeze-dried açai powder, both of which contain only the minimal sugar from the fruit itself. Look in the frozen foods section at the grocery store for single-serving unsweetened açai packets or buy the freeze-dried powder online (NOW Foods has a great option).

Makes 1 serving

Vanilla collagen protein powder containing 20 to 30 grams protein
2 tablespoons chia seeds
1 cup full-fat coconut milk
1 packet frozen açai, or 1 tablespoon açai powder
¼ cup frozen blueberries
¼ cup frozen or uncooked cauliflower rice (optional for a thicker base; see page 315)
Optional topping: 1 tablespoon hemp hearts or Coconutty Cereal (page 244)

Place all the ingredients except the toppings in a high-speed blender and blend to your desired consistency. Serve in a bowl, topped if desired.

REMINDER: If you're looking for other inspiration this morning (or any other time, for that matter), you can always browse through the rest of this plan or find something in the Girl on the Go or Plant-Based Devotee plans. They're full of Fab Four Smoothies and other breakfast recipes that you'll love, such as Fab Four Chia Seed Pudding (page 184), Cinnamon Protein Pancakes (page 191), and Warm Triple Seed Faux-meal (page 340). Feel free to mix and match as you see fit. They're all rooted in the Fab Four, and one plan might work better for you on a given day.

LUNCH

GREEN GODDESS SALAD

Whip up a simple, clean Green Goddess salad.

Makes 1 serving

DRESSING

½ cup extra virgin olive oil

2 tablespoons freshly squeezed lemon juice

1 tablespoon apple cider vinegar (optional for added tang)

2 tablespoons minced chives

2 tablespoons roughly chopped green onion

¼ cup chopped cilantro

¼ cup chopped fresh flat-leaf parsley

¼ teaspoon mustard seed powder

SALAD

4 cups mixed greens

1 cup nonstarchy vegetables (such as cucumber, broccoli, or asparagus), sliced

½ avocado, diced

¼ cup mâche or celery leaves (optional for added phytochemicals)

3 ounces protein of your choice (optional)

1 teaspoon chopped tarragon (optional)

1. Combine all the dressing ingredients in a small bowl and whisk to mix.

2. Plate the mixed greens and sliced vegetables, then top with the avocado. If you like, add the the mâche or celery leaves and the protein. Drizzle with 2 tablespoons of the dressing. Top with the tarragon if desired.

3. The extra dressing will keep in a covered jar in the refrigerator for about a week.

WEEKEND WARRIOR: For many of my clients who are moms, working out during the week can be a real challenge. If you have a full-time job, there might never be an hour to spare. Even if you don't have a traditional nine-to-five, your free time can vanish before your eyes. Then, on the weekend, when there's actually time to get to and from the gym or a class, a lot of my clients say they feel guilty or selfish about not spending every moment they can with their kids. It's something I've experienced myself as a new mom. But I also know how I feel when I give my body that forty-five, sixty, or ninety minutes of attention: refreshed, energized, and in a calmer place where I can handle all the curveballs that may be coming my way. If you have a spouse or partner who has the same busy schedule and also wants to work out, one idea is to trade off weekends. You take the first and third Saturday, and your spouse or partner gets the second and fourth. Put it on the family calendar so everyone knows. On your off weeks, try to wake up thirty minutes early on Saturday or Sunday and bank a quick at-home workout from an app. Another idea is to swap your usual dinner and a movie date night for a workout date night. If the babysitter is already coming, book a class together and grab a healthy meal afterward.

DINNER

COCONUT TZATZIKI CHICKEN SKEWERS WITH COCONUT YOGURT TZATZIKI AND CUCUMBER SALAD

Go Greek with dairy-free coconut tzatziki. The marinade can be used for up to 20 ounces of chicken, so if you want to have leftovers for lunch tomorrow, just double the chicken.

Makes 2 servings

1 cup coconut milk
1 tablespoon freshly squeezed lemon juice
1 teaspoon pink Himalayan salt

½ teaspoon freshly ground black pepper

½ teaspoon ground turmeric

½ teaspoon cayenne

½ teaspoon ground ginger

½ teaspoon chile flakes

8 to 10 ounces chicken breast, cut into 2-inch cubes (double the amount for leftovers)

Coconut Yogurt Tzatziki for dipping (recipe follows)

Cucumber Salad (recipe follows)

1. In a medium bowl, whisk the coconut milk, lemon juice, salt, pepper, and spices. Add the chicken and stir to coat. Refrigerate for 2 to 4 hours.

2. When you're ready to cook, prepare your grill.

3. Skewer the chicken cubes and grill them for 10 to 15 minutes, rotating them regularly to cook all sides.

4. Serve the chicken with the tzatziki for dipping (or drizzle it on top) and with cucumber salad alongside.

COCONUT YOGURT TZATZIKI

½ large cucumber, grated

1 cup coconut yogurt (see Tip)

¼ cup chopped fresh dill

1 tablespoon freshly squeezed lemon juice

1 tablespoon extra virgin olive oil

Pink Himalayan salt and freshly ground black pepper

Place the cucumber in a cheesecloth or thin towel and gently squeeze to remove some of the water. In a small bowl, stir all the ingredients together.

TIP: Many coconut yogurts have high amounts of added sugar, so be mindful and read the nutrition facts carefully. I usually buy plain coconut yogurt with the fewest ingredients. A few brands I like are COYO, New Earth Superfoods, CocoYo,

(continued)

Anita's, and The Coconut Cult. You can also make your own homemade coconut yogurt (see page 243). In addition to making this tzatziki, you can flavor coconut yogurt with produce such as macerated raspberries for a bridge snack.

DARK CHOCOLATE

I prefer chocolate that is made with limited ingredients and that uses monk fruit, stevia, or erythritol as its sweetener instead of sugar. Another thing to look for is how the bar was processed, which should be listed on the packaging or wrapper. A few brands that meet those standards are The Good Chocolate, Hu, and ChocZero. Try to avoid chocolate processed with alkali (alkalized chocolate or Dutch processing). Alkalization processing decreases polyphenols and flavanols, the antioxidants that make dark chocolate good for you!

CUCUMBER SALAD

1 tablespoon avocado oil
1 tablespoon white wine vinegar
Pinch of pink Himalayan salt and freshly ground black pepper
½ large cucumber, thinly sliced
¼ cup thinly sliced red onion
2 tablespoons chopped fresh dill

In a medium bowl, whisk the avocado oil, vinegar, salt, and pepper. Add the cucumber, onion, and dill. Toss to coat. You can prepare and chill the salad for up to 2 hours before serving.

DESSERT: If you want something decadent or "Not So Fab" Four tonight, tell yourself it's a choice, not a cheat. Cheat meals or days imply that you're breaking some sort of rule or regimen. Food freedom and body love mean accepting your decisions and knowing that you can always regain your balance at the next meal with the Fab Four. You can always pop a cube of Freezer Fudge (page 214), break off a piece of dark chocolate (see the box), or whip up some Dark Chocolate Avocado Mousse (page 349).

Day 7—Weekend Day

BREAKFAST

EGGS BENEDICT

One of my favorite brunch foods is eggs Benedict. With a few healthy swaps, you can enjoy a cleaner version of the same tried-and-true recipe: grass-fed butter is rich in CLA; pasture-raised eggs are higher in omega-3s; a base of a high-fiber, gluten-free English muffin or bread will offer lower net carbohydrates; a sugar-free, pasture-raised Canadian bacon won't spike your blood sugar; and adding spinach is an easy way to incorporate fibrous greens.

Makes 4 servings

HOLLANDAISE
¾ cup (1½ sticks) unsalted butter (I like Kerrygold)
3 large pasture-raised egg yolks
1½ teaspoons freshly squeezed lemon juice
¼ teaspoon cayenne or hot paprika (optional)
Kosher salt and freshly ground black pepper

OPEN-FACED SANDWICH
8 large pasture-raised eggs
1 tablespoon distilled white vinegar
8 slices sugar-free Canadian bacon (I like US Wellness Meats)
4 handfuls of fresh spinach
4 English muffins (I like Mikey's—or use Barely Bread rolls)
¼ cup minced chives
1 tablespoon chopped fresh dill
1 tablespoon chopped fresh tarragon
1 tablespoon chopped fresh parsley
Pink Himalayan salt and freshly ground black pepper

(continued)

DECLUTTERING

Before our son, Sebastian, arrived, I completed a massive purge and decluttering of our home to make room for all things baby. It felt incredible. I was in nesting mode, and afterward I felt much calmer and more comfortable in our space. When you let go, you give yourself room to grow. It also can help you destress. (A 2012 study out of UCLA found that mothers who described their house as messy had higher cortisol levels.) You might not have time for a full spring cleaning, but if you have a spare hour, try tackling something today. One recommendation: your pantry, refrigerator, or maybe the entire kitchen. What better way to kick-start healthier decisions than by clearing out old food so you have room for new? Or take a fresh look at a dresser, closet, or room that's been calling your name. Bonus points (and good karma) for donating to Goodwill or a local charity, or giving any unexpired food to a food bank.

1. To make the Hollandaise, in a small saucepan over medium heat, melt and cook the butter until it's foamy but not yet beginning to brown, 3 to 4 minutes.

2. Place the egg yolks and 2 teaspoons filtered water in a blender. Start blending and, working very slowly, stream in the hot butter until it's incorporated. Blend in the lemon juice, cayenne, and a pinch each of salt and pepper. Transfer the Hollandaise to a small bowl and place plastic wrap directly on the surface so it doesn't form a skin. Set aside at room temperature.

3. To make the open-faced sandwich, first poach the eggs: fill a saucepan with a couple inches of filtered water. Add the vinegar and heat the pan over medium heat until bubbles appear on the bottom of the pan (you want to barely reach a simmer). Crack an egg into a small bowl, tip the bowl edge close to the surface of the water, and slowly slip the egg into the water. Use a slotted wooden spoon to gently push the egg white toward the yolk. Check the egg after 4 minutes, lifting it out of the water to feel the white for firmness. Cook to your desired consistency, then use the slotted spoon to remove the eggs from the water and transfer to a paper towel-lined plate.

4. In a frying pan over medium-high heat, cook the Canadian bacon until golden brown, about 3 minutes per side. Place the bacon on a paper towel-lined plate. Add the spinach to the pan and cook until it's lightly wilted, 1 to 2 minutes. Set aside.

5. To assemble the dish, split and toast the English muffins. Layer each half with 1 slice Canadian bacon, half a handful of spinach, 1 poached egg, and 1 tablespoon Hollandaise. Sprinkle each with a pinch of herbs and salt and pepper.

LUNCH: Try my Ribboned Rainbow Salad over Sprouted Sunflower Seed Hummus (see the Plant-Based Devotee plan, page 288). Optional: add 3 ounces of leftover skewered chicken from Day 6 to your wrap.

DINNER

ITALIAN MEATBALL SOUP WITH ZOODLES

Sunday night is another time when a warm, comforting meal sounds particularly good. This meatball soup is a savory and healthy way to wrap up the weekend. Zoodles are a healthy swap for pasta noodles and add fiber and greens to your dinner.

Makes 4 servings

MEATBALLS

1 pound ground turkey breast
¼ cup ground flax meal
¼ cup finely chopped fresh parsley
1 egg
¼ cup minced yellow onion
1 garlic clove, minced
¼ teaspoon pink Himalayan salt

SOUP

2 teaspoons extra virgin olive oil
½ cup chopped yellow onion
1 cup ¼-inch-diced peeled carrots
½ cup ¼-inch-diced celery
2 garlic cloves, minced
8 cups chicken bone broth or reduced-sodium chicken broth
2 (14.5-ounce) cans petite diced tomatoes
1 rosemary sprig

(continued)

2 bay leaves
1 tablespoon minced fresh basil
1 tablespoon chopped fresh parsley
2 zucchinis, zoodled
2 summer squash, zoodled
Pink Himalayan salt and freshly ground black pepper

1. Preheat the oven to 400°F.
2. To make the meatballs, place all the ingredients in a large bowl. Gently hand mix just until they are combined—don't overmix. Form 1-inch meatballs and place them on a baking sheet. Bake for 12 minutes, until cooked through.
3. To prepare the soup, in a Dutch oven over medium-high heat, heat the olive oil. Add the onion, carrots, celery, and garlic and sauté until tender and fragrant, 4 to 6 minutes. Add the broth, tomatoes, rosemary, bay leaves, basil, and parsley. Cover, bring to a simmer over medium-high, turn the heat to low, and simmer for 30 minutes.
4. Remove the bay leaves and rosemary. Add the meatballs and zoodles, cover and simmer for 5 minutes, until the meatballs and zoodles are heated through. Season with salt and pepper to taste and serve.

PICTURE IT: Life is always more inspired with visualization. Building a mood or vision board can help motivate and encourage. Even the act itself can be cathartic. If you have kids, it can be a fun activity for the whole family, so everyone can support each other's hopes and dreams. Fill your board with pictures, words, people, places, memories, and anything else that speaks to you. It could be a goal you want to achieve, a passion you want to reawaken, or just a creative way to break out of a funk. Look at your board every day and visualize what it holds coming to life.

Day 8—Weekday

BREAKFAST

TURMERIC ALMOND BLISS FAB FOUR SMOOTHIE

This week we're going to try two Fab Four Smoothie recipes with turmeric. Turmeric is an anti-inflammatory herb with a variety of health benefits, including supporting liver function and skin health. Let's start with Turmeric Almond Bliss.

Vanilla coconut collagen protein powder containing 20 to 30 grams protein
1 tablespoon almond butter
1 tablespoon flaxseeds
Handful of spinach
1 tablespoon ground turmeric or turmeric blend (I like GoldynGlow's Energy
   Blend with Maca)
¼ cup organic raspberries (optional)
1 to 2 cups unsweetened almond milk

Place all the ingredients in a high-speed blender and blend to your desired consistency.

MONDAY MOVEMENT: If last week's at-home workout schedule suited you, feel free to run it back and do it again. If it wasn't your jam, mix it up this week. Here are a few ideas for how:

- **DON'T GO SOLO:** Some of us need a friend, a trainer, or the communal energy of a class to get motivated and moving. Set up gym time with a friend, book a session with a personal trainer, or sign up for a class or group boot camp. It can help you stay accountable and prevent you from skipping days.
- **SCHEDULE IT:** It sounds simple, but blocking out a specific day and time can improve your consistency. Calendar your gym time, book your personal training session, or sign up for class in advance. Be realistic and adjust if necessary.

CONSIDER TEACHER TRAINING

If you love yoga, Pilates, Spin, health coaching, or another type of wellness practice, one thing to consider is to sign up for teacher or coach training. It could be just what you need to step outside your comfort zone. It might even be your secret calling. Leading and inspiring others while doing something you love could reignite the passion in your life, and helping others reach their goals could reinvigorate your approach to health and fitness. The more inspired you are the more you inspire others. The world needs your help to effect change. It can also be a way to get yourself out there and develop more self-confidence speaking in front of a group. Even if you don't end up teaching or coaching, going through training will help you improve your practice and form, and you'll log a healthy number of hours.

If you find yourself snoozing through your 6 A.M. Spin class or having to cancel on your workouts, pick a new day or time.

- **COMMIT FINANCIALLY:** If you pay upfront for a gym membership, class series, or trainer package, or even buy a piece of home workout equipment, you'll give yourself a financial incentive to use it. Go through your household budget and see if there's room to make it happen.
- **FIND A CHALLENGE:** Instagram, Facebook, and fitness apps are full of workout challenges that you can join for free. Do a little research and find one that sounds motivating to you. Or form your own challenge with a group of friends. Even if you're competing, be sure to root for each other!

LUNCH: If you have leftover Italian Meatball Soup with Zoodles from dinner last night, warm up a bowl. If you're not in the mood, build a Fab Four salad at home or from the salad bar at your grocery store. See page 150 for some tips.

DINNER: If you enjoyed Meatless Monday last week, try another clean take on a comforting Italian dish. One choice is my Stacked Eggplant Parmesan (see the Plant-Based Devotee plan, page 308). If cooking just isn't in the cards today, choose a healthy takeout option from your self-made body-loving menu (see the Girl on the Go plan, page 185). Making your own takeout menu is an easy way to guide yourself (and your family) to healthier decisions on a weekly basis. All you have to do is take a few minutes and make a list of the clean, healthy dishes available from your favorite restaurants. Then, the next time you're ordering takeout, use it to steer yourself in a healthy direction.

JOURNALING: If (like me) you've thought about starting a journal a thousand times but never actually put pen to paper, make a commitment to yourself to try this week. Whether it's first thing in the morning, midday when you can find ten minutes of peace and quiet, or in the evening after your kids go to bed, make journaling a daily ritual this week. See the Plant-Based Devotee plan, page 343.

Day 9—Weekday

BREAKFAST

SOUTHWEST SCRAMBLE

Mix up your routine. Enjoy eggs for breakfast and a smoothie for lunch today. A Southwest-style scramble is a simple staple. If you choose to use salsa or hot sauce on your scramble, be sure to choose options with no sugar added.

Makes 2 servings

6 pasture-raised organic eggs
1 tablespoon ghee
¼ cup chopped green bell pepper
2 tablespoons minced yellow onion
2 tablespoons cilantro or other microgreens (see Tip; or use regular cilantro)
3 baby heirloom tomatoes, thinly sliced
Salsa, guacamole, diced avocado, or hot sauce (optional)

1. Whisk the eggs in a bowl.
2. In a frying pan over medium-high heat, melt the ghee. Add the bell pepper and onion and sauté until the onion is translucent, 3 minutes. Pour in the eggs and scramble them gently, stirring occasionally with a spatula until cooked through.

(continued)

3. Plate the scramble with cilantro microgreens and tomatoes. Serve with salsa, guacamole, chopped avocado, or hot sauce if desired.

TIP: Microgreens are small, week-old plants that can serve up higher nutrient density than their full-grown counterparts. Cilantro microgreens are high in beta-carotene and lutein, antioxidants that support skin health. Any microgreen from your grocery or farmers' market will work in this recipe; just remember that they have a milder taste than the full-grown plant.

LUNCH

DETOX WINTER MINT FAB FOUR SMOOTHIE

Need a breather from cooking or meal prep? Keep it simple with a Fab Four Smoothie for lunch. One new recipe I'm really loving year-round is Detox Winter Mint. The triple dose of greens (spinach or leafy greens, mint, and greens powder) gives it a super boost of functional antioxidants.

Vanilla protein powder containing 20 to 30 grams protein
1 tablespoon MCT oil
2 tablespoons acacia fiber (I use NOW Foods)
Handful of spinach or dark "super" leafy greens (I like the OrganicGirl brand)
Handful of fresh mint
1 tablespoon greens powder (I like NOW Foods Green Phytofoods)
1 to 2 cups unsweetened almond milk

Place all the ingredients in a high-speed blender and blend to your desired consistency.

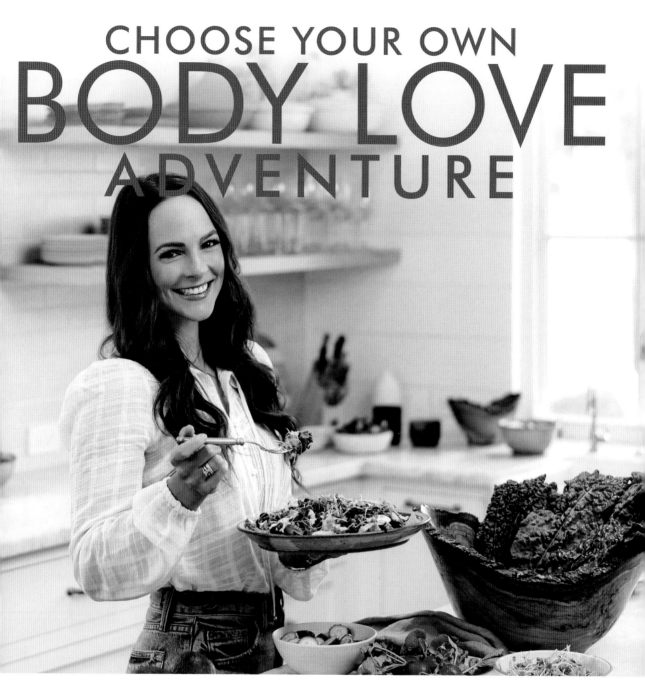

CHOOSE YOUR OWN
BODY LOVE
ADVENTURE

The Fab Four—my system of making sure you get enough protein, fat, fiber, and greens—is a light structure lifestyle that positively reinforces healthy eating habits every day no matter what life throws at you. You may be a Girl on the Go today, and a Domestic Goddess when life slows down, or maybe you're wondering how to be a Plant-Based Devotee or have an event for which you want to be Red-Carpet Ready.

She might jet-set for work, have a packed social life, or be a working mama who needs healthy, quick meals for herself and her family. Either way, the Girl on the Go prioritizes her health but doesn't want to spend hours doing it. This plan offers simple wellness tips plus quick meals made in 30 minutes or less to keep your routine efficient.

Cookies and Cream Fab Four Smoothie (page 163)

No time? Blend your smoothie the night before and store it in a stainless-steel water bottle in your fridge. The fiber in your smoothie will thicken overnight, so add a splash of nut milk in the morning to thin it, shake, and go.

Flaky Tuna and Toasted Walnut Salad

(page 181)

Canned salmon, mackerel, tuna, sardines, and anchovies are simple protein staples that will encourage you to make semi-homemade meals instead of ordering takeout. Here's a quick checklist to help you get the good stuff:

- Is it water-packed? (This will help you avoid oxidized oils.)
- Is it wild and sustainably caught?
- If you're buying tuna, is it chunk light or skipjack? (These varieties are the lowest in mercury.)
- Is it in a pouch or BPA-free can to avoid endocrine-disrupting chemicals (EDCs)?

Coconut Cauliflower Rice with Sweet Coconut Chicken and Broccoli

(page 182)

A new category to look for when purchasing chicken is "heritage." According to the Livestock Conservancy, a heritage chicken is hatched from a heritage egg sired by a breed that meets the American Poultry Association Standard of Perfection, established prior to the mid-twentieth century. Standard chickens are slow-growing, and naturally mated, and have a long, productive outdoor life. To be labeled *heritage*, the chicken must include the variety and breed name on the label. Heritage chickens and their eggs contain higher levels of omega-3 and vitamins A and E.

GO

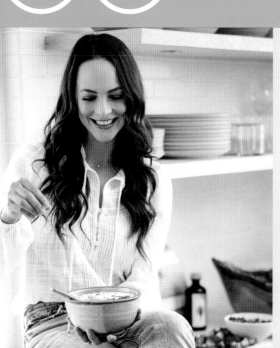

Every little bit counts!

The research shows that short 10-minute bursts of intense exercise before breakfast, lunch, and dinner have greater impact on blood sugar levels than one longer, 30-minute workout before dinner. This style of exercising, coined "Exercise Snacking," is perfect for the Girl on the Go. Take the stairs to the office in the morning, walk to pick up lunch, and do a quick strength circuit on your living room floor when you get home.

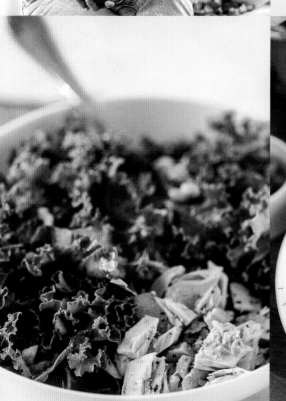

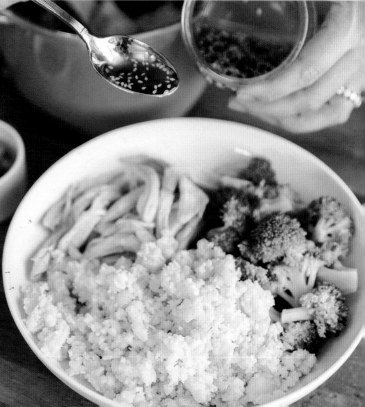

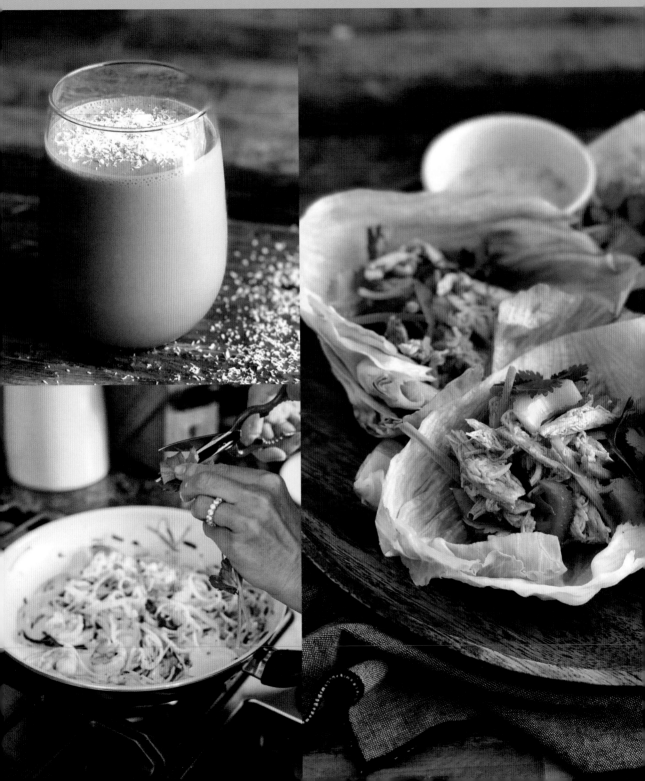

Cinnamon Coconut
Fab Four Smoothie

(page 144)

Spices can be potent superfoods—as long as they haven't gone bad in your cabinet. Keep a permanent marker in your cabinet set your own expiration date one year from the date of purchase. A 2016 review of eleven cinnamon studies confirmed that cinnamon supports glucose control by decreasing fasting blood glucose levels, so there's plenty of incentive to eat it all before it expires!

Take a Breath

Breathwork can decrease anxiety, increase focus, reduce cravings, and promote digestion. If you are looking for a reminder to keep reaping these benefits, download the breathwork app State, which was created by my friends Brian Mackenzie, a human optimization coach, and Dr. Andrew Huberman, a professor of neuroscience at Stanford. Their app is a beautifully simple way to drastically change your biological state with breathing exercises.

Shrimp Scampi
and Zoodles

(page 165)

The most nutrient-dense proteins can help the Girl on the Go (or any client, for that matter) prevent deficiencies. My favorites include liver, red meat, and shellfish because they offer up key micronutrients like copper, zinc, magnesium, and vitamins A, D, B_{12}, and B_6. Bonus: shrimp and ground beef are both quick proteins to sauté.

Buffalo Chicken
Lettuce Cups (page 254)

Beware of hidden sugar! Clean condiments support the Girl on the Go in making dishes delicious with minimal steps. Three often-sugar-filled condiments to replace today are barbecue sauce, ketchup, and soy sauce. Primal Kitchen BBQ sauce and ketchup and Thrive Market Coconut Amino Sauce are good options.

DOMESTIC

The Domestic Goddess is a woman—urban or suburban—whose home is her sanctuary and whose kitchen is her happy place. She also knows it's important to take the time needed to care for herself. So she kicks her wellness routine into high gear with thoughtful and wholesome nutrition, all while making fitness fun and self-care a sensational staple.

Almond Bliss Fab Four Smoothie

(page 237)

Collagen protein, used in this recipe, is a great way to round out your amino acid profile, because it provides the nonessential amino acid glycine. The body needs on average 10 grams of glycine a day to synthesize new collagen internally, but research suggests we make only 3 grams daily. More important, there are claims that meat-eating diets can mean shorter life-spans due to high levels of the amino acid methionine, but that risk is eradicated when diets are high in glycine. Up your glycine intake by consuming collagen protein, gelatin, bone broth, pork rinds, eggs, or pastured chicken skin.

Southwest Scramble

(page 239)

Don't avoid eggs because of their cholesterol; if you eat lower amounts of cholesterol, your body will just produce its own and for the more than 70 percent of us who aren't hyper-responders, three eggs a day won't have an effect on total or LDL ("bad") cholesterol—and will serve up a multivitamin's worth of B vitamins.

Super Green Kale Chips

(page 273)

The best strategy for increasing the anti-inflammatory benefits of sulforaphane is by pairing your cooked cruciferous vegetables with a dehydrated or raw cruciferous vegetable to help ensure you are consuming a viable source of myrosinase. (See pages 107–108 to learn more.)

GODDESS

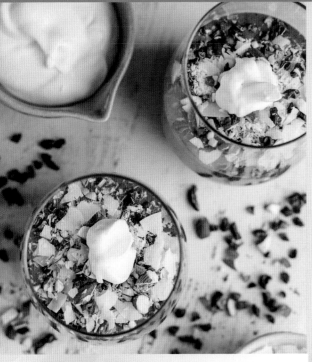

Lights On

Red-light therapy boosts mitochondrial energy production and regeneration, increases collagen production, and decreases inflammation. It's great for reducing joint pain, preparing the body for sleep, and repairing muscles post-workout. For the Domestic Goddess looking to invest in her sanctuary, Joovv offers a number of at home units red-light therapy units in a range of sizes and prices.

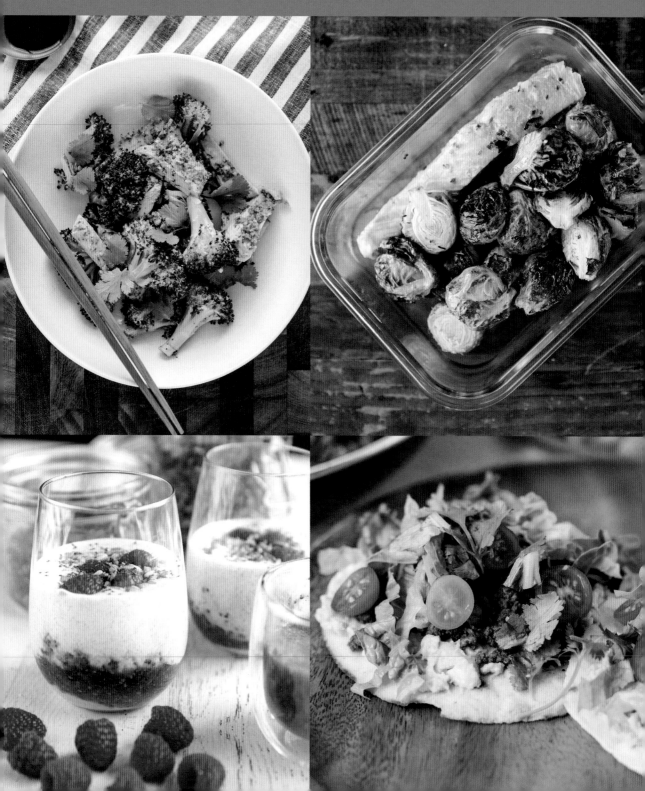

Lime Cilantro Chicken and Broccoli

(page 247)

Mix up simple sheet-pan dinners! Make any dressing a marinade by swapping in avocado oil for olive oil. Try this hack with my Lemon Tahini Dressing (page 158), Green Goddess Dressing (page 229), or dairy-free Presto Pesto (page 286). The lime-cilantro spread used in this recipe is referred to as "the sauce" in the LeVeque house and promises to give your chicken a savory nutty coating.

Sun Butter and Jelly Swirl Fab Four Smoothie

(page 261)

A blender chia jam is a fun way to layer in fiber and a punch of flavor without the sugar of traditional jams.

Garlic Salmon and Brussels Sprouts

(page 263)

This salmon reheats well, but store it in a glass container to lower your exposure to EDCs like BPA and phthalates found in plastic. As a reminder, never heat in plastic in the microwave or allow plastic drinking bottles to be left in direct sunlight or a warm location. See Endocrine-Disrupting Chemicals on page 46.

Ground Beef Tostada Salad

(page 252)

A build-your-own bar gives friends and family the ability to create the meal of their dreams without the stigma of being high maintenance. Not to mention, a build-your-own-tostada bar will encourage family members to pile on the fiber and greens. Get creative with this basic recipe by adding sliced beets, radish, cucumber, and pepper options.

MIX AND

My hope is that you feel inspired by these plans, find it easy to incorporate these tips and tricks into your lifestyle, and are motivated to love on your body with self-care, a sweaty workout, or even just a few minutes of breathwork. Don't feel like you have to be locked in to any one archetype. Get inspired by your favorite tips, then mix and match! Add animal protein to a vegetarian dish or swap in beans for meat to make it plant-based. Push yourself to try something new.

Cook once, eat many times!

A great hack for leftover beans and soups is to freeze them in 2-ounce silicon baby food molds. You can quickly defrost one or two of them for a protein bridge snack or main meal.

When in doubt, think protein!

Up the protein of your Shrimp Louie Salad (page 206) with a pasture-raised hard-boiled egg. If you are buying a salad out and the protein seems small (3 ounces or less) opt for double protein to prevent mindless snacking later.

Add zest with herbs and citrus!

Change up the flavors of the Mexican Chicken Vegetable Soup (page 178) with herbs, citrus, and toppings. Instead of cilantro, lime, jalapeño, and onion, top this soup with basil, a squeeze of lemon juice, and olives.

Shut it down!

Your computer, your phone, and your body. You can't catch up on missed sleep, and new research shows that just one night of short sleep duration can induce insulin resistance. If you want to have your cake and eat it too, go to bed!

MATCH

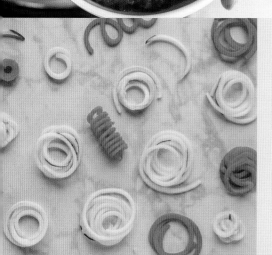

Changing the shape can change the experience!

Vegetables can be shredded, turned into noodles, cubed, or riced and mixing it up can increase intake. Take a minute to think about your favorite comforting meal. Is there a processed starch that could be replaced with a vegetable?

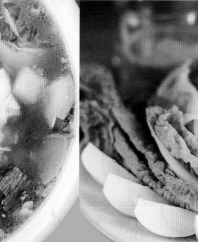

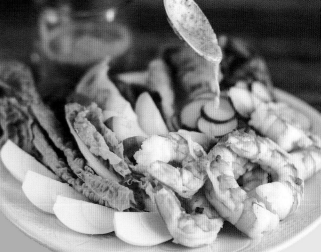

PLANT-BASED

For the girl devoted to eating a predominately plant-based diet, this plan helps balance each plate to keep blood sugar stable and hunger calm with a substantial bridge snack to tide you over. The Plant-Based Devotee also knows that rounding out her daily menu with other plant-based staples, from supplements to self-care, is crucial to living a fully plant-loving lifestyle.

Green Fab Four Smoothie Bowl (page 204)

You might have heard that chewing your smoothie will prime your body for digestion by releasing salivary amylase, an enzyme that breaks down carbohydrates. Yes, chewing increases enzyme release, but seeing, tasting, and smelling your food will do the same. So instead of stressing about chewing your smoothie, take a minute to slow down and be present while you eat. Support your digestion and slow down your sip by topping your smoothie in a bowl with hemp hearts, coconut, and almonds that will slow you down so you can really enjoy your meal.

Cauliflower Rice Tabbouleh (page 315)

Get your choline! It's is responsible for helping to prevent nonalcoholic fatty liver disease (NAFLD) because it's the raw material needed to make very-low-density lipoprotein (VLDL), the vehicle that transports fat out of the liver. Nonalcoholic fatty liver disease—a disease state in which fat accumulation occurs in the liver of those who drink very little or no alcohol at all—is sadly on the rise in all age groups. That's all the more reason to include great sources of choline in your diet, such as eggs, almonds, and cruciferous vegetables like cauliflower, broccoli, and Brussels sprouts.

Roasted Black Bean Vegan Burger (page 323)

I can't wait for you to try this grain-free veggie burger! It serves up 10 grams of fiber and 15 grams of protein. It's also the perfect meatless Monday for a Domestic Goddess and a quick freeze and heat for my Girl on the Go. Make a double batch and freeze the leftovers!

DEVOTEE

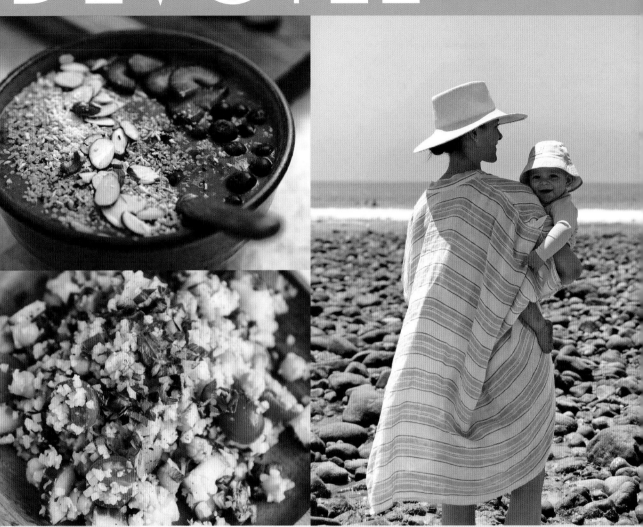

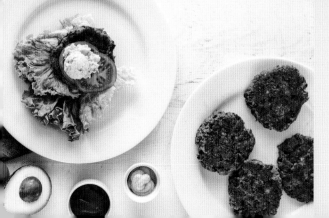

Vitamin D + Sea

Hit the beach with your babies to synthesize the sunshine vitamin! Ten to fifteen minutes of sun exposure midday three times a week is the most effective way to boost and maintain healthy levels of vitamin D.

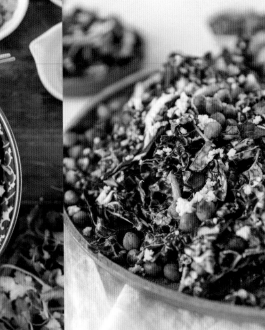

Cuddle up!

Cuddling decreases cortisol, lowers blood pressure, and triggers the release of oxytocin. Hugs all around.

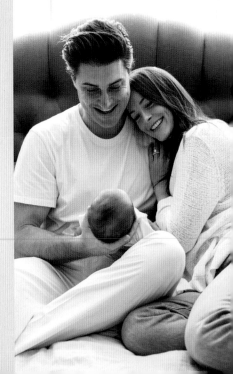

Almond Pad Thai with Shirataki Noodles

(page 300)

Shirataki noodles are made of soluble fiber called glucomannan from the konjac plant, which slows digestion and promotes satiety. They have little to no effect on glucose, and glucomannan has been known to lower in glucose levels in healthy and insulin-resistant patients.

Drink Trace Minerals

Over three quarters of the United States population is deficient in magnesium. One of the best ways to increase your magnesium intake is by adding trace mineral drops back into filtered water or by purchasing spring water. Spring water comes from underground springs and retains its mineral content without the most typical contaminants.

Chocolate Fab Four Smoothie

(page 171)

Low on protein? Crush cravings with a Chocolate Fab Four Smoothie! Protein is the most satisfying macronutrient and decreases sugar cravings.

Vegan Kale Caesar with Crispy Smoked Chickpeas

(page 306)

Cruciferous vegetables are loaded with phytochemicals that protect against cancer and support detoxification pathways, but you may have also been warned to avoid them for optimal thyroid health. Cruciferous vegetables contain organic compounds called oxalates, which, like phytic acid (see page 50), are considered anti-nutrients because they bind to minerals, preventing absorption. Specifically for thyroid health, oxylates or oxalic acid can prevent the absorption of iodine, which is needed to produce thyroid hormone. Before you throw the baby out with the bathwater, simply ensuring adequate iodine and cruciferous vegetable intake can provide your body all their benefits without depriving it of other nutrients. A few iodine-rich foods to add to your daily diet include fish, shellfish, or sea vegetables like seaweed snacks or kelp granules.

Chlorophyll Mint Fab Four Smoothie (page 336)

Mix up the base liquid of your smoothie using the homemade lemonades and spa waters on page 288.

Preparing for an event? A short timeline doesn't require a drastic diet or lifestyle change. A simple, clean, and consistent routine can help this Red-Carpet Ready gal prepare for any special event without deprivation. Instead, stack up tips and tricks for supercharged results.

Fruit-Free and Fab Four!

Start your day with a pre-breakfast workout to increase human growth hormone and testosterone to burn fat and follow up your workout with a fruit-free Fab Four Smoothie to fuel up with the lowest sugar intake.

Delicious and Nourishing

Satisfy your protein needs and support digestion with a bone broth vegetable soup and add wild salmon to the Green Goddess Salad (page 229) for the perfect dose of omega-3 and greens to support supple skin.

Every Day's a New Day with Body Love!

My life's mission is to help simplify the science of nutrition so you feel empowered to take control of your health. My hope is that by the time you finish this book you'll feel confident in your food choices, educated on how to satisfy and nourish your body, and equipped with the tools to hit your goals while consistently eating healthy—and hopefully, you'll never diet again!

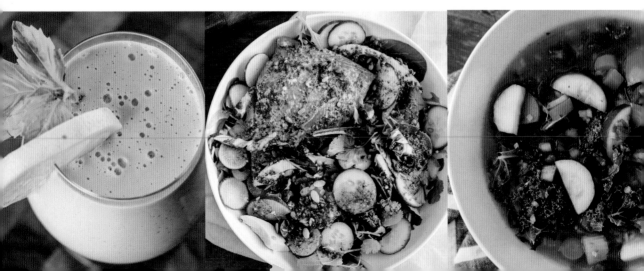

DINNER

GRAIN-FREE VEGGIE-LOADED ENCHILADAS

Mix up Taco Tuesday with these grain-free, vegetable-rich enchiladas.

Makes 4 servings

ROASTED VEGETABLES
1 yellow squash, cut into ½-inch dice
1 red pepper, cut into ½-inch dice
1 medium red onion, roughly chopped
1 small head broccoli, roughly chopped
1 small head cauliflower, roughly chopped
2 tablespoons avocado oil, plus more for the baking dish
Pink Himalayan salt and freshly ground black pepper

HOMEMADE ENCHILADA SAUCE
2 tablespoons avocado oil
1 to 2 teaspoons unmodified potato starch, or 1 to 2 tablespoons coconut flour
1 tablespoon chipotle powder
¼ cup chili powder
½ teaspoon garlic powder
¼ teaspoon ground cumin
½ teaspoon dried oregano
2 cups chicken bone broth or chicken stock

ENCHILADAS
Avocado oil
8 grain-free or organic corn tortillas (I like Siete brand)
2 cups shredded chicken (see Easy Peasy Shredded Chicken, page 254, or use a precooked rotisserie chicken)
2 cups shredded organic pasture-raised cheese
Garnishes: fresh cilantro, diced avocado or guacamole, salsa

(continued)

1. To prepare the roasted vegetables, preheat the oven to 400°F.
2. Spread the vegetables evenly on a rimmed baking sheet, drizzle with the avocado oil, and season with salt and pepper. Hand toss to coat evenly. Roast for 30 minutes, until lightly browned and fork tender. Set aside and lower the oven heat to 350°F.
3. Meanwhile, make the enchilada sauce. In a medium saucepan over medium heat, combine all the ingredients except the chicken broth, whisking to remove any lumps. Continue whisking as you slowly add the broth. Bring to a simmer and cook for 10 minutes, until thickened slightly. (The sauce can also be made ahead a couple days and refrigerated.)
4. To assemble the enchiladas, coat a 9-by-12-inch baking dish with avocado oil. Lay the tortillas out on a clean cutting board and spread the center of each with 1 to 2 tablespoons enchilada sauce. Layer on the shredded chicken, roasted vegetables, and 1 cup of the cheese, evenly distributing them among the tortillas.
5. Roll to close the enchiladas and arrange them seam side down in the baking dish. Spread the remaining enchilada sauce and sprinkle the remaining 1 cup of cheese over the enchiladas.
6. Bake for 10 minutes, until the cheese is melted and the tortillas are warm and lightly toasted on the edges. Serve garnished with cilantro, diced avocado or guacamole, and salsa.

Day 10—Weekday

BREAKFAST

QUICK INSTANT POT COCONUT YOGURT

One of my culinary inspirations and go-to LA bakeries is Sweet Laurel. Their cookbook and social media (@sweetlaurelbakery and @laurelgallucci) are full of amazing recipes that are grain-free, gluten-free, dairy-free, and without refined sugars. One recipe I love, and have adapted here to work in an Instant Pot, is Sweet Laurel's Coconut Yogurt. My favorite way to enjoy it is with my Coconutty Cereal.

Makes 2 servings

One 13.5-ounce can organic coconut milk, regular (no guar gum)
One 13.5-ounce can organic coconut cream
2 or 3 prebiotic-free probiotic capsules (see Tip)
Coconutty Cereal (recipe follows)

1. Pour the coconut milk and coconut cream into an Instant Pot and whisk to combine. Secure the lid and press "Yogurt." Toggle until "boil" is displayed.
2. When it is boiling, the Instant Pot will beep. Open the lid and check that the coconut mixture is at 115°F. Open the probiotic capsules, pour their contents into the pot, and whisk to combine.
3. Secure the lid, push the "Yogurt" button again, and set the time to 16 hours. When the time is up, open the lid. Pour the yogurt into sterilized glass containers with lids and set in the fridge to thicken.
4. Top with coconutty cereal.

TIP: The probiotics must be prebiotic-free, or the fermentation will not happen properly. One option is Clinical GI Probiotic Veg capsules from NOW Foods.

COCONUTTY CEREAL

Makes 12 servings

1 cup raw walnuts
1 cup raw pecans
1 cup raw almonds
1 cup raw cashews
2 tablespoons coconut oil, melted
1 tablespoon honey
1 cup coconut flakes
½ cup hemp hearts
1 teaspoon pink Himalayan salt

1. Preheat the oven to 220°F.
2. Place the nuts in a food processor and pulse to create small chunks. (Or put them in a sealed, heavy-duty freezer bag and use a mallet to pound them to your desired chunk size.) In a large bowl, mix the coconut oil, honey, coconut flakes, hemp hearts, salt, and nut chunks. Transfer the mixture to a baking sheet.
3. Bake for 30 minutes, until the nuts are dry and toasted. Let the mixture cool, then store it at room temperature in an airtight container.

LUNCH: Choose a healthy takeout option from your self-made body-loving menu (see the Girl on the Go plan, page 185).

DINNER

BUTTERY LIME COD WITH SLAW

When it comes to fish, I tend to default to salmon. To help mix it up, try this super-quick cod dish served over slaw.

Makes 4 servings

4 (4-ounce) skinless wild cod fillets
1 teaspoon pink Himalayan salt
2 tablespoons unsalted butter (I like Kerrygold)
1 teaspoon lime zest
3 cups finely shredded red cabbage
1 carrot, peeled and shredded
1 green onion, thinly sliced
1 tablespoon freshly squeezed lime juice
1 tablespoon extra virgin olive oil
½ teaspoon freshly ground black pepper
2 tablespoons chopped fresh cilantro

1. Sprinkle the cod with ½ teaspoon of the salt.
2. In a large skillet over medium-high heat, melt the butter with the lime zest. Lay the cod fillets in the pan and pan-fry until golden and cooked through, 3 to 4 minutes per side.
3. In a medium bowl, mix the cabbage, carrot, green onion, lime juice, olive oil, remaining ½ teaspoon salt, and pepper. The slaw can be made 3 to 6 hours ahead of time and stored in the refrigerator to chill and allow the flavors to mix.
4. Plate the slaw and top it with the cod fillets and a sprinkling of cilantro.

OPTIONAL BREAKFAST PREP: Fab Four Chia Seed Pudding (see the Girl on the Go plan, page 184).

Day 11—Weekday

MORNING MOVEMENT: Choose a thirty- to sixty-minute workout that involves weight lifting, kettlebells, resistance, or strength training. A couple of class options include yoga with weights or a HIIT class (which combines aerobic and anaerobic exercise). Strength training helps tone, tighten, and build lean muscle mass. You want to get an anaerobic workout that makes your muscles sore. This can help increase insulin sensitivity, lower blood sugar levels, and increase your metabolism.

BREAKFAST

ANTI-INFLAMMATORY VANILLA SPICE FAB FOUR SMOOTHIE

If you prepped Fab Four Chia Seed Pudding last night, dig in this morning. If not, try this aromatic vanilla smoothie. Spices aren't just for cooking and baking; this smoothie incorporates cinnamon, cloves, turmeric, and black pepper into a warming combination.

Vanilla collagen protein powder containing 20 to 30 grams protein
1 tablespoon MCT oil
2 tablespoons acacia fiber (I use NOW Foods)
Handful of spinach
1 teaspoon ground cinnamon (preferably freshly grated Ceylon; see Tip)
½ teaspoon ground cloves
½ teaspoon ground turmeric
Pinch of freshly ground black pepper
1 to 2 cups unsweetened coconut milk

Place all the ingredients in a high-speed blender and blend to your desired consistency.

TIP: Cinnamon can add a functional boost and has been linked to improved metabolic markers, reduced blood sugar spikes, and increased insulin sensitivity. My favorite type of cinnamon is Ceylon, because this variety contains a lower amount of coumarin, a natural flavor found in plants that in large quantities has been linked to liver damage. A study in the *Journal of Agriculture and Food Chemistry* found that cassia cinnamon contained up to sixty-three times more coumarin than Ceylon cinnamon. Also, grating the cinnamon yourself offers the richest flavor and the highest nutritional value. You can buy Ceylon cinnamon sticks and ground Ceylon at most grocery stores.

LUNCH: Egg Salad over Arugula with Jilz Crackerz (see the Girl on the Go plan, page 167).

DINNER

LIME CILANTRO CHICKEN AND BROCCOLI

Chicken and broccoli may sound like a ho-hum dish, but you can make it finger-licking with the right marinade and dipping sauce. My version does just that and will have you craving more. It's also a good example of how you can easily combine healthy fats as part of a dipping sauce (this recipe uses cashews and avocado oil).

Makes 2 servings

MARINADE/DIPPING SAUCE
1 tablespoon freshly squeezed lime juice
½ cup packed cilantro leaves
1 cup unsalted cashews, dry-roasted, raw, or toasted (see Tip, page 323)
¼ cup avocado oil
4 garlic cloves, roughly chopped
1 tablespoon tamari

(continued)

1 tablespoon coconut aminos

1 jalapeño pepper, stemmed, seeded, and roughly chopped

CHICKEN AND BROCCOLI

2 boneless, skinless chicken breasts, pounded thin (see Tip)

1 large broccoli head, cut into florets

2 tablespoons avocado oil

1. Preheat the oven to 475°F.

2. In a food processor, pulse all the marinade/dipping sauce ingredients to a pesto consistency. Reserve half to serve as a dipping sauce.

3. Place the chicken on a parchment-lined baking sheet and coat it with the marinade. Coat the broccoli with avocado oil, then spread it on the baking sheet with the chicken. Bake for 7 minutes, flip the chicken breasts and broccoli florets, and bake for 7 more minutes, until the chicken is cooked through and the broccoli is lightly browned.

4. Serve immediately with the dipping sauce.

TIP: Looking to put dinner on the table in a flash? I pound my chicken breasts thin to speed up the cooking process. Place a breast inside a sealable heavy-duty freezer bag and seal the bag, removing as much air as possible. Pound the chicken to an even ¼-inch thickness using the flat side of a meat mallet or a rolling pin.

PHONE A FRIEND: Texting has seemingly replaced talking, and catching up on social media has seemingly replaced really catching up. But your phone is still a phone. Try using it tonight to connect with a friend or family member. Dopamine is released when we hear, see, or touch another person. You might be surprised how good it makes you feel to actually talk to someone on the phone again. Or, better yet, use that phone call to get a coffee, lunch, or workout on the books. Nothing replaces real, in-person face time . . . not even FaceTime.

Day 12—Weekday

BREAKFAST

ALMOND BLISS FAB FOUR SMOOTHIE

Every sip of this new Fab Four Smoothie is a little bit of bliss. The combination of vanilla, coconut, almond, and cacao will have your taste buds dancing.

Vanilla collagen protein powder containing 20 to 30 grams protein
1 tablespoon almond butter
2 tablespoons chia seeds
1 tablespoon coconut flakes
1 tablespoon cacao nibs
Handful of spinach
1 to 2 cups unsweetened almond milk

Place all the ingredients in a high-speed blender and blend to your desired consistency.

LUNCH: Try my quick and easy Flaky Tuna and Toasted Walnut Salad (see the Girl on the Go plan, page 181).

DINNER

KOREAN BARBECUE STEAK WITH
SPICY BOK CHOY

Permission to get your nom on with this Korean-style steak served with sautéed bok choy. You can serve it over cauliflower rice (see page 315) or the real stuff, like California basmati rice, which has been tested to have lower levels of arsenic than other types.

Makes 2 to 4 servings

¼ cup coconut aminos
2 teaspoons toasted sesame oil (see Tip)
½ cup sliced green onions (white and pale green parts), plus ¼ cup sliced green parts
1 tablespoon minced garlic
1 tablespoon minced fresh ginger
3 tablespoons sesame seeds, toasted (see Tip, page 182)
1 pound flank steak, cut across the grain into thin slices (ideally ⅛ inch thick)
1 tablespoon algae oil
Spicy Bok Choy, for serving (recipe follows)

1. In a medium bowl, whisk together the coconut aminos, sesame oil, ½ cup white and pale green onions, garlic, ginger, and 2 tablespoons of the sesame seeds. Add the steak and toss to coat, then set aside to marinate for 15 minutes.

2. In a large cast-iron skillet over high heat, heat the algae oil until shimmering, then add the steak in a single layer and stir-fry for 5 minutes, until browned.

3. Transfer to a platter and sprinkle with the remaining ¼ cup green onions and remaining 1 tablespoon of sesame seeds. Serve with spicy bok choy.

TIP: Toasted sesame oil is produced from toasted sesame seeds, and it can add delicious flavor to Asian-inspired dishes. However, when the seeds are toasted at too high a temperature, their oils can go bad. Also, many brands use chemical extraction techniques. Opt for a slow-roasted and expeller-pressed sesame oil to preserve the nutrients and fatty acids, such as Napa Valley Naturals organic toasted sesame oil. Store it in the fridge for optimal freshness.

SPICY BOK CHOY

Makes 2 servings

1 tablespoon coconut oil
2 garlic cloves, minced
1 tablespoon minced fresh ginger
1 tablespoon tamari
1 teaspoon red pepper flakes
4 bunches baby bok choy, cleaned and ends trimmed

1. In a large skillet with a lid, heat the coconut oil over medium-high heat. Add the garlic, ginger, tamari, red pepper flakes, and 1 tablespoon of water and cook, stirring constantly, until fragrant, about 1 minute.
2. Add the bok choy and stir carefully to coat it with oil. Put the lid on and cook for about 2 minutes, until the bok choy is crisp-tender, stirring occasionally. Store in the fridge for up to 2 days.

ROLL IT OUT: In recent years, I've really taken to foam rolling to help improve my fascia health, lymphatic drainage, and alignment. Fasciae, also known as connective tissue, are found throughout the body. They wrap and protect the muscles and organs and are also where our nerves lie. The problem is fasciae can store toxins and thicken and harden when they aren't exercised correctly, which can result in poor alignment, limited flexibility, nerve constriction, poor blood flow, weak lymphatic drainage, and even cellulite.

My go-to expert is Lauren Roxburgh. I feel like a million bucks after seeing her for check-ins, and I use her exercises and rollers almost every day at home. Lauren has a great online program with videos and her own rollers that you can use as part of a daily foam rolling routine.

Day 13—Weekend Day

BREAKFAST

TROPICAL TREAT FAB FOUR SMOOTHIE

Here's another new Fab Four Smoothie recipe that will take your taste buds on a tropical vacation. The combination of coconut, pineapple, and vanilla is reminiscent of a piña colada. It's also the perfect recipe to incorporate the creamy almond and macadamia nut butter blend I created with Wild Friends.

Vanilla coconut collagen protein powder containing 20 to 30 grams protein
1 tablespoon Wild Friends Almond Macadamia Be Well Blend
2 tablespoons chia seeds
Handful of spinach
¼ cup pineapple (fresh or frozen)
1 to 2 cups unsweetened almond milk
1 tablespoon organic shredded coconut (optional)

Place all the ingredients but the coconut in a high-speed blender and blend to your desired consistency. Top with the shredded coconut if desired.

LUNCH: When brunch is late and lunch is later, a mezze platter (aka snack tray) may hold you over until dinner. Just be sure to plate up the Fab Four with food like vegetable crudités, hummus, raw nuts, and olives. Turkey, avocado, and lettuce rollups are another fun addition.

AFTERNOON MOVEMENT: Here are a few ideas for some light Saturday movement. The goal is to get outside and not turn into an all-day couch potato: (1) go for a thirty-minute walk; (2) find a bit of nature and go for a hike; or (3) be a tourist in your own city, visit a museum, or explore an up-and-coming neighborhood—those steps will add up fast.

DINNER

SHEET PAN MACKEREL AND RED POTATOES

This herb-scented preparation is another tasty fish dish that is different from your standard salmon.

Makes 4 servings

4 fresh mackerel, gutted and cleaned
2 lemons, sliced
2 rosemary sprigs, halved
8 bay leaves
6 teaspoons extra virgin olive oil
1 cup halved small red potatoes

1. Preheat the oven to 375°F.

2. Place the mackerel on a parchment-lined baking sheet. Into each fish, insert 2 lemon slices, a piece of rosemary, and 2 bay leaves. Using a sharp knife, carefully slash the skin of the mackerels on a diagonal, then drizzle with 3 teaspoons of the olive oil. Place the potatoes around the fish and drizzle with the remaining olive oil.

3. Roast for 10 minutes, turn the fish, and continue roasting for another 10 minutes, or until the fish is cooked through and the potatoes are fork tender.

Day 14—Weekend Day

BREAKFAST: Make some Super Seeded Pancakes by loading up your favorite gluten-free pancake mix (I like Birch Benders) with 1 tablespoon chia seeds, 1 tablespoon flaxseeds, 1½ teaspoons poppy seeds, and 1½ teaspoons ground cinnamon (see Tip, page 247). The seeds will add fat and fiber, and the cinnamon will add a hint of sweetness.

253

LUNCH

BUFFALO CHICKEN LETTUCE CUPS

If football is on in your house or you're going to a friend's to watch a game, steer the viewing party in a clean (but tasty) direction with these chicken snacks.

Makes 4 servings

Easy Peasy Shredded Chicken (recipe follows), or precooked rotisserie chicken, shredded
¼ cup Buffalo sauce (I like New Primal Medium, or see Tip)
16 iceberg lettuce leaves
2 celery stalks, diced small
½ cup shredded carrot

In a medium bowl, toss the chicken with the Buffalo sauce. Make 8 lettuce cups using 2 leaves per cup and fill them with the chicken, celery, and shredded carrot.

TIP: When shopping for Buffalo sauce, look for an option that has no added or refined sugar, that is free of industrial seed oils, and that is dairy-free.

EASY PEASY SHREDDED CHICKEN

This past summer, my friend the New York Times best-selling cookbook author Danielle Walker taught me how to pressure cook a whole chicken in an Instant Pot. She even throws the bones back in (after the chicken is cooked) and cooks them again to make her bone broth. So clever and resourceful! Danielle is a phenomenal resource for clean, whole food meals made from scratch, and I recommend you check out the bone broth version of this recipe and her books, blog, and social media @againstallgrain.

Makes 4 servings

1 (3- to 4-pound) whole chicken
½ cup filtered water (or vegetable or chicken broth)

1. Place the chicken and water in the Instant Pot, close the lid, and lock it into place. Check that the valve is sealed and select manual high pressure for 25 to 30 minutes (30 minutes for a 4-pound bird).

2. Let the pressure release naturally, open the lid, and place the chicken on a cutting board to shred. Discard the skin, save the bones for broth or discard them, shred the chicken, and store it in a glass container with a lid for 3 to 4 days in the refrigerator.

DINNER

CHICKEN POTATO SOUP

This is a warm, filling recipe for the fall or winter.

Makes 4 servings

4 bacon slices, diced
1 large white onion, cut into ¼-inch dice
4 large garlic cloves, thinly sliced
1 cup ¼-inch-thick carrot slices
1 cup ¼-inch-thick celery slices
2 tablespoons Italian seasoning (I like Simply Organic) or 2 teaspoons each dried thyme, oregano, and parsley
3 cups baby potatoes
8 cups chicken bone broth or chicken stock
4 cups cooked chicken breast, shredded (see Easy Peasy Shredded Chicken, opposite, or use a precooked rotisserie chicken)
2 cups coarsely chopped baby spinach

(continued)

1. In a large pot over medium heat, cook the bacon. When the fat is rendered (cooked out) and the bacon bits are crisp, remove the bacon and set aside. Add the onion and garlic to the fat in the pan and sauté until the onion is translucent, 3 to 4 minutes. Add the carrot, celery, and seasoning and sauté for 2 to 3 minutes, until tender.

2. Add the potatoes and broth, bring the mixture to a simmer, and cook for 15 minutes, until the potatoes are tender. Using a wooden spoon, smash some of the potatoes to thicken the broth.

3. Add the chicken and spinach and let simmer for 4 minutes, until the chicken is warmed through. Serve warm with the bacon bit topping.

SUNDAY SELF-CARE: Taking care of your body means you're taking care of yourself. Your skin, face, eyebrows, nails, and even your back all love attention, and a little love can go a long way to making you look and feel vibrant and refreshed. Give yourself the spa treatment. Use a scrub, apply a face mask, give your eyebrows a quick cleanup, book a manicure or pedicure, splurge for a full massage, or book time at an infrared sauna. (If your kids gave you "coupons" for your birthday or Mother's Day, this could also be the perfect time to cash in on the back rub they owe you.)

Looking for a DIY face mask? Try one of these antimicrobial honey masks to hydrate and clean. Combine the ingredients and apply the mask to a clean, dry face. Leave on for 3 to 5 minutes. Rinse off and apply moisturizer.

WARMING AND HYDRATING HONEY AND CINNAMON FACE MASK

1 tablespoon manuka honey
½ teaspoon ground cinnamon
1 to 4 drops rosehip oil

BRIGHTENING HONEY AND LEMON FACE MASK

Don't use this mask after exfoliating or with open cuts because the lemon will sting.

1 tablespoon manuka honey
2 tablespoons lemon juice

Day 15—Weekday

MONDAY MOVEMENT: How do you want to move this week? Maybe it's time to try something new and push yourself. One option is to hit it hard with a HIIT workout. High-intensity interval training combines aerobic and anaerobic exercise over a short period of time (usually less than thirty minutes). Among other benefits, it can help lower insulin resistance and improve metabolism, which are both great for weight loss. Google a well-reviewed HIIT class near you and sign up.

BREAKFAST: Revisit Day 1 and make yourself a Fab Four Smoothie Bowl (page 203). Choose any flavor you want.

LUNCH: Soup makes great leftovers, so warm up a bowl of Chicken Potato Soup (page 255). Add a side salad of your choosing.

DINNER: On this Meatless Monday, try the Spaghetti Squash Chow Mein from the Plant-Based Devotee plan, page 320. Optional: add 4 ounces of shrimp.

EVENING SELF-CARE: Enjoy a night at home luxuriating in a Boosted Bath (see the Red-Carpet Ready plan, page 266). If you hit it hard with a HIIT workout this morning, it's the perfect end to the day.

Day 16—Weekday

MORNING MOVEMENT: To balance yesterday's more intense HIIT workout, let's do some light cardio this morning and go for a brisk thirty- to forty-five-minute walk. Engage your whole body and find an up-tempo pace so you break a good sweat.

BREAKFAST

MATCHA CHIA SEED PUDDING

Matcha Chia Seed Pudding is a green way to start your day. Matcha contains the phytochemical EGCG, which increases the production of glutathione, one of our most potent antioxidants.

Makes 1 serving

¼ cup chia seeds
1½ cups unsweetened vanilla almond milk
Vanilla protein powder containing 20 to 30 grams protein
1 tablespoon matcha powder
1 tablespoon coconut butter

1. Place the chia seeds in a mason jar (or other glass container with a screw-down lid). Combine the almond milk, protein powder, matcha powder, and coconut butter in a high-speed blender and blend, then pour the mixture over the chia seeds and screw the lid on tight. Shake to mix in the chia seeds and place in the refrigerator.

2. After 20 minutes, shake lightly again (to remix the chia seeds) and return to the refrigerator. The pudding will be ready to eat in 1 to 2 hours, but it will have the best consistency if you leave it overnight.

LUNCH

GREEK CHICKEN SALAD

When you make this salad, you might want to mix up a double batch of the vinaigrette dressing to use later in the week.

Makes 2 servings

DRESSING

¼ cup extra virgin olive oil or avocado oil
Juice of 1 lemon
1 tablespoon red wine vinegar
2 large garlic cloves, minced
2 tablespoons dried oregano
1 teaspoon pink Himalayan salt
Freshly ground black pepper

SALAD

2 chicken breasts, cooked and sliced
2 romaine hearts, rinsed and chopped
4 small Persian cucumbers or ½ English cucumber, diced
2 cups cherry or grape tomatoes
½ green pepper, thinly sliced
½ red onion, thinly sliced
½ cup pitted Kalamata olives
1 avocado, thinly sliced

In a large bowl, whisk all the dressing ingredients together. Add the salad ingredients and toss to coat.

(continued)

DINNER

GROUND BEEF TOSTADA SALAD

Mix up Taco Tuesday with this delectable beef tostada salad.

Makes 4 servings

1 pound ground beef
2 tablespoons chili powder
2 tablespoons smoked paprika
1½ teaspoons garlic powder
¾ teaspoon red pepper flakes
1 teaspoon pink Himalayan salt, plus more to taste
8 cups shredded romaine lettuce
1 cup halved grape tomatoes
½ cup cilantro leaves
1 orange bell pepper, cut into ¼-inch dice
1 tablespoon avocado oil
Juice of 1 lime
2 avocados
1 garlic clove, minced
4 Siete almond flour tortillas (or another grain-free tortilla)

1. Place the beef in a skillet and cook it over medium-high heat until browned and cooked through, 7 to 10 minutes, breaking it into smaller pieces with a wooden spoon as it cooks. If you prefer drier meat, drain some of the fat from the skillet. Add the chili powder, paprika, garlic powder, chile flakes, and 1 teaspoon salt to the skillet. Stir the seasonings into the meat and cook for 2 to 3 minutes to combine and heat through.

2. In a large bowl, toss the romaine, tomatoes, cilantro, and bell pepper with the avocado oil and half of the lime juice. In a medium bowl, mash the avocado with the garlic and the remaining lime juice. Salt to taste. In a medium skillet over medium heat, toast the tortillas one at a time until both sides are crispy.

3. To serve, layer the tortillas with avocado smash, ground beef, and the romaine mixture.

TECH-FREE TUESDAY: Try going tech-free tonight. Read, have a game night, break out a puzzle, journal, write someone a real letter, or just talk to a friend or your spouse, partner, or kids. Even if it's just for an hour or two, let all your screens stay dark. Create your own comedy, awaken your imagination, and connect IRL with those you love. My husband likes to call it Talk O'clock.

Day 17—Weekday

MORNING MOVEMENT: Download or stream a workout on your phone. Choose one that focuses on strength or resistance training with weights, kettlebells, or your own body weight. You can also head to the gym and do yoga with weights or another HIIT class.

BREAKFAST

SUN BUTTER AND JELLY SWIRL FAB FOUR SMOOTHIE

This is a riff on old-fashioned PB&J, but with sunflower butter, which is a seed butter and thus a great option for people with allergies to peanuts or tree nuts. I've provided directions for giving your glass a playful looking swirl of PB intertwined with J, but you can also blend everything at once in the usual way.

Vanilla protein powder containing 20 to 30 grams protein
2 tablespoons sunflower butter

(continued)

2 tablespoons chia seeds

1 to 2 cups unsweetened vanilla almond milk

¼ cup frozen red raspberries

¼ cup filtered water

1. Make the "PB": combine the protein powder, sunflower butter, 1 tablespoon of the chia seeds, and almond milk in a high-speed blender and blend to your desired consistency. Pour the mixture into a glass. Rinse out the blender.

2. Add the "J": place the raspberries, water, and remaining 1 tablespoon chia seeds in the blender and blend to your desired consistency. Pour the mixture into your glass.

3. Swirl the contents once with a spoon or metal straw.

LUNCH

TURKEY CHOPPED SALAD

Here's my streamlined take on a chopped salad.

Makes 1 serving

1 tablespoon extra virgin olive oil

1 tablespoon apple cider or red wine vinegar

¼ teaspoon Dijon mustard (optional)

4 ounces chopped roasted turkey (I like Applegate Organic smoked turkey breast)

½ cup ¼-inch-diced cucumber

½ cup ¼-inch-diced tomato

¼ cup quartered radishes

2 tablespoons thinly sliced peperoncini peppers

¼ cup sprouts (optional)

¼ avocado, cubed

Pink Himalayan salt and freshly ground black pepper to taste

In a medium bowl, whisk the oil, vinegar, and, if desired, the mustard together until emulsified. Add the remaining ingredients and toss to combine.

APPLE CIDER VINEGAR: In a study performed on mice, apple cider vinegar (ACV) improved glucose uptake into the liver and muscles. This suggests that ACV could potentially help balance blood sugar and increase insulin sensitivity in humans. I try to incorporate it into at least two meals per week.

DINNER

GARLIC SALMON AND BRUSSELS SPROUTS

Make it a Wild Wednesday with wild salmon. To make it even wilder, buy the Brussels sprouts on the stalk—they're fun to cut off. This recipe is protein efficient and full of healthy fats and phytochemicals.

Makes 4 to 6 servings

1 pound Brussels sprouts, trimmed and halved
6 garlic cloves, minced
6 tablespoons extra virgin olive oil
2 tablespoons dried oregano
2 teaspoons pink Himalayan salt
1 teaspoon freshly ground black pepper
6 (4-ounce) wild salmon fillets
1 lemon, thinly sliced

1. Preheat the oven to 450°F.
2. In a large bowl, combine the Brussels sprouts, garlic, olive oil, oregano, salt, and pepper. Mix to coat the Brussels sprouts evenly. Using a slotted spoon, transfer the Brussels sprouts to a rimmed baking sheet, leaving the garlic oil in the bowl. Roast the Brussels sprouts for 15 minutes, stirring once or twice during cooking.

(continued)

3. Move the Brussels sprouts to make room for the salmon fillets on the pan. Drizzle the salmon with the reserved garlic oil, cover each fillet with a slice of lemon, and return the pan to the oven for 10 to 12 minutes, until the salmon is cooked through.

REMINDER: After a plant is picked, it begins to break down and use its own stored nutrients to sustain itself, which translates into fewer nutrients for you and me. This is called the cellular respiration rate, and each kind of fruit or vegetables has a different rate. Brussels sprouts have a rapid cellular respiration rate, so try to eat them as close as possible to their pick date. Even though they store well, you're better off not letting them linger.

Day 18—Weekday

BREAKFAST

CREAMY MOCHA FAB FOUR SMOOTHIE

Blast off with this creamy coffee-infused smoothie.

Collagen protein powder (plain or chocolate) containing 20 to 30 grams protein
½ cup cold-brew coffee
1 teaspoon grass-fed butter (such as Kerrygold)
1 teaspoon MCT oil
1 tablespoon acacia fiber (I use NOW Foods)
½ teaspoon ground cinnamon (see Tip, page 247)
½ teaspoon raw cacao powder (if you used plain protein powder)
1½ cups coconut milk

Place all the ingredients in a high-speed blender and blend to your desired consistency.

LUNCH

PEANUT KALE SALAD

I love this salad combining peanuts and kale. You can top it with your choice of protein. It goes great with chicken and salmon.

Makes 2 to 4 servings

Pink Himalayan salt
1 large bunch kale, stemmed and chopped
¼ cup peanut butter (see page 73)
2 teaspoons lite seasoned rice vinegar (a third less sodium and sugar)
2 teaspoons coconut aminos (or 1 teaspoon each coconut aminos and tamari)
1 teaspoon minced fresh ginger
1 small garlic clove, minced
3 to 4 tablespoons hot filtered water
¼ red onion, thinly sliced
¼ cup dry-roasted peanuts, chopped, for garnish

1. In a large pot over high heat, bring water and a pinch of salt to a rolling boil. Prepare a bowl of ice water. Blanch the kale for 2 minutes, remove it with tongs, and shock it in the ice water. When cool, squeeze the excess water from the kale.

2. While the water is coming to a boil, in a large bowl, whisk together the peanut butter, rice vinegar, aminos, ginger, garlic, and hot water.

3. Add the kale, onion, and peanuts to the bowl with the dressing and toss well to coat.

DINNER: Try a new recipe from the Girl on the Go plan or Plant-Based Devotee plan. Or if you don't feel like cooking tonight, pick something from your body-loving takeout menu (see the Girl on the Go plan, page 185).

BREW A HOT TEA: The ritual of sipping hot tea in the evening can help reduce cravings, calm the body, and even support sounder sleep. See the Plant-Based Devotee plan, page 287.

Day 19—Weekday

BREAKFAST

SWEET AND SAVORY BASIL FAB FOUR SMOOTHIE

This sweet and savory smoothie was a happy accident. It was developed during a fridge forage when the only nut or seed butter I had was tahini.

Vanilla protein powder containing 20 to 30 grams protein
¼ avocado
1 tablespoon tahini
1 tablespoon acacia fiber (I use NOW Foods)
Handful of fresh basil leaves (or basil microgreens)
Juice of ½ lemon
1 teaspoon powdered holy basil (see Tip)
1 to 2 cups unsweetened almond milk

Place all the ingredients in a high-speed blender and blend to your desired consistency.

TIP: Holy basil, an adaptogenic herb from the mint family, adds a functional boost. It has been called the Mother Medicine of Nature and the Queen of Herbs and has been known to have anti-inflammatory, antibacterial, and antistress benefits. You can buy it in powdered form either online or in health food stores.

LUNCH: Choose a healthy takeout option from your self-made body-loving menu (see the Girl on the Go plan, page 185).

DINNER: Make personal pizzas tonight, but try using a cauliflower crust. It has more fiber, lower net carbohydrates, and is gluten-free. I like Cali'flour Foods (they have a vegan option, too) and Outer Aisle Gourmet. The cooking directions will be listed on the package. Here are a few body-loving sauce, cheese, and topping combinations for inspiration.

- **SUPER VEGGIE:** black olives, green olives, mushrooms, green pepper, spinach, and basil; shredded mozzarella (or a vegan nut-based option); and marinara sauce. Add toasted hemp hearts when the pizza comes out of the oven.
- **PESTO:** zucchini, squash, eggplant, roasted red pepper, shredded mozzarella (or a vegan nut-based option), and homemade Classic Basil Presto Pesto (Plant-Based Devotee plan, page 286)
- **BARBECUE CHICKEN:** red onion, cilantro, cooked shredded chicken (see page 254), shredded mozzarella, and unsweetened BBQ Sauce
- **SAUSAGE AND PEPPERONI:** sausage, pepperoni, green pepper, shredded mozzarella, and marinara sauce

TRY IT AGAIN SOMEWHERE NEW: Your opinion of a workout might be based on trying it one time, with a specific teacher, on a specific day, at a specific location. If you didn't have the best experience but you're still interested in that type of workout, try it again somewhere new. Not all studios, teachers, or classes are going to be a fit or match your personal preference. Consistency will happen when you find what you love, and what you love might take you a few different classes, studios, and teachers to zero in on.

One of my early clients, Lainey, age thirty-six, wanted full-service nutrition and training, and I happily obliged. In one of our first meetings, she was vocal about not wanting to do yoga because the one class she had been to was too slow. We tried a few other types of workouts, but she didn't like them. I asked her to try yoga again, this time at a studio that played music and had an upbeat flow. I recommended two studios, and the second one clicked. She loved it. After three months, she was doing headstands and advanced standing poses. She became a regular, and to this day yoga is still her go-to workout. All because she was willing to try it again somewhere new.

Day 20—Weekend Day

BREAKFAST

SWEET POTATO HASH AND EGG BAKE

This hash made with sweet potatoes is a hearty, nutrient-dense way to start your weekend.

Makes 2 servings

2 tablespoons avocado oil
½ cup ¼-inch-diced sweet potato
½ cup ¼-inch-diced parsnip
½ cup ¼-inch-diced white onion
1 garlic clove, minced
2 cups chopped stemmed kale
Kosher salt and freshly ground black pepper
8 large organic eggs
3 tablespoons grated sharp cheddar cheese (optional)

1. Preheat the oven to 350°F.
2. In a large oven-safe skillet over medium heat, heat 1 tablespoon of the avocado oil. Add the sweet potato and parsnip to the skillet, stirring to coat them in oil. Transfer the skillet to the oven and roast for 20 minutes.
3. Meanwhile, heat the remaining 1 tablespoon of avocado oil in a small skillet over medium heat. Add the onion and sauté until tender but not brown, about 6 minutes. Add the garlic and a small amount of the kale at a time, stirring until each begins to wilt before adding the next. Sprinkle with salt and pepper. Sauté until the pan liquid has evaporated. Set aside.
4. In a large bowl, whisk the eggs with half of the cheese (if using) and ¼ teaspoon each salt and pepper. Set aside.
5. When the skillet comes out of the oven, stir in the garlic-onion-kale mixture. Add the egg mixture and stir to distribute it evenly. Cover the skillet, turn the

heat on the stovetop to medium-low, and cook until the eggs are almost set but still moist in the center, about 4 minutes.

6. Sprinkle the remaining cheese over top. Turn on the broiler and broil just until the eggs are set in the center and the cheese is beginning to brown, about 1 minute. Watch closely!

LUNCH

LETTUCE-WRAPPED PAN-FRIED SLIDERS AND ROASTED ROOT FRIES

This is a cleaner, leaner alternative to your typical burger-and-fries combination. You'll get the same satisfaction but with more fiber, lower net carbohydrates, and the use of a cleaner cooking oil (avocado oil).

Makes 4 servings

2 cups ½-inch-diced peeled root vegetables (sweet potato, carrot, and parsnip)
1 tablespoon avocado oil
1½ teaspoons pink Himalayan salt
1 pound grass-fed ground beef
1 tablespoon Worcestershire sauce
1 garlic clove, minced
8 lettuce leaf cups (romaine, butter, or red leaf)
1 ripe tomato, cut into 8 thin slices
Toppings: sliced avocado, unsweetened organic ketchup, and organic yellow mustard

1. Preheat the oven to 450°F.
2. In a medium bowl, toss the root vegetables with the oil and ½ teaspoon of the salt. Spread the veggies in a single layer on a rimmed baking sheet and

(continued)

roast until golden and crisp, about thirty-five minutes, turning them halfway through.

3. In a medium bowl, mix the beef, Worcestershire, garlic, and remaining 1 teaspoon salt. Mold the mixture into 8 slider patties. In a large skillet over medium heat, cook the patties for 2 to 3 minutes per side, until the desired doneness is reached.

4. Wrap the sliders in lettuce and add your choice of toppings. Serve with the roasted veggies alongside.

DINNER

FRESH SHRIMP SPRING ROLLS WITH ALMOND BUTTER DIPPING SAUCE

This recipe is one of my new favorites. You can buy precooked shrimp or use my simple recipe from Day 1 (see page 206) to cook your own.

Makes 2 servings

ALMOND BUTTER DIPPING SAUCE
2 tablespoons almond butter
2 tablespoons coconut aminos
Juice of ½ small lime (about 2 tablespoons)
1 garlic clove, minced
1 teaspoon sriracha, or to taste
1 teaspoon red pepper flakes
2 tablespoons hemp hearts

SHRIMP ROLLS
5 (8-inch) round rice paper wrappers
10 Boston or red-leaf lettuce leaves, cut in half lengthwise, with any thick stems removed
⅓ cup shredded carrots

⅓ cup thinly shredded red cabbage

⅓ cup fresh bean sprouts

5 cooked jumbo shrimp, peeled, deveined, and cut in half lengthwise

10 fresh mint leaves

¼ cup chopped cilantro

1. To make the almond butter dipping sauce, combine all the sauce ingredients except the hemp hearts in a medium bowl. Whisk, adding 2 to 3 tablespoons water, until the sauce reaches your desired consistency. Top with the hemp hearts to add a little protein.

2. To make the shrimp rolls, fill a large bowl with lukewarm water and set a damp dish towel on a cutting board. Immerse 1 rice paper sheet into the water for 15 to 20 seconds. Remove the sheet, shaking off the excess water, and lay it flat on the dampened cloth. Lay 2 lettuce leaves on the center of the rice paper. On the lettuce, place 1 tablespoon carrots, 1 tablespoon cabbage, 1 tablespoon bean sprouts, 2 shrimp halves, 2 mint leaves, and a sprinkling of cilantro. Roll the rice paper sheet around the shrimp and veggies into a tight burrito shape. Repeat with the other 4 rice papers.

3. Slice the rolls in half and serve immediately with the almond dipping sauce.

Day 21—Weekend Day

BREAKFAST: Loaded Avocado Toast with Poached Eggs and Microgreens: toast two slices of bread, spread half an avocado on each piece, add 1 or 2 poached eggs (see page 234), and top with microgreens of your choice.

For the toast, you can opt for a low-net-carbohydrate bread like Barely Bread or a gluten-free fermented sourdough like Bread SRSLY or Coco Bakes, or make your own ketogenic Macadamia Nut Bread (page 272).

MACADAMIA NUT BREAD

Makes 1 loaf

Ghee or coconut oil, for the pan
½ cup whole raw macadamia nuts
½ cup whole raw cashew nuts
5 eggs
1 rounded teaspoon baking soda
1 cup coconut butter, softened
½ teaspoon sea salt
2 tablespoons freshly squeezed lemon juice

1. Preheat the oven to 350°F and grease a standard loaf pan with ghee or coconut oil.
2. In a food processor, blend the nuts into a chunky butter (a texture between chunky and smooth). While running the food processor, break 1 egg at a time and drop it down the chute. Wait until each egg is fully incorporated before adding the next. With the food processor still running, add the baking soda to fully combine. Turn off the machine, add the coconut butter and sea salt, and pulse (or turn on low) just a few times to mix. Add the lemon juice and pulse to combine.
3. Scrape the batter into the prepared loaf pan and bake for 35 minutes, until lightly brown on top. Let cool on the counter. Store the loaf in the refrigerator and slice as needed. Enjoy fresh or toasted.

LUNCH: Asian Crunch Salad (see the Plant-Based Devotee plan, page 311) with 4 cups shredded cooked chicken to up the protein (see the Easy Peasy Shredded Chicken recipe on page 254, or use a precooked rotisserie chicken).

SUNDAY FUNDAY: Get outside this afternoon. Fifteen minutes of sun exposure can allow your body to make the active form of vitamin D. Just be sure to wear sunscreen. Opt for brands that use zinc oxide (a mineral that is a physical blocker) and that are chemical-free. If you're looking for a bridge snack to bring along, try these Super Green Kale Chips.

SUPER GREEN KALE CHIPS

Makes 2 servings

½ bunch green kale, stemmed and torn into chip-size pieces
½ teaspoon extra virgin olive oil
¼ teaspoon Dr. Cowan's Threefold Blend Powder (see Tip)
⅛ teaspoon seasoned salt (I like M Salt) or pink Himalayan salt

1. Preheat the oven to 300°F.
2. Dry the kale completely and spread it in one layer on a rimmed baking sheet. Pour the olive oil onto your clean hands and massage the kale all over. Dust the kale with the vegetable powder and salt.
3. Bake until the edges of the kale are brown but not burned, 10 to 15 minutes. Store in a glass container in the pantry for up to a week.

TIP: Vegetable powders provide a sneaky way to get your family eating more vegetables, and because they are dehydrated, they retain a lot of their vitamins and minerals. My favorite brand, Dr. Cowan's, includes savory green vegetable powders with an addictive umami flavor that can be used to season roasted vegetables and proteins in addition to these kale chips. A little goes a long way, too, so the jars last for a few months.

DINNER

CHICKEN POT PIE SOUP WITH TAPIOCA FLOUR BISCUITS

The biscuits in this recipe are a healthy play on piecrust and give you a soft crunch and something to dip into the soup.

Makes 2 or 3 servings

¼ cup ghee
1 small yellow onion, cut into ¼-inch dice
2 celery stalks, cut into ¼-inch dice
2 carrots, cut into ¼-inch dice
½ cup frozen peas
1 bay leaf
3 garlic cloves, minced
4 small red potatoes, quartered
¼ cup extra-fine almond flour (or other gluten-free flour)
1 (24-ounce) package organic chicken bone broth
1½ cups unsweetened, unflavored almond milk
2 teaspoons chopped fresh thyme leaves
2 cups shredded cooked chicken (see Easy Peasy Shredded Chicken, page 254, or use precooked rotisserie chicken)
Pink Himalayan salt and freshly ground black pepper
1 tablespoon chopped fresh Italian parsley for garnish
Tapioca Flour Biscuits (recipe follows)

1. In a large pot, melt the ghee over medium heat. Add the onion, celery, carrots, peas, and bay leaf and sauté for 5 minutes, until the vegetables are softened.

2. Add the garlic, potatoes, and almond flour and cook for 2 minutes, stirring often, until the flour dissolves.

3. Stir in the chicken broth, almond milk, and thyme, bring the mixture to a simmer, then lower the heat and simmer for 20 minutes. Remove the bay leaf

and add the chicken. Season with salt and pepper to taste and serve garnished with chopped parsley along with the biscuits.

TAPIOCA FLOUR BISCUITS

Makes 14 to 16 biscuits

$^2/_3$ cup tapioca flour
1 cup extra-fine almond flour
$^1/_3$ cup coconut flour
2 teaspoons baking powder
$^1/_4$ teaspoon sea salt (I like Real Salt) or pink Himalayan salt
$^1/_3$ cup ghee or coconut oil, melted
2 eggs

1. Preheat the oven to 375°F and line a baking sheet with parchment paper. In a large bowl, combine all the flours, the baking powder, and the salt. Add the ghee and eggs and whisk lightly until smooth.
2. For each biscuit, scoop out 2 tablespoons of dough and form it into a thin, flat, biscuit shape. (Thinner is better, about ½ inch thick.)
3. Place the biscuits on the prepared pan and bake for 15 minutes, until lightly browned.
4. You can freeze the leftover biscuits for up to 3 months, but make sure they're at room temperature before freezing. To enjoy them again, just defrost on your kitchen counter and toast in the toaster or toaster oven, or in the oven at 350°F until warm, about 5 minutes.

GO FOR A FLOAT: Have you tried isolation or flotation therapy, where a comforting, zero-gravity environment is created in single-person, warm-water-filled tubs? An unhurried Sunday soak might be just what you need to prepare for the week ahead. See the Plant-Based Devotee plan, page 309, for more details.

8

PLANT-BASED DEVOTEE

BE TRUE TO YOURSELF AND THRIVE

AS I SAID IN the introduction, I'm a choose-your-own-adventure type of nutritionist. I want to help my clients live the lifestyles of their choice while still helping them reach their goals. The beauty of the Fab Four (and the science behind it) is that it allows you to do just that. Regardless of your lifestyle preference, the guiding principle is the same: to prioritize protein, fat, fiber, and greens at every meal. It's light structure that gives you the flexibility to eat and live the way you want.

One of the most common questions I received after *Body Love* was how to live the Fab Four lifestyle as a vegetarian or vegan. It is already largely plant-based, encouraging you to fill more than half your plate with whole food fats, nonstarchy fiber-rich vegetables, and leafy greens. But many readers wanted a deeper dive into plant-based proteins along with other Fab Four tips and tools designed for vegetarians or vegans. This type of feedback was encouraging because it meant I was reaching a broad spectrum of eaters who wanted to make the Fab Four their own.

I want to give everyone the science, tools, and guidance they need to live the way they want. It's what I do every day in my practice as a nutritionist and health coach.

I work with many people who are committed to a plant-based lifestyle (along with plenty who are plant-based much or most of the time). I've been touched by the passion and commitment they have for living and eating the way they do, which is why I chose the term *Plant-Based Devotee* to describe this archetype. Whatever your reasons are for choosing a vegetarian or vegan lifestyle, please know that I respect your decision and that I'm here to support your journey. I want to help you truly thrive. So, let me officially welcome you to the *Body Love* family. This chapter is for you, as well as anyone else looking for plant-based inspiration to add to their Fab Four repertoire.

At the outset, I want to highlight a few key things to be mindful of as a vegetarian or vegan.

The main issue that can arise with a plant-based lifestyle is developing nutrient deficiencies. The most common deficiency I see in my practice is with protein, which is not found in the same abundance or density in plant-based sources as in animal sources. Insufficient protein intake can make you feel hungry and affect your ability to maintain muscle mass. When I ask my plant-based clients to track their daily protein intake, many are below 0.5 gram per pound of body weight, or the minimum I want them to eat per day (see page 30). In the plan in this chapter, I've tried to create meals that offer adequate amounts of protein. However, depending on your unique body chemistry, weight, and other health factors, you might need to do something to add more protein to your day. One tool I use to help clients who are struggling to meet the minimum is to add an afternoon bridge snack, typically in the form of a Fab Four Smoothie (see Bridge Your Protein Gap with a Fab Four Smoothie, opposite).

Plants also lack certain vitamins and minerals found in animal proteins and other animal-based foods. A few other common deficiencies can include iron, B vitamins (B_{12} in particular), and vitamin D. In addition, I find that many of my Plant-Based Devotee clients tend to eat a limited number of foods, and that affects the range of nutrients they consume. Anyone eating an imbalanced diet runs a similar risk, but nutrient deficiencies can become a real health issue for vegetarians and vegans.

It's critical that you seek the advice and counsel of your physician or a functional medical doctor when it comes to nutrient deficiencies. They can call for a deficiency panel (a blood test), read and interpret your test results, and recommend specific supplements or multivitamins. From my perspective, there are a few things to focus on:

- Try to eat at least 0.5 gram of protein per pound of body weight per day.
- Source the most nutrient-dense foods you can.
- Introduce variety and color to your plate whenever possible.
- Use vitamin and mineral supplements on your doctor's advice if necessary.
- Add an afternoon Fab Four Smoothie if you're low on protein for the day.

Next, you need to be mindful of your sources of plant-based protein. I encourage you to return to chapter 1, page 47, which lays out my approach to plant-based proteins in more detail. Generally speaking, I prefer nuts, seeds, and beans/legumes for my Plant-Based Devotee clients. Although grains such as quinoa, buckwheat, and amaranth contain protein, they're mostly starchy carbohydrates. If you rely on them too heavily, you will continuously spike your blood sugar. Excessive grain consumption can lead to elevated insulin levels, imbalanced hunger hormones, and an erratic blood sugar curve. Just because you're a vegetarian

BRIDGE YOUR PROTEIN GAP WITH A FAB FOUR SMOOTHIE

A Fab Four Smoothie is a fast, nutritious, and scrumptious way to add 20 to 30 grams of protein to the day. A quick hack for this would be to double the recipe for your morning smoothie, then drink half for breakfast and take the other half with you in an insulated or stainless steel bottle (to keep it cold) for later. If you get hungry within two hours of a meal, feel lethargic or lack energy, or a quick calculation of your protein intake shows you're low for the day, you can give your bottle a shake and sip on your bridge smoothie.

GAIN INSIGHT WITH AN APP

Download the app called Cronometer. You enter the food you eat, and it returns a detailed breakdown of the nutritional content. I love this app because it positively reinforces eating nutrient-dense foods. As the day and week progress, it aggregates that data so you can see exactly which vitamins, minerals, and macronutrients you might not be getting enough of. It's not a substitute for consulting a physician or functional medical doctor, but it can give you some basic information about what you're eating and where you might be lacking nutritionally.

ADD COLORFUL VARIETY

Just like some of my clients' meals, I've noticed that some plant-based social media accounts and blogs are severely lacking in color. Often the meals pictured are a monotone of beige, brown, and white food (such as the vegan versions of waffles, pancakes, pasta, wraps, quinoa bowls, and baked goods). As you will recall from chapter 4, leafy greens and colorful vegetables are a key source of phytochemicals, vitamins, minerals, fiber, and water. If you're inspired by a dish or recipe in your feed but see that it lacks color, modify it by adding something from the fiber and greens chart on pages 93–101. That colorful variety is valuable. Remember, fill half your plate with fiber and greens.

PLANT-BASED "MEATS"

There are a lot of new plant-based "meats" on the market. Though they may seem like a quick way to reach your daily protein requirement, I generally advise my clients to avoid them. The ingredient list can include soy protein, gluten protein, and bad industrial seed oils. Recently, one major brand tested positive for glyphosate (a toxic pesticide) and its metabolite (AMPA) at several parts per billion. Research has shown that as little as a fraction of a part per billion can negatively affect over 4,000 genes, so this finding is very troubling.

or vegan doesn't mean you can't develop blood sugar–related health issues such as type 2 diabetes, metabolic syndrome, and PCOS. My view is that you should generally keep grains to ¼ to ½ cup per meal. If you have a specific weight loss or body composition goal, I would also keep grain consumption to once per day. As for soybeans and tofu, I don't recommend them because glyphosate residue and phytoestrogens within soy products are endocrine disruptors and have been linked to various health problems, including thyroid, reproduction, and skin issues.

From my standpoint as a nutritionist, eating enough protein is the most challenging part of a plant-based lifestyle. One of the easiest ways to boost your protein intake is with a Fab Four Smoothie. Between your protein powder, a fat like nut butter or avocado, and a few tablespoons of chia or flaxseeds, you can easily get 20 to 30 grams of protein to start your day.

Another key concept to be aware of is bioavailability. Plant-Based Devotees should take steps to limit the amount of so-called antinutrients in their food. Phytic acid and lectins are referred to as antinutrients because they block the absorption of vitamins and minerals. They may also cause digestive and other issues. Phytic acid is an enzyme inhibitor that binds with zinc, iron, and calcium in the gastrointestinal tract, making these minerals inaccessible. It is found in nuts, seeds, and beans/legumes.

Lectins are found in the skins or shells of plants and are especially problematic for people with poor gut health. They are highest in whole grains and beans/legumes. Ideally, you should soak your nuts and sprout your seeds, beans/legumes, and grains to help eliminate phytic acid and lectins, since these foods can make up so much of a plant-based diet. As you read through the plan in this chapter, you'll see recipes that can help you incorporate these techniques into your everyday cooking. (For techniques for soaking and sprouting and more information on bioavailability, see chapter 1, page 51, and chapter 4, page 114.)

TIP: You can always make sprouted beans and grains in bulk and then freeze them in ice cube trays. If you're looking for a little more substance for any meal, simply pop out a serving, defrost, and add it to the dish.

HOW TO SPROUT QUINOA

Quinoa is a healthy alternative to rice and also a complete protein. Although I don't recommend eating it at every single meal, it's still a good option for my plant-based clients. I always recommend sprouting quinoa.

1. Rinse the quinoa and place it in a glass sprouting jar with a breathable mesh lid. Add room temperature filtered water (enough to cover) and ½ teaspoon pink Himalayan sea salt. Screw the lid in place.

2. Let soak. A good rule of thumb is about 8 hours, but you can go as long as 12 hours (overnight) or as few as 4 hours.

3. Drain and discard the soak water by pouring it out through the mesh lid.

4. Refill with room temperature filtered water and rinse well by gently shaking the jar. Drain and discard the water through the mesh lid again.

5. Invert the jar and lay it at an angle so that air can circulate and excess water can fully drain out, about 5 minutes. Place the jar upright. Repeat this step three or four times per day for two to three days.

(continued)

6. Within a couple days, the quinoa should begin to sprout. Let the sprouts grow to at least ¼ inch and up to 2 inches.

7. Rinse the sprouts well and store them in an airtight jar with a solid lid in the refrigerator. Enjoy them within 2 to 3 days and eat the whole thing—the quinoa and the sprout.

PLAN OVERVIEW

THE FAB FOUR SMOOTHIE IS A UNIVERSAL FORMULA

Every single Fab Four Smoothie recipe in this book and in *Body Love* can be made vegetarian or vegan. All you have to do is use a plant-based protein powder. That's it. If you want more recipe inspiration, flip back to the Girl on the Go and Domestic Goddess plans. Together they offer twenty-one unique, great-tasting flavors to choose from. *Body Love* has fifty flavors as well.

In the plan and sample days that follow, I'll give you a bunch of delicious recipes, practical tips, and guidance for a plant-based Fab Four lifestyle. My hope is that you can find both the inspiration and information to live and eat the way you want. I want all my Plant-Based Devotees out there to stay healthy, nourished, and hit their goals. The plan will help you thrive, reduce nutrient deficiencies, balance your plate to stay full, and increase the bioavailability and diversity of the nutrients you consume.

The plan also comes with delicious new Fab Four Smoothie recipes such as Sweet Spiced Carrot Cake (page 284), Matcha Limeade Green (page 295), Ginger Lemonade (page 302), Blackberry Kale (page 310), Brainiac (page 318), Super Seed (page 321), Raspberry Lemonade (page 325), Chlorophyll Mint (page 336), and Coconut Turmeric (page 344).

Day 1—Weekday

MORNING MOVEMENT: Choose a thirty- to sixty-minute workout that involves weight lifting, kettlebells, resistance, or strength training. A couple of class options include yoga with weights or a HIIT class (which combines aerobic and anaerobic exercise). Strength training helps tone, tighten, and build lean muscle mass. The point is to get an anaerobic workout that makes your muscles sore. This can help increase insulin sensitivity, lower blood sugar levels, and increase your metabolism.

TIP: If you tend to hit snooze more than you would like to admit, you might be battling the effects of sleep inertia, a physiological state of slower cognition and motor skills right when you wake up. Feeling groggy, foggy, and a little clumsy obviously isn't ideal for a weight training day! If you're a serial snoozer, consider purchasing a wake-up-light alarm clock, which uses light instead of sound to help you wake up more naturally. It will gradually get brighter, simulating the sunrise, and in the process can help lessen the effects of sleep inertia. The light slowly syncs to your circadian rhythm so you wake up alert and ready to work out. You can find a bunch of affordable light alarm clocks online.

BREAKFAST: The beauty of my smoothie formula is that it works for any lifestyle, from keto to paleo to raw vegan and everything in between. For any Fab Four Smoothie recipe, you simply swap the protein powder to fit your preference. For my Plant-Based Devotees, I prefer certified organic pea protein and minimal plant-based blends. See page 61 for more details.

ANAEROBIC EXERCISE CAN HELP MAINTAIN MUSCLE MASS

To help build and maintain muscle mass, vegetarians and vegans who might be consuming lower amounts of protein should regularly incorporate anaerobic exercises into their workout routine, such as weight lifting, kettle-bells, resistance, or strength training. A couple of class options include yoga with weights or a HIIT class (which combines aerobic and anaerobic exercise). You want to exert your muscles and make them sore. These types of workouts have been found to increase IGF1 gene expression with an increased protein synthesis after two to four hours. In other words, if you lift weights, the hormone IGF1 can help you retain and build new muscle. Anaerobic exercise and lean muscle mass also help increase insulin sensitivity, lower blood sugar levels, and increase your metabolism. In the plan in this chapter, there are three suggested strength training days: Day 1 kicks things off strong; Day 8 suggests working out with a friend, partner, or trainer if you need added motivation; and Day 15 gives you a home-based option.

BREAKFAST

SWEET SPICED CARROT CAKE FAB FOUR SMOOTHIE

Let's kick things off with a new recipe inspired by sweet, spice-scented carrot cake.

Vanilla protein powder containing 20 to 30 grams protein
1 tablespoon almond butter
1 tablespoon flaxseeds
1 cup chopped raw carrots
1½ teaspoons ground cinnamon (see Tip, page 247)
1 to 2 cups unsweetened almond milk

Place all the ingredients in a high-speed blender and blend to your desired consistency.

LUNCH

AVOCADO BEAN SALAD

This is a great plant-based alternative to egg salad. White beans easily take on the herb and red onion flavors, and an avocado can replace egg-based mayonnaise. It makes a great lunch served over a bed of arugula, with a few gluten-free crackers or a slice of gluten-free toast.

TIP: If you do make this recipe in bulk, squeeze a little lemon juice on top to keep the avocado from turning brown.

Makes 2 servings

2 avocados, diced
⅓ cup finely chopped parsley
⅓ cup finely chopped dill

⅓ cup finely chopped chives

2 celery stalks, finely chopped

2 tablespoons finely chopped red onion, soaked for 5 minutes in cold water, drained and rinsed

2 tablespoons vegan mayonnaise (optional)

1 cup canned or cooked white beans, drained and rinsed (see page 52)

Pink Himalayan salt and freshly ground black pepper

In a large bowl, combine the avocado, parsley, dill, chives, celery, onion, and mayonnaise (if using). Slowly stir in the white beans and gently smash them until blended. Season to taste with salt and pepper.

DINNER

PESTO ZOODLES AND HEMP HEARTS

This clean, simple recipe can be served warm or at room temperature. The pesto flavor is up to you—the recipe can be customized five different ways.

Makes 1 serving

1 zucchini, zoodled

½ cup heirloom cherry tomatoes

1 tablespoon extra virgin olive oil

3 tablespoons Presto Pesto (flavor of choice; recipe follows)

2 tablespoons hemp hearts

1. To serve warm, in a large pan over medium-low heat, sauté the zoodles and tomatoes in the oil for 5 minutes, until the zoodles are tender and the tomatoes are blistered. Turn off the heat, stir in the pesto, and sprinkle with hemp hearts.

2. To serve at room temperature, combine all the ingredients in a medium bowl. Let the mixture marinate for 5 to 10 minutes before serving.

(continued)

PRESTO PESTO

Making homemade pesto is quick and easy. This is my body-loving formula, which you can customize as you wish. The nuts, oils, and herbs are up to you.

2 garlic cloves, minced
¼ cup nuts (see below)
2 cups herbs or greens (see below)
Juice of ½ lemon (optional)
¼ to ½ cup finely grated or crumbled cheese (optional)
½ cup oil (see below)
Red pepper flakes, minced jalapeño, or freshly ground black pepper (optional)

CLASSIC BASIL: Use pine nuts, basil, and extra virgin olive oil.
POPEYE: Use shelled pistachios, spinach, and avocado oil (optional cheese: Parmigiano-Reggiano).
SPICY TACO: Use walnuts, cilantro, and extra virgin olive oil (optional cheese: cotija).
CRUCIFEROUS PUNCH: Use cashews, arugula, and extra virgin olive oil (optional cheese: pecorino).
FRESH HERB: Use pine nuts, mint and basil, and extra virgin olive oil.

1. Pulse the garlic in a food processor to mince it. Let sit for 10 to 15 minutes (see Reminder).
2. Add the nuts and herbs of your choice and, if you're using them, the lemon juice and cheese.
3. Turn on the food processor and pour the oil and spices of your choice (if using) through the chute. Process until the mixture is in small, fine chunks. Refrigerate if you don't use it immediately.

REMINDER: If a recipe calls for garlic, mince or chop the garlic, then let it rest for ten or fifteen minutes. This will allow for the production of allicin, a phytochemical responsible for garlic's anti-inflammatory, anticancer, and immune-boosting properties.

REMINDER: Mixing up your plant-based protein throughout the day can help ensure you're getting a variety of amino acids. As stated in chapter 1, I don't think you need to rigidly pair proteins at every single meal. Pairing is done to create a *complete* protein meal, or one with all nine essential amino acids. However, your liver absorbs essential amino acids, and as long as you're eating a mix of proteins throughout the day, studies have shown that you don't need to pair proteins at every single meal. The key is not to get stuck eating one source over and over. If you had a bean/legume lunch, try to use nuts or seeds at dinner, and generally rotate through all three.

BREW A HOT TEA: One way I wind down at the end of the day is to brew a hot herbal tea after dinner. The ritual of sipping steaming, comforting tea in the evening can help reduce cravings, calm the body, and even support sounder sleep. Three to try include chamomile, which contains apigenin, an antioxidant that promotes sleep; valerian root, which increases levels of GABA, a neurotransmitter needed for sleep (the smell of valerian root can turn some people off, so you can also take GABA in supplement form); and lavender, which has a relaxing aroma.

> **BACK TO BODY LOVE**
>
> For additional Fab Four sauces, dressings, and dips that are vegetarian or vegan, you can always go back to *Body Love*, which has simple recipes like Pistachio Mint Pesto, Cilantro Pesto, Chimichurri Sauce, Lemon Aioli, Roasted Garlic Cashew Cream Sauce, Fab Four Vinaigrette, Dill Ranch Dressing, Lemon Vinaigrette, Homemade Hummus, and Avocado Hummus.

Day 2—Weekday

BREAKFAST: Spices are a great way to increase the nutritional density of your Fab Four Smoothie. Yesterday we incorporated cinnamon. Today let's add ground cloves, turmeric, and black pepper to make a warming Anti-Inflammatory Vanilla Spice Fab Four Smoothie. See the recipe in the Domestic Goddess plan, page 246.

LUNCH

RIBBONED RAINBOW SALAD OVER SPROUTED SUNFLOWER SEED HUMMUS

This dish is a perfect example of what I mean when I encourage you to add colorful variety to your plate.

Makes 1 serving

1 teaspoon apple cider vinegar
1 tablespoon extra virgin olive oil
1 zucchini or summer squash
1 heirloom carrot
1 cucumber
2 cups arugula
1 watermelon radish, thinly sliced
1 tablespoon hemp hearts
Sprouted Sunflower Seed Hummus (recipe follows)

1. In a large bowl, whisk the vinegar and olive oil to emulsify.
2. Using a vegetable peeler, peel the squash, carrot, and cucumber into long ribbons. Add the arugula, radish, vegetable ribbons, and hemp hearts to the dressing and toss to coat thoroughly. Serve over 2 to 4 tablespoons of Sprouted Sunflower Seed Hummus.

SPROUTED SUNFLOWER SEED HUMMUS

Makes about 1¼ cups

Hummus doesn't always need to be made with beans, and I'm excited about this seed-based variation.

1 cup raw, unsalted sunflower seeds (I like NOW Foods brand)
1 to 2 garlic cloves
2 tablespoons tahini
Juice of ½ lemon
Pink Himalayan salt
2 tablespoons extra virgin olive oil
⅛ teaspoon cayenne pepper (optional)

1. Soak the sunflower seeds overnight in a half-gallon sprouting jar (you can find this online; NOW Foods has a good option). The next day, drain and rinse through the mesh lid until the water runs clear, then leave on the counter to sprout. When the first small sprouts start to form after 8 to 12 hours, it's time to make the hummus. Rinse and drain the sprouts. (If you don't see any sprouts forming, drain the jar and let it sit on the counter for a second night. Repeat the drain and rinse process the next day.)

2. Pulse the garlic in the food processor to mince it. Let it sit for 10 to 15 minutes (see Reminder, page 286). Add the sprouted sunflower seeds, tahini, lemon juice, and a pinch of salt. Turn on the food processor and pour the olive oil slowly through the chute, then add another pinch of salt and the cayenne (if you like your hummus spicy hot). Process until smooth. If you prefer a fluffier hummus, add a small amount of cold filtered water (from 2 tablespoons to ½ cup) until your desired consistency is reached.

DINNER

SPICY VEGAN BLACK BEAN TACOS

Increase the phytochemical content of your Taco Tuesday by making a black bean and vegetable filling.

Makes 2 servings

BLACK BEAN AND VEGETABLE FILLING

1 teaspoon extra virgin olive oil

1 garlic clove, minced

½ yellow or red onion, finely diced

2 cups mixed ¼-inch-diced vegetables (my favorite mix: carrot, zucchini, squash, and cauliflower)

1½ cups canned black beans, drained and rinsed, or Pressure-Cooked Dry Beans (recipe follows)

1½ teaspoons chili powder

½ teaspoon smoked paprika

½ teaspoon ground cumin

¼ teaspoon pink Himalayan salt

¼ teaspoon freshly ground black pepper

⅛ teaspoon cayenne pepper

¼ cup filtered water

TACO ASSEMBLY

8 to 10 Bibb or iceberg lettuce leaves

1 avocado, smashed

¼ cup heirloom tomatoes, halved

¼ cup salsa of choice

1. In a large skillet over medium heat, heat the olive oil until shimmering. Add the garlic and onion and sauté until soft, 4 to 5 minutes. Add the diced vegetables and sauté for 4 to 5 minutes, until fork tender. Add the black beans, all the spices, and the water and stir to coat. Cook, stirring occasionally, until the

beans are heated through and any water from the vegetables has evaporated, 2 to 3 minutes. Serve chunky or pulse in a food processor for 30 seconds to make smoother.

2. To assemble the tacos, spoon the filling into the lettuce "shells" and top with the avocado, tomato, and salsa.

PRESSURE-COOKED DRY BEANS

Whenever you cook dry beans, it's important to take steps to reduce their antinutrient content. One way is soaking; for details about how and why, see chapter 1, page 50. Another great option is to use a pressure cooker. Pressure-cooking reduces antinutrients in under an hour and is an affordable way to prepare beans in bulk.

Makes 6 to 8 servings

1 pound dry beans, rinsed
1 tablespoon extra virgin olive oil
2 garlic cloves
1 bay leaf
½ white onion (optional)
1 teaspoon pink Himalayan salt
8 cups filtered water

Combine all the ingredients in a pressure cooker or Instant Pot that's at least 10-quart size. Cook on high pressure for 30 minutes (for black and pinto beans) or 40 minutes (for chickpeas) and let the pressure release naturally. Rinse and drain the beans and remove and discard the bay leaf, onion, and garlic.

KITCHEN JAM: Self-care can be as simple as remembering to turn on some music while you make dinner. Like good food, good music has a way of calming and comforting us. Tonight, pair Taco Tuesday with a kitchen jam. If today was trying, pick a song that soothes you. If today was easy breezy, have some fun. Or pick a song that takes you back to a special memory. Don't be shy, you're allowed to sing out loud and dance, too. If you need a reminder, put a portable speaker near your prep area.

Day 3—Weekday

MORNING MOVEMENT: Breathe, sweat, and clear your mind with a yoga class. Personally, I love a Vinyasa class where the music is bumping and the playlist is filled with an inspiring mix of pop, hip-hop, rock, and R&B. If you're hyperflexible (either naturally or because you practice a lot), it can be tempting to show off a little and extend into super-deep poses. Instead, try to focus on your alignment and engaging the proper muscles to support the pose. It will yield better body composition results, prevent injury, and help keep that ego in check! (If you're not into yoga, the principle remains the same with other kinds of exercise, which can all become ego-driven if you're not careful.)

BREAKFAST: Mix up the fat in your smoothie by using extra virgin olive oil instead of a nut butter. EVOO is brain-healthy and anti-inflammatory. The perfect recipe to try this in is my Dark Chocolate Olive Oil Sea Salt (see the Girl on the Go plan, page 189).

LUNCH

CREAMY COCONUT BROCCOLI SOUP WITH WATERCRESS AND SPICY PEPITAS

One way to add to your daily intake of phytonutrients is to garnish your favorite soup or dip with a leafy green such as watercress or a microgreen variety. Another garnishing trick is to use a flavorful roasted seed mix like the spicy one in this recipe. It will not only repli-

cate a crouton crunch, but the added protein and fat from the mix will help keep you full and fueled.

Makes 4 to 6 servings

2 tablespoons extra virgin olive oil
2 garlic cloves, peeled and crushed
2 shallots, finely chopped
1 broccoli head, trimmed and cut into florets
½ cup ¼-inch-diced celery
½ cup ¼-inch-diced carrot (optional)
3 cups vegetable stock
½ cup full-fat coconut milk
2 tablespoons nutritional yeast
1 teaspoon pink Himalayan salt
½ teaspoon freshly ground black pepper
Toppings: handful of watercress and 2 tablespoons Go Raw Spicy Fiesta Sprouted
    Seed Mix (pepitas and sunflower seeds)

1. In a medium saucepan over medium heat, heat the olive oil until shimmering. Add the garlic and shallots and sauté until soft, 4 to 5 minutes. Add the broccoli, celery, carrot (if using), and stock and bring to a rolling boil. Cover, turn the heat to low, and simmer for 10 minutes, until the vegetables are fork tender. Stir in the coconut milk, nutritional yeast, salt, and pepper. Using an immersion blender, puree to the desired consistency.
2. Top with the watercress and sprouted seed mix.

TIP: Flavor is always important, but texture also plays a role in making a meal enjoyable. If you don't use the sprouted seed mix suggested above, try roasting or pan-frying cooked chickpeas to add a warm, crispy texture. Use a clean cooking oil (such as avocado) and your favorite spices.

DINNER

VEGAN CAULIFLOWER RICE BOWL WITH AVOCADO AND CRISPY HARISSA CHICKPEAS

This vegan rice bowl is topped with buttery avocado and spiced, crispy chickpeas. The textures and spice add interest to every bite.

Makes 1 serving

½ cup canned or cooked chickpeas (page 291), drained and rinsed
1 tablespoon avocado oil
1 tablespoon organic harissa seasoning (or 1½ teaspoons smoked paprika)
2 cups chopped stemmed kale
1 garlic clove, minced
1 cup cooked cauliflower rice (see page 315)
½ avocado, sliced or diced

1. Pat the chickpeas dry with a paper towel. In a skillet over medium heat, combine the oil, chickpeas, and harissa. Cook for 4 to 6 minutes, stirring often to crisp all sides of the chickpeas. Using a slotted spoon, move the chickpeas to a plate covered with a paper towel.
2. Add the kale and garlic to the pan and cook until the kale is wilted, 2 to 3 minutes, stirring often.
3. Layer the cauliflower rice, crispy chickpeas, kale, and avocado in a bowl, and enjoy warm.

PHONES DOWN: Raise your hand if you're not proud of the amount of time you spend on your phone and social media. I'm not, and I'd venture to bet you aren't either. And recent research from the Centers for Disease Control isn't pretty, with smartphone use being linked to a 12 percent increase in anxiety and depression.

Taking one night off won't resolve the issue, but I think it's a good practice to put your phone down for some portion of the night, even if it's only twenty or thirty minutes. There's no shortage of healthy, productive, and creative ways to spend that time. If you want to break your phone habit (or addiction), one resource to check out is the book *How to Break Up with Your Phone* by Catherine Price. And if social media is giving you anxiety, making you feel depressed, or negatively affecting you mentally or emotionally, please seek help from a mental health professional. Our feeds are such a huge part of our lives today that they can create problems just as big. One resource to help you find someone to talk to is www.womenshealth.gov/mental-health. I've gone to therapy during a few difficult periods in my life, and I've found it immensely helpful.

Day 4—Weekday

BREAKFAST

MATCHA LIMEADE GREEN FAB FOUR SMOOTHIE

Try using an herbal tea, spa water, or homemade lemonade or limeade as the liquid in your smoothie, like in this pretty green smoothie. It will increase your water consumption, lower your intake of gums and emulsifiers from nut milks, and might save you a few bucks.

Vanilla protein powder containing 20 to 30 grams protein
½ small avocado
1 tablespoon chia seeds
Handful of spinach
2 cups Matcha Limeade (page 296)

Place all the ingredients in a high-speed blender and blend to your desired consistency.

(continued)

HOMEMADE LEMONADES AND SPA WATERS

Below are five homemade lemonades and spa waters that are a breeze to make—just stir all the ingredients together. You can keep them in a pitcher in the refrigerator or use them in a Fab Four Smoothie like Matcha Limeade Green (page 295), Ginger Lemonade (page 302), Raspberry Lemonade (page 325), or Chlorophyll Mint (page 336).

Makes 2 to 3 servings

MATCHA LIMEADE
2 teaspoons matcha green tea powder
Juice of 2 or 3 limes
4 to 5 cups filtered water
Stevia or monk fruit sweetener to taste (optional)

APPLE CIDER VINEGAR LEMONADE
2 tablespoons apple cider vinegar
Juice of 2 or 3 lemons
4 to 5 cups filtered water
Stevia or monk fruit sweetener to taste (optional)

SILICA ACV LEMON WATER
1 teaspoon food-grade diatomaceous earth (don't worry, it's flavorless)
1/2 teaspoon apple cider vinegar
Juice of 1 lemon
4 to 5 cups filtered water

CHLOROPHYLL MINT WATER
1 teaspoon NOW Foods Liquid Chlorophyll
Handful of peppermint leaves
4 to 5 cups filtered water

SPA WATER BLENDS
1 cup sliced fruit or herbs in your preferred combination (such as lemon, cucumber, and mint; strawberry and basil; or orange and grapefruit)
4 to 5 cups filtered water

LUNCH

NUTTY VEGGIE ROLLS

If you're having salad fatigue, one way to mix up your routine is by packaging your greens as a wrap. Some wrapper ideas include collard greens, a coconut wrap, or rice paper, as in this veggie roll. It is an easy homemade version of what you might see at a sushi bar, and it packs a nice protein punch, too, courtesy of the nut-based sauce—it contributes about 15 grams all on its own!—and hemp hearts.

Makes 2 servings

NUTTY SAUCE
2 tablespoons almond or peanut butter
2 tablespoons coconut aminos
Juice of ½ small lime (about 2 tablespoons)
1 garlic clove, minced
1 teaspoon sriracha, or to taste
1 teaspoon red pepper flakes
3 tablespoons hemp hearts
2 to 3 tablespoons filtered water

VEGGIE ROLLS
4 round rice paper wrappers
4 romaine leaves
1 cup shredded carrots
1 cup thinly sliced cucumber
½ avocado, cut into 4 slices

1. To make the sauce, combine all the ingredients in a medium bowl, starting with 2 tablespoons filtered water, and whisk until smooth. If you want a thinner consistency, stir in up to 1 tablespoon additional water.

2. To make the rolls, fill a large bowl with lukewarm water and set a damp dish towel

(continued)

on a cutting board. Immerse 1 rice paper sheet in the water for 15 to 20 seconds. Remove, shake off the excess water, and lay it flat on towel. Place 1 piece of the lettuce in the center of the rice paper. On the lettuce, place ¼ cup each of the carrots and cucumber and 1 slice of the avocado. Tightly roll the paper around the veggies. Repeat with the remaining three wrappers.

3. Serve the rolls with the sauce.

DINNER

BLACK LENTIL KALI MASOOR DAL

Digestive spices like cumin, coriander, and turmeric make the perfect pairing for beans and legumes, which have the potential to make some people feel bloated (see Bean Bloat, opposite). This dish made with black lentils is full of spices and was inspired by the many delicious flavors of India.

Makes 2 servings

2 tablespoons extra virgin olive oil (or grass-fed butter or ghee)
1 medium yellow onion, finely chopped
1 tablespoon finely chopped fresh ginger
2 garlic cloves, finely chopped
½ teaspoon ground cumin
1 teaspoon ground chili powder
1 teaspoon ground coriander
¼ teaspoon ground turmeric
½ teaspoon garam masala
1 cup finely diced or pureed tomatoes
1 teaspoon pink Himalayan salt
1½ cups dried black lentils
3 cups filtered water
Optional toppings: 1 tablespoon coconut cream, fresh cilantro

1. In a pressure cooker or Instant Pot on medium heat, heat the oil and sauté the onion, ginger, and garlic until the onion is translucent, about 2 minutes. Add the cumin, chili powder, coriander, turmeric, and garam masala and stir until aromatic, about 1 minute. Add the tomatoes and salt and cook, stirring, until the water evaporates and you see oil on the bottom of the pressure cooker. Add the lentils and water and stir to combine.

2. Secure the lid with the release valve closed. Cook on manual for 20 minutes, then do a natural release.

3. Serve the dal in a bowl with your choice of toppings.

> ## BEAN BLOAT
>
> Do beans cause you to bloat or give you digestive discomfort? To help ease the situation, try soaking them or cooking them in a pressure cooker. You can also season and cook them with digestive spices (such as cumin, coriander, ginger, turmeric, and fennel) or try using a piece of seaweed in the cooking water. Some beans/legumes (such as lentils and mung beans) are lower in starch and sugar, which might also help.

Day 5—Weekday

JUST MOVE: The workout tools and tips listed in this book are here to help you find the type of workout(s) you will love and commit to. We can debate the pros and cons of every type of workout, but one is always better than none! Keep it simple today and just go for a brisk walk. Aim for at least twenty-five minutes.

BREAKFAST: Before the weekend starts, reap the detoxifying benefits of broccoli sprouts and celery with my favorite new detox smoothie, the Super Green Machine (see the Girl on the Go plan, page 174).

LUNCH

BRAINIAC SALAD

Take advantage of some of the most brain-healthy plant-based foods found in nature with this supercharged salad.

Makes 1 serving

1 tablespoon extra virgin olive oil
1 tablespoon freshly squeezed lemon juice
2 cups baby spinach
2 cups baby kale
½ avocado, diced
¼ cup blueberries
1 tablespoon hemp hearts
1 tablespoon chopped walnuts

In a salad bowl, whisk the olive oil and lemon juice. Top with the other ingredients and toss to coat.

DINNER

ALMOND PAD THAI WITH SHIRATAKI NOODLES

Eating a plant-based diet doesn't prevent metabolic syndrome, insulin resistance, or diabetes. I've worked with vegetarian and vegan clients who have been diagnosed with such conditions. Every case is different, but in general if you overeat processed, acellular carbohydrates, you put yourself at risk. I urge my clients to fill their plates with fiber and greens first and then incorporate lower-carbohydrate-density options for better blood sugar balance. For example, swap out pasta for zoodled vegetables—or use shirataki noodles, as in this tasty dish. Shirataki noodles are healthy noodles made from the glucomannan (fiber) of the konjac plant.

Makes 2 servings

2 tablespoons coconut oil

2 cups broccoli florets

2 cups shredded peeled carrots

½ red pepper, thinly sliced

½ cup peas

6 tablespoons coconut aminos

2 tablespoons smooth almond butter

2 tablespoons filtered water

1 (7-ounce) package Miracle Noodle Fettuccine Shirataki Noodles, prepared according to package instructions

¼ cup thinly sliced green onions

2 tablespoons sesame seeds

1. In a large skillet over medium-high heat, heat the coconut oil. Add the broccoli, carrots, red pepper, and peas and sauté until tender, 6 to 8 minutes.

2. Whisk the coconut aminos, almond butter, and water in a small bowl.

3. Add the shirataki noodles and amino blend to the skillet and mix to incorporate. Top with the green onions and sesame seeds.

PRACTICE GRATITUDE: Each week is its own adventure . . . or roller coaster. Whether the past five days have been smooth sailing or filled with one challenge after another, take a moment to reflect on what you're thankful and grateful for in your life. See the Girl on the Go plan, page 170.

Day 6—Weekend Day

FRESH-AIR CARDIO: Find some fresh air and get outside for a thirty- to sixty-minute run, hike, or bike ride. If it's the middle of winter or the weather is poor, don't let that stop you from logging some type of cardio workout. A few indoor options: use the elliptical machine at the gym, take a class on your favorite app, or sign up for a Spin class.

BREAKFAST

GINGER LEMONADE FAB FOUR SMOOTHIE

Use the Apple Cider Vinegar Lemonade recipe from Day 4 to make this smoothie.

Vanilla protein powder containing 20 to 30 grams protein
1 tablespoon cashew butter
1 tablespoon acacia fiber (I use NOW Foods)
1 teaspoon ground ginger
Juice of ½ lemon
Handful of spinach
2 cups Apple Cider Vinegar Lemonade (page 296)

Place all the ingredients in a high-speed blender and blend to your desired consistency.

LUNCH

FALAFEL COLLARD WRAP

This yummy wrap offers another great use for the Sprouted Sunflower Seed Hummus you made on Day 2. Falafel is good protein to add to a wrap or salad, and it can also be dipped into a fat-based sauce.

Makes 6 servings

FALAFEL

1½ cups pressure-cooked chickpeas, drained and rinsed (see Tip, page 291)

2 tablespoons tahini

1 tablespoon sprouted chickpea flour or milled chia seeds (I use Thrive Market or NOW Foods)

2 garlic cloves, minced

½ cup fresh Italian parsley

½ cup fresh cilantro

1 tablespoon lemon juice

¼ teaspoon ground cumin

¼ teaspoon ground coriander

1 teaspoon pink Himalayan salt

WRAP

1 collard leaf, cleaned and trimmed

2 tablespoons diced tomato

1 tablespoon diced red onion

¼ red pepper, sliced into thin strips

1 tablespoon Sprouted Sunflower Seed Hummus (page 289)

1 tablespoon Classic Basil Pesto (page 286)

1. Preheat the oven to 400°F. Line a baking sheet with parchment paper.
2. In a food processor, combine all the falafel ingredients and process until smooth. Form the mixture into 12 small balls and place them on the prepared

(continued)

sheet. Bake for 15 to 20 minutes, turning them halfway through, until slightly browned.

3. To assemble the wrap, lay out a collard leaf and place 2 falafel balls on it. Layer on the tomato, onion, red pepper, hummus, and pesto. Roll tightly and serve.

4. You can store the extra falafel balls in the refrigerator in a sealable glass container for up to 4 days or in the freezer for up to 6 months.

DINNER

VEGETABLE AND CAULIFLOWER RICE SOUP

Making a batch—or maybe a double batch—of a warming, hearty, and fiber-rich vegetable soup like this one over the weekend is a great way to set yourself up for success during the week. It can be a bridge snack to help you avoid processed snack foods, or quickly heated for a last-minute weeknight dinner, or frozen for the future to prevent "Not So Fab" takeout orders.

Makes 4 servings

2 tablespoons extra virgin olive oil
½ yellow onion, cut into ¼-inch dice
4 garlic cloves, minced
2 cups ½-inch-diced celery
2 cups small broccoli florets
2 cups ½-inch-diced zucchini
2 cups ½-inch-diced carrots
1 yellow and 1 red bell pepper, cut into ½-inch dice
1 (12-ounce) bag frozen or uncooked cauliflower rice (see page 315)
2 (1-quart) boxes organic vegetable broth
1 (13-ounce) box crushed tomatoes
2 cups finely chopped kale

Pink Himalayan salt

1 teaspoon smoked paprika (optional)

1 teaspoon dried parsley, or 2 tablespoons freshly minced parsley (optional)

1 teaspoon ground cumin (optional)

1 teaspoon chili powder (optional)

1. In a large pot over medium-low heat, heat the olive oil. Add the onion and garlic and sweat (cook without coloring) until tender. Add the celery, broccoli, zucchini, carrots, peppers, and the cauliflower rice, increase the heat to medium, and cook for 6 to 8 minutes, or until the vegetables are fork tender, stirring occasionally. Add the broth and bring to a boil, then turn down the heat to a simmer and cook for 6 to 8 minutes.

2. Blend half of the crushed tomatoes into a puree and pour them into the soup to thicken the broth. Add the remaining crushed tomatoes to the soup to add chunks. Stir in the kale and simmer for 1 to 2 minutes to wilt, then season to taste with salt. If you like more spice, add the smoked paprika, parsley, cumin, and chili powder.

TIP: Some of my clients are predominately plant-based, but they will from time to time incorporate collagen and bone broth. If you fall into this camp, consider swapping out your vegetable broth for chicken bone broth, which contains the amino acids glycine and proline.

CONDIMENT COLLECTION: Overhauling your kitchen and pantry doesn't need to happen overnight, but removing the sugary condiments you've collected is a great place to start. Attack those fridge doors and write a grocery list of BWBK-approved condiments to stock up on.

Day 7—Weekend Day

BREAKFAST: If you're vegetarian and in the mood for a warm egg breakfast, try one of these dishes from the Domestic Goddess plan: Farmers' Market Frittata (page 210), Eggs Benedict (page 233), Southwest Scramble (page 239), Sweet Potato Hash and Egg Bake (page 268), or Loaded Avocado Toast with Poached Eggs and Microgreens (page 271).

If you're vegan, choose a Fab Four Smoothie or make one into a bowl. Flip through the other plans and try something new. All you have to do is use your plant-based protein powder. Here's a sampling of what you'll find:

GIRL ON THE GO: Green Ginger (page 161), Cookies and Cream (page 163), Chocolate Walnut (page 171), Super Green Machine (page 174), Pecan Pie (page 177), Happy Gut (page 181), and Dark Chocolate Olive Oil Sea Salt (page 189).

DOMESTIC GODDESS: Green Smoothie Bowl (page 204), Triple Chocolate Crunch (page 218), Green Goddess (page 221), Turmeric Almond Bliss (page 237), Anti-Inflammatory Vanilla Spice (page 246), Creamy Mocha (page 264), and Sweet and Savory Basil (page 266).

LUNCH

VEGAN KALE CAESAR WITH CRISPY SMOKED CHICKPEAS

This vegan kale salad, with its creamy dressing and crispy toppings of chickpeas and garlicky nuts, is a satisfying twist on a classic Caesar salad.

Makes 1 serving

CRISPY CHICKPEAS
2 tablespoons avocado oil
½ cup cooked or canned chickpeas, rinsed and patted dry

½ teaspoon smoked paprika
Pink Himalayan salt and freshly ground black pepper

GARLICKY NUT CRUMBLES
1 garlic clove
1 tablespoon extra virgin olive oil
2 tablespoons raw cashew nuts
2 tablespoons hemp hearts
Pink Himalayan salt

SALAD AND DRESSING
2 tablespoons vegan mayonnaise
1 tablespoon freshly squeezed lemon juice
½ teaspoon Dijon mustard
½ teaspoon garlic powder
2 cups chopped stemmed kale
½ cup chopped radicchio
Optional topping: shredded nut cheese of choice

1. To prepare the crispy chickpeas, in a large skillet, heat the oil until shimmering over medium-high heat. Rub the chickpeas with the smoked paprika and fry them, stirring occasionally, until they're crispy, 3 to 5 minutes. Transfer them to a paper towel-lined plate and let them cool and dry. Season with salt and pepper. (Another option is to bake the seasoned chickpeas on a baking sheet at 350°F for 30 minutes, stirring halfway through.)

2. To make the garlicky nut crumbles, in a food processor, pulse the garlic, olive oil, and cashews to combine. Sprinkle with the hemp hearts and a pinch of salt, and hand mix. You can store any extra crumbles in a sealed glass container in the refrigerator for up to a week.

3. To assemble the salad and dressing, in a large bowl, whisk the mayonnaise, lemon juice, mustard, and garlic powder. Add the kale and radicchio and toss to coat. Add the fried chickpeas and nut crumbles and toss again. Top with a nut cheese of your choice if desired.

DINNER

STACKED EGGPLANT PARMESAN

My husband loves Italian dishes, especially on a Sunday night. This is one clean recipe he's requested on multiple occasions.

Makes 2 servings

1 to 2 teaspoons unmodified potato starch (see page 91)

1 tablespoon pink Himalayan salt

2 eggs, whisked (for vegetarians) or ½ cup aquafaba (for vegans; see Tip)

2 cups gluten-free panko bread crumbs

2 tablespoons Simply Organic Italian seasoning (or 2 teaspoons each dried thyme, oregano, and parsley)

2 medium Japanese eggplants, cut into ½-inch slices and patted dry

2 tablespoons avocado oil

2 cups marinara or arrabbiata sauce (I like Rao's or Thrive Market brands)

1 cup Parmesan or soft nut cheese (I like Kite Hill)

¼ cup fresh basil leaves

2 tablespoons dried oregano

2 tablespoons minced fresh parsley

1 tablespoon extra virgin olive oil

1 teaspoon Maldon salt or other big flaky salt

1. Preheat the oven to 350°F.

2. In a small bowl, mix the potato starch and salt. In a second small bowl, whisk the eggs or aquafaba. In a third small bowl, combine the panko and Italian seasonings. Dust the eggplant slices with the starch mixture to absorb any moisture, dredge them in the egg, and coat them in the bread crumb mixture.

3. In a medium skillet over medium heat, heat the avocado oil until shimmering. Working in batches and not crowding the pan, fry the eggplant slices for 1 to

2 minutes per side, until crisp, then transfer to a baking sheet. Transfer the pan to the oven and bake for 10 to 15 minutes.

4. While the eggplant is baking, heat the marinara. Mix the cheese in a bowl with the basil, oregano, and parsley.

5. To serve, stack 2 eggplant slices with the cheese/nut cheese mixture and marinara. Drizzle the top with the olive oil and sprinkle with the salt.

TIP: Aquafaba, the liquid from inside a box or can of chickpeas, is a great substitute when vegans need egg whites for dredging. A standard can of chickpeas contains ½ to ¾ cup of aquafaba, plenty for this dish. You can also use aquafaba in place of egg whites in other recipes. Here is a simple conversion chart to follow:

1 egg = 3 tablespoons aquafaba
1 egg white = 2 tablespoons aquafaba
1 whipped egg white = 4 ounces aquafaba whipped with ¼ teaspoon cream of tartar

GO FOR A FLOAT: Have you heard of isolation or flotation therapy? Single-person tubs or pods are filled with water and Epsom salts and kept around 100°F to create a warm, zero-gravity environment. Then you climb in and soak. In this quiet, distraction-free, and weightless state, cortisol levels decrease and the brain can enter into a theta brain wave state, which is typically experienced in deep sleep or meditation, but can also occur right before we fall asleep or wake up. Theta brainwaves have been linked with creativity, intuition, and relaxation, making this the perfect slow Sunday soak to prepare you for the coming week.

Day 8—Weekday

SWEAT SUPPORT: Asking for help is a strength, not a weakness, and relying on your favorite trainer, workout buddy, or significant other to help get you to the gym or a class a few Mondays in a row might be all it takes to get you going on your own. Let's start this week strong with another thirty- to sixty-minute workout featuring weight lifting, kettlebells, resistance, or strength training. A couple of class options include yoga with weights or a HIIT class. The goal is to build and maintain lean muscle mass, which can help increase insulin sensitivity, lower blood sugar levels, and increase your metabolism.

BREAKFAST

BLACKBERRY KALE FAB FOUR SMOOTHIE

Spinach is my go-to leafy green for a Fab Four Smoothie, but I also incorporate kale from time to time (and sometimes it's the only leafy green left in the refrigerator). Just be sure to use only the leaves, not the stems. Also, you can use baby kale if you find kale to be bitter.

Vanilla protein powder containing 20 to 30 grams protein
½ small avocado
1 tablespoon chia seeds
Handful of kale
¼ cup frozen blackberries
1 to 1½ cups unsweetened vanilla almond milk or water

Place all the ingredients in a high-speed blender and blend to your desired consistency.

LUNCH

ASIAN CRUNCH SALAD

In this salad featuring Asian flavors, I use kumquats instead of mandarin oranges. Kumquats are high in fiber, vitamin C, and riboflavin.

Makes 4 servings

DRESSING
2 tablespoons avocado oil
1 garlic clove, minced
1 teaspoon minced fresh ginger
1 tablespoon lite seasoned rice vinegar
1 tablespoon coconut aminos
Juice of ½ lime

SALAD
1 napa cabbage head, thinly sliced
1 red pepper, thinly sliced
2 cups thinly sliced cucumber
1 cup shredded carrots
¼ cup thinly sliced red onion
4 kumquats, thinly sliced
½ cup chopped cilantro
¼ cup sliced green onions
⅓ cup slivered almonds
¼ cup sesame seeds
Optional toppings: 1 sliced avocado and ¼ cup chickpeas

In a large bowl, whisk the dressing ingredients. Add the salad ingredients and toss well to coat. To add more protein and fat, add the avocado and chickpeas if desired.

DINNER

SPINACH, ARTICHOKE, AND WHITE BEAN CASSEROLE

Try this wholesome casserole. It's loaded with the Fab Four, flavored with fresh herbs, and will fill you up like a casserole should.

Makes 2 to 3 servings

1 tablespoon extra virgin olive oil
1 medium yellow onion, cut into ¼-inch dice
3 garlic cloves, minced
1 (14-ounce) jar artichoke hearts in water, drained and chopped
2 cups packed roughly chopped spinach
2 cups packed roughly chopped kale
1½ cups cooked cannellini beans or 1 (15-ounce) can, drained and rinsed
¼ cup cashews
Juice of 1 lemon
2 to 3 tablespoons nutritional yeast (optional)
¼ cup filtered water
1 teaspoon chopped fresh thyme
1 teaspoon chopped fresh basil
1 teaspoon chopped fresh oregano
Toasted hemp hearts
Red pepper flakes

1. Preheat the oven to 400°F.
2. In an ovensafe skillet over medium heat, heat the olive oil. Sauté the onion until translucent, 3 to 4 minutes. Add the garlic and sauté for 2 minutes. Add the artichokes, spinach, and kale and stir to warm the greens through and wilt them. Stir in 1 cup of the beans and remove the pan from the heat.

3. In a food processor, combine the cashews, remaining ½ cup of beans, lemon juice, nutritional yeast (if using), water, and roughly half of the thyme, basil, and oregano. Blend until smooth and creamy, then stir into the skillet mixture.

4. Transfer the skillet to the oven and bake for 12 minutes, until hot throughout and the top layer is slightly browned.

5. Sprinkle with the remaining herbs, toasted hemp hearts, and red pepper flakes.

TIP: As mentioned in chapters 3 and 4, consistently eating fibrous vegetables is a phenomenal way to promote gut health. Artichokes are high in resistant starch and can help speed up the growth of healthy gut bacteria.

MOODY MONDAY: Are you suffering from a bad case of the Mondays? One way to process those emotions and the residual stress of the day (sans wine) is breathwork. For more, see the Domestic Goddess plan, page 209.

Day 9—Weekday

WALK IT OUT: It always surprises me how many miles I walk on my trips to New York, but the minute I land in Los Angeles, I automatically jump in my car to go anywhere, including an errand that's right around the corner. Movement is a mind-set. See if you can shift into gear by walking somewhere today. A few simple ideas: take the stairs when you have the opportunity, walk to lunch instead of ordering it to a conference room or your desk, tackle an errand or two on foot, or walk to a coffee shop for the afternoon if you work from home.

BREAKFAST

EASY-BAKE 'NOLA

This is the perfect topping for your favorite custom-designed Fab Four Smoothie Bowl (for how, see the Domestic Goddess plan, page 204).

Makes about twenty ¼-cup servings

2 cups whole raw Marcona almonds or natural almonds
1 cup roughly chopped pecans
1 cup roughly chopped walnuts
1 cup hemp hearts
¾ cup unsweetened coconut flakes
¼ cup ground flaxseed meal
6 tablespoons coconut oil
4 drops of organic liquid monk fruit sweetener (or 2 tablespoons maple syrup)
1 teaspoon pure vanilla extract
1 teaspoon ground cinnamon
½ teaspoon ground cloves
½ teaspoon ground ginger
½ teaspoon kosher salt or pink Himalayan salt

1. To skin the almonds, place them in a medium bowl, cover them with room temperature water, and let them soak for 1 to 2 hours. Drain and rinse the almonds in cold water. Carefully squeeze the almonds to remove them from the loosened skins. Let them dry completely, then roughly chop.
2. Preheat the oven to 275°F.
3. In a large bowl, mix all the ingredients together. Spread the mixture on a rimmed baking sheet. Bake for 60 minutes, stirring with a spatula every 20 minutes. Let the mixture cool completely, then store it in an airtight container.

LUNCH

CAULIFLOWER RICE TABBOULEH

This tabbouleh is leaner and lighter, because I've replaced the traditional grains with gluten-free, nutrient-rich cauliflower rice.

Makes 1 serving

2 cups cooked cauliflower rice (see Cauliflower Rice)
3 tablespoons chickpeas
3 tablespoons finely diced cucumber
3 tablespoons quartered cherry tomatoes
3 tablespoons finely chopped red onion
3 tablespoons finely chopped fresh mint
3 tablespoons finely chopped fresh parsley
Juice of ½ lemon
1 tablespoon red wine vinegar
2 tablespoons extra virgin olive oil
Pink Himalayan salt and freshly ground black pepper

1. Place the cauliflower rice in a large bowl. Add the chickpeas, cucumber, tomatoes, onion, mint, and parsley and mix well.

2. In a small bowl, whisk the lemon juice, vinegar, and olive oil. Season with salt and pepper. Pour 2 to 3 tablespoons of this dressing over the cauliflower mixture and stir to coat.

CAULIFLOWER RICE

Cauliflower rice is a fiber-rich grain alternative that has lower net carbohydrates and lower carbohydrate density than white or brown rice. Cauliflower is a cruciferous vegetable and a good source of sulforaphane, a phytochemical

(continued)

that activates genes responsible for detoxification, reducing inflammations, and cell defense (see the chart on page 93 for more details).

It's easy to purchase cauliflower rice premade in the freezer department of your grocery store and cook it according to the instructions on the bag. You can also make it quickly yourself by pulsing raw cauliflower florets in a food processor until a rice-like size is reached. A medium head of cauliflower will yield about 4 cups of rice. Then to cook it, in a large skillet over medium heat, combine 1 tablespoon of avocado oil and up to 4 cups cauliflower rice. Cook for 5 to 7 minutes, stirring occasionally, until it's cooked through.

Some of the recipes in this book call for frozen or uncooked cauliflower rice, while others call for cooked. Either way, it's up to you whether you want to start with store-bought frozen or homemade. (You can also make broccoli rice using this recipe.)

DINNER

SHEET-PAN-ROASTED VEGETABLES

Roasted vegetables make a warm, comforting, and easy plant-focused base for delicious meals. The formula is simple: 4 to 5 cups of nonstarchy vegetables; 1 cup of starchy vegetables (optional); and 2 tablespoons of high-heat cooking oil. Try one of the variations below and then add a plant-based protein of your choice.

Makes 2 servings

VEGAN TERIYAKI
2 tablespoons coconut oil
1 cup sliced trimmed mushrooms
1 cup broccoli florets
1 cup quartered trimmed Brussels sprouts
1 cup ¼-inch-diced red onion
1 cup ¼-inch-cubed Japanese yam
Topping: vegan teriyaki sauce (my favorite is Thrive Market Coconut Aminos)

ITALIAN

2 tablespoons avocado oil (or extra virgin olive oil)

1 cup ½-inch-diced zucchini

1 cup broccoli florets

1 cup ½-inch-thick red pepper strips

1 cup cherry or Roma tomatoes

1 yellow onion, quartered

1 cup small red-skin potatoes

Toppings: pesto, olives, or capers

FAJITA

2 tablespoons avocado oil

2 cups ½-inch-thick red pepper strips (or yellow and orange mixed)

1 cup ½-inch-thick green pepper strips

1 cup ½-inch-thick white onion slices

1 cup cauliflower florets

Toppings: avocado, guacamole, or salsa

ASIAN

2 tablespoons algae oil, avocado oil, or coconut oil

1 cup ½-inch-thick matchstick carrots

1 cup snap peas

1 cup ½-inch-sliced mushrooms

1 cup ½-inch-thick red pepper strips

1 cup chopped green onion

¼ kabocha squash, peeled and cut into ¼-inch-thick slices

Toppings: hemp hearts, sesame seeds, or coconut aminos

1. Preheat the oven to 375°F.

2. Drizzle a baking sheet with the oil. Spread the vegetables across the pan and toss to coat. Roast for 20 to 30 minutes, turning the vegetables halfway through, until they're slightly browned on the edges. Top with your toppings of choice.

TIP: To help different types of vegetables roast at a similar rate, chop all the non-starchy/less dense vegetables into the same size pieces and chop all of the starchy/denser vegetables to be *half* that size.

OIL PULLING: According to this ancient Ayurvedic technique, swishing coconut oil around in your mouth can help promote gum and dental health, and potentially alleviate certain skin issues. I'm not aware of any major studies to support some of these claims, but the fatty acid profile of coconut oil (caprylic, capric, and lauric acid) is antibacterial and antifungal, which might help explain some people's results. If you want to give oil pulling a try, start with ½ teaspoon of coconut oil and swish it around in your mouth for 2 to 3 minutes. If you see positive results (or enjoy doing it), you can work your way up to 1 tablespoon and a swishing time of 15 minutes. Some people swear by oil pulling and do it every day. I fall more in the occasional category (when I feel like my teeth and gums need some love!) and usually try to swish for 10 minutes. I listen to podcasts to help pass the time. Just remember, this remedy isn't a proven cure-all, and you still need to brush your teeth and floss every day!

Day 10—Weekday

MORNING MOVEMENT: Choose a thirty- to sixty-minute cardio workout such as a run, bike ride, Spin class, or class on your favorite app. An upbeat Vinyasa yoga class or HIIT class can also get your blood pumping if running, cycling, or dancing isn't your cup of tea.

BREAKFAST

BRAINIAC FAB FOUR SMOOTHIE

Similar to the Brainiac Salad from Day 5, this Fab Four Smoothie includes some of the most brain-healthy plant-based foods found in nature, such as spinach, kale, blueberries, extra virgin olive oil, and walnuts.

Vanilla protein powder containing 20 to 30 grams protein
1 tablespoon extra virgin olive oil
¼ avocado
1 tablespoon chia seeds
Small handful of spinach
Small handful of baby kale
¼ cup blueberries
1½ cups walnut milk

Place all the ingredients in a high-speed blender and blend to your desired consistency.

LUNCH: Whip up a clean, quick, and simple Green Goddess Salad (see the Domestic Goddess plan, page 229).

TIP: The next time you buy celery, add the leaves to your salad. Celery leaves contain antioxidants and beneficial enzymes, as well as potassium, folate, and vitamins K, C, and B_6.

DINNER

SPAGHETTI SQUASH CHOW MEIN

Makes 2 servings

This is a clean, lower-carbohydrate version of the popular Chinese-style dish.

1 large spaghetti squash
¼ cup coconut aminos
3 garlic cloves, minced
4 drops of organic liquid monk fruit (or 1 tablespoon coconut sugar)
2 teaspoons grated fresh ginger
¼ teaspoon freshly ground white pepper
2 tablespoons extra virgin olive oil
1 yellow onion, cut into ¼-inch dice
3 celery stalks, sliced diagonally
2 cups shredded cabbage
½ cup shredded carrot
½ cup toasted hemp hearts
2 tablespoons sesame seeds

1. Cut the squash crosswise, seed it, and pressure-cook it for 7 minutes on rapid release. (You can also roast the squash inverted on a baking sheet in a 400°F oven for 40 to 50 minutes, until tender.) Use a fork to scrape the stringy squash flesh into a bowl.

2. In a medium bowl, whisk the coconut aminos, garlic, sweetener of choice, ginger, and white pepper; set aside.

3. In a large skillet over medium-high heat, heat the olive oil. Add the onion and celery and sauté until tender, 3 to 4 minutes. Stir in the cabbage and carrot and cook until heated through, about 1 minute. Stir in the spaghetti squash and the sauce mixture and cook until well combined and heated through, about 2 minutes. Top with the hemp and sesame seeds.

REMINDER: Don't heat or cook with an oil above the temperature at which it begins to smoke. If you do, the oil will begin to oxidize and release harmful free radicals and other compounds. See page 79 for guidelines on smoke point and using different cooking oils.

SPIKY STRESS RELIEF: Part of my wind-down routine a couple times per week is to roll my feet on a spiky massage ball or to lie back on a spiky acupressure mat. Both techniques can help calm your nervous system, relieve muscle tension, ease aches and pains, and help you relax. See the Girl on the Go plan, page 173, and the Domestic Goddess plan, page 217, for more details.

Day 11—Weekday

BREAKFAST

SUPER SEED FAB FOUR SMOOTHIE

Seeds abound in this chocolate smoothie. Some of my plant-based clients always default to nuts and nut butters, so this is a tasty way to mix it up. Sunflower butter is a seed butter and thus a great option for people with allergies to peanuts or tree nuts. It has a creamy, nutlike flavor that tastes great with chocolate. The chia, flax, hemp hearts, and flax milk add fiber, fat, and more protein.

Chocolate protein powder containing 20 to 30 grams protein
1 tablespoon sunflower butter
1 tablespoon chia seeds
1 tablespoon flaxseeds
1 tablespoon hemp hearts
Handful of spinach
1 cup flax milk (or unsweetened coconut milk)

Place all the ingredients in a high-speed blender and blend to your desired consistency.

LUNCH

SPICY CASHEW SPREAD

A homemade sprouted raw spread or fermented cheese can be a good protein base for a sandwich or wrap. Store-bought options can get pricey and may contain bad oils, soy protein isolates, gluten protein, and excess emulsifiers and gums to make them taste like a specific food. Try making this version instead. It uses whole foods and savory seasonings to nourish and delight.

Makes 9 servings

1 cup plus 2 tablespoons filtered water
½ cup sun-dried tomatoes
3 cups raw cashews (see Tip)
1 tablespoon freshly squeezed lemon juice
1 garlic clove, minced
½ teaspoon pink Himalayan salt
1 red bell pepper
1 tablespoon chili powder
1 teaspoon paprika or smoked paprika
½ teaspoon cumin seed
¼ cup diced yellow onion
1 carrot
1 jalapeño, stemmed

1. Warm 1 cup of the water. In a medium bowl, combine the sun-dried tomatoes and the warm water and let soak for 5 minutes.
2. Place the cashews in a food processor and pulse them into a semifine meal. Transfer the meal to a large bowl.
3. Drain the tomatoes and add them to the food processor along with the remaining 2 tablespoons water and all the other ingredients. Blend until a paste-like consistency is reached. Transfer the paste to the bowl containing the cashews and use a spatula to combine the ingredients thoroughly.

4. Serve the spread with crackers and crudités, or roll it in a collard wrap with sliced vegetables and avocado, or add it to your favorite Mexican dish, such as lettuce-cup tacos or a veggie burrito. Store it in a glass container in the refrigerator for 2 to 3 days.

TIP: Cashews can be replaced with walnuts or sprouted seed mix.

INCREMENTAL ELEVATION: Elevating your plant-based lifestyle doesn't require wholesale changes all at once. We all have our go-to recipes and favorite dishes, the ones we've been cooking or enjoying for years. It can take time to make the changes you want, so take the pressure off yourself and find ways to get there incrementally. You could modify one of your favorite recipes, eat one less soy or tofu dish per week, learn to make something new like a dip or dressing, or use a simple technique like soaking and sprouting. Over time, small changes can add up to a new lifestyle and help you elevate every day.

DINNER

ROASTED BLACK BEAN VEGAN BURGERS

If you prefer, you can serve these veggie patties over an arugula salad tossed with a squeeze of lemon, drizzle of olive oil, and salt. Or double up the veggies by offering a side dish of Roasted Root Fries (see the Domestic Goddess plan, page 269).

Makes 4 servings

1 tablespoon avocado oil
1 tablespoon chili powder
1 tablespoon ground cumin

(continued)

1½ teaspoons smoked paprika

3 garlic cloves, minced

8 ounces shiitake mushrooms

1 carrot, roughly chopped

1 green pepper, roughly chopped

½ yellow onion, finely diced

2 cups canned black beans, drained and rinsed, or Pressure Cooked Dry Beans
(page 291)

2 tablespoons unsweetened organic ketchup (I like Primal Kitchen)

½ cup walnuts

¼ cup flax meal

2 cups packed spinach

¼ cup aquafaba (see Tip, page 309) or 2 flax eggs (see page 331)

8 romaine, butter, or red-leaf lettuce leaf cups

Toppings of choice: avocado, tomato, grilled onion, fresh thinly sliced red onion,
sautéed sliced mushrooms, fried egg

Condiments of choice: sugar-free alternatives like Primal Kitchen ketchup,
mustard, barbecue, or Thousand Island sauce

1. Preheat the oven to 400°F.

2. In a large bowl, whisk the avocado oil, chili powder, cumin, smoked paprika, and garlic. Add the mushrooms, carrot, green pepper, and onion and toss to coat. Spread the seasoned vegetables on a baking sheet and roast for 20 minutes (flipping at 10 minutes) to caramelize them and remove most of the water.

3. Meanwhile, spread the beans on a separate baking sheet and roast them along with the vegetables for 10 minutes, until they're dried out a bit (some will split open).

4. In a food processor, pulse the roasted vegetables with the ketchup, walnuts, flax meal, and spinach. Take care not to overprocess; you want the veggies in tiny chunks about the size of bread crumbs.

5. In a large bowl, combine the roasted beans, aquafaba, and vegetable-nut mix and hand-mix gently but thoroughly. Form the mixture into 4 patties.

6. Pan-fry the patties in a large skillet over medium heat for 4 minutes per side, until warm and set.

7. Wrap each burger in 2 lettuce leaf cups and add your choice of toppings and condiments.

ROLL IT OUT: Try foam rolling at home—I do it several times a week. It's a quick, easy, and body-loving routine that not only feels great but also can help improve fascia health, lymphatic drainage, and alignment. Fasciae are the connective tissues that wrap and protect the muscles, organs, and nerves. See the Domestic Goddess plan, page 251.

Day 12—Weekday

MORNING MOVEMENT: End the week on a strong note with a thirty- to sixty-minute workout of your choice. It can be cardio, anaerobic (weights), or both. You break through plateaus only when you elevate expectations, push yourself, and persevere. Push for the end of your week and don't be afraid to up the intensity. Speaking of which, especially if you haven't done it yet, today might be a great time to try a HIIT class (high-intensity interval training).

BREAKFAST

RASPBERRY LEMONADE FAB FOUR SMOOTHIE

Use the Silica ACV Lemon Water recipe from Day 4 to make this refreshing raspberry citrus smoothie.

Vanilla protein powder containing 20 to 30 grams protein

¼ avocado

(continued)

1 tablespoon chia seeds
¼ cup raspberries (fresh or frozen)
Handful of spinach
Juice of ½ lemon (optional)
2 cups Silica ACV Lemon Water (page 296)

Place all the ingredients in a high-speed blender, adding the lemon juice if you prefer more lemon flavor, and blend to your desired consistency.

TIP: Raspberries contain beneficial phytochemicals and are also fiber-rich, which results in lower net carbohydrates and lower carbohydrate density. If you used fresh raspberries in this smoothie recipe, you can use any remaining raspberries from the basket the next day (or the day after) as part of a bridge snack or dessert:

- **BRIDGE SNACK:** ¼ cup raspberries with 1 tablespoon nut butter makes for a delicious and deconstructed take on PB&J.

- **DESSERT:** ¼ cup raspberries with either 1 teaspoon cacao nibs or a piece of body-loving dark chocolate (see page 232) offers an indulgent nibble.

LUNCH

MEXICAN CHOPPED SALAD WITH CILANTRO VINAIGRETTE

Keep it simple with this Mexican chopped salad. It's a palate pleaser that takes hardly any time to make, and you'll have leftover dressing to use later in the week.

Makes 1 serving

SALAD
4 cups chopped romaine lettuce
⅛ red onion, thinly sliced

½ cup sliced tomatoes

¼ cup canned black beans, drained and rinsed, or Pressure-Cooked Dry Beans
(page 291)

2 tablespoons pumpkin seeds (I like NOW Foods and Go Raw brands)

½ avocado

CILANTRO VINAIGRETTE

2 cups cilantro leaves

½ cup avocado oil

1 tablespoon champagne vinegar

1 tablespoon freshly squeezed lime juice

1 garlic clove, minced

½ teaspoon pink Himalayan salt

1. Combine the salad ingredients in a medium bowl.

2. Blend all the vinaigrette ingredients in a high-speed blender until smooth.

3. Dress the salad with 2 tablespoons (or your preferred amount) of the vinaigrette
and toss to coat.

DINNER

ROASTED CAULIFLOWER MEDALLIONS WITH ROMESCO SAUCE

*Romesco sauce needs almost no tweaking for the Fab Four. The characteristic red pepper,
tomato, garlic, almonds, and other ingredients form a combination that bursts with flavor,
almost like a red pepper pesto.*

Makes 4 to 6 servings

ROMESCO SAUCE

2 red peppers, stemmed and seeded

4 tomatoes on the vine

(continued)

2 large garlic cloves, peeled

½ cup raw whole or Marcona almonds

1 teaspoon chili powder or red pepper flakes

1 tablespoon chopped fresh parsley

1 teaspoon paprika (use smoked paprika for a smokier flavor)

Pink Himalayan salt and freshly ground black pepper

2 tablespoons sherry vinegar (optional)

¼ to ½ cup extra virgin olive oil

CAULIFLOWER MEDALLIONS

1 large cauliflower head

¼ cup avocado oil

Pink Himalayan salt and freshly ground black pepper

½ cup chopped pitted Kalamata olives

¼ cup chopped fresh parsley

1. Preheat the oven to 450°F.

2. To make the romesco sauce, place the red peppers and tomatoes on a baking sheet and roast for 15 to 20 minutes, until slightly charred on one side. Transfer to a bowl and let them cool. Lower the oven heat to 425°F.

3. Meanwhile, in a food processor fitted with a steel blade, pulse the garlic cloves until minced; set aside for 10 to 15 minutes (see page 115).

4. Place the almonds in a skillet and toast them over medium-low heat for 2 to 3 minutes, stirring often, until browned and fragrant; set aside.

5. Hand-peel the cooled peppers and tomatoes and deseed the tomatoes. Using a spatula, scrape the minced garlic down into the bottom of the food processor (it will be stuck on the sides). Add the toasted almonds and chili powder and process into a paste. Add the red pepper, tomatoes, parsley, paprika, and salt and pepper to taste, and process until smooth. With the machine running, add the vinegar (if using) and the olive oil, pouring in a slow stream until the sauce is at your desired consistency.

6. To make the cauliflower medallions, trim the stem of the cauliflower and

remove any leaves. Set the head upright on a cutting board and carefully cut it vertically into ½- to ¾-inch-thick medallions. Place the medallions on a rimmed baking sheet, drizzle with avocado oil, season with salt and pepper, and roast for 20 minutes, until lightly browned and tender, turning the medallions over about halfway through.

7. Serve the cauliflower medallions with Romesco sauce, garnished with Kalamata olives and parsley.

Day 13—Weekend Day

BREAKFAST: Let's borrow a breakfast tool from the Girl on the Go plan. Ready? Right now, without looking anything up, build a Fab Four Smoothie using your favorite protein, fat, fiber, and greens. The idea is for you to get comfortable with the formula so you don't always need to be looking at a recipe. This way, you'll understand the components so you'll know what to order at a smoothie bar or restaurant.

FIND NATURE: We have a physiological need for natural sunlight (vitamin D), and in my opinion, a deep human need for nature as well. We spend so much of our lives indoors or in front of screens that's it's important to reconnect with the natural world. A few ideas: plan a walk or hike, invite some friends to the beach or go swimming at a lake, or set yourself up on a blanket on a lovely, green park lawn. See the Girl on the Go Plan, page 154.

LUNCH: I love recommending a coconut-milk-based curry for my plant-based clients. It's a comforting dish with a healthy dose of MCTs (healthy fats) and anti-inflammatory spices like curry and turmeric. Use my Curry in a Hurry Sauce recipe (subtract the fish sauce and add salt to taste) from the Girl on the Go plan, page 169. You can enjoy it over ½ cup sprouted quinoa or cooked cauliflower rice (see page 315), or 2 to 4 cups steamed, roasted, or sautéed vegetables. Add ¼ cup pan-fried chickpeas to your curry or top it with a few tablespoons of seeds for crunch.

FEELING SNACKY?: A vegetarian or vegan mezze platter (snack tray) may hold you over until dinner. Just be sure to plate up the Fab Four, like vegetable crudités, hummus, raw nuts, and olives. If you need more, add a cup of soup from the freezer. A few recipes you can make an extra batch of and freeze: Creamy Coconut Broccoli (page 292), Vegetable and Cauliflower Rice (page 304), Tomato (page 331), or Kale Detox (page 355).

DINNER: Make a Super Veggie or Pesto personal pizza tonight using cauliflower crust. See the Domestic Goddess plan, page 267.

KOMBUCHA

Kombucha is a fermented tea that contains probiotic bacteria. It has become very popular, and you'll see a variety of options and flavors available at most grocery stores. However, on its own, kombucha is not a meal replacement drink or snack, and in my opinion it shouldn't be for everyday consumption.

The best fermented foods are those in which the bacteria eat the naturally occurring sugars present in the food. Kombucha is different because there isn't any naturally occurring sugar in brewed tea. This means that sugar needs to be added in order for the bacteria (known as a symbiotic culture of bacteria and yeast, aka "scoby"—google a photo of it) to have something to ferment (eat and break down). It depends on the manufacturer, but generally kombucha is fermented once with a cup of granulated sugar and then a second time with more than a cup of fruit juice. The end product may contain excess sugar, alcohol, candida, yeast, and acetaldehyde (a toxic by-product).

If drinking kombucha leaves you feeling buzzed or anxious or makes you crave carbohydrates two to three hours later, it's not a great morning or midday option for you. Personally, I consider it an occasional treat. I like the effervescence and enjoy it with an evening meal or when I'm tempted to indulge in an adult beverage midweek. It's a great replacement for alcohol when your partner brings home an IPA.

PROBIOTIC-RICH FOODS

If you're looking to increase your intake of probiotics with fermented foods, here are a few things and brands to look for:

1. Does the product contain protein, fat, or fiber? (Dairy- and soy-free are preferred.)

2. Did they need to add sugar to grow the bacteria? (Preferably not.)

3. Vegetables: I like sauerkraut and kimchi from Farmhouse Culture and Wildbrine.

4. Coconut yogurt: I like Anita's, COYO, New Earth Superfoods, CocoYo, and The Coconut Cult.

Day 14—Weekend Day

BREAKFAST: Whip up some Cinnamon Protein Pancakes (see the Girl on the Go plan, page 191). To make a vegan version, use a vegan egg substitute, such as aquafaba (see Tip, page 309) or a flax egg: for each egg needed, mix 1 tablespoon ground flaxseeds with 3 tablespoons water and let the mixture sit in the refrigerator until thickened, about 15 minutes.

LUNCH

TOMATO SOUP

Makes 2 servings

Tomato soup is a classic. I love adding a crunchy side, and my favorite for this soup is to create little stacks made by spreading flax crackers with Sprouted Sunflower Seed Hummus (page 289) and topping them with slices of cucumber. These stacks add a little Fab Four personality and boost the protein, fat, fiber, and greens. Another option would be to add a side of my Super Green Kale Chips (page 273). (continued)

2 tablespoons extra virgin olive oil
4 garlic cloves, peeled
¼ cup chopped white onion
4 cups peeled, seeded, and chopped tomatoes (see Tip)
2 cups organic vegetable broth (or chicken bone broth if you partake)
¼ cup cashews
1 teaspoon pink Himalayan salt

1. In a stockpot over medium heat, combine the olive oil, garlic, and onion and sauté, stirring continuously, for 3 to 5 minutes, until the onion is translucent and the garlic is aromatic.

2. Add the tomatoes and broth, bring to a boil, lower the heat, and simmer for 20 minutes.

3. Turn off the heat, add the cashews, and let the soup cool slightly as the cashews soak for 5 to 10 minutes. The longer the cashews soak, the easier they are to blend, but if you have a powerful blender, you don't need as much time.

4. Using a hand blender, blend the soup into a puree (or use a high-speed blender, work in batches, and return the soup to the pot). Season with salt.

TIP: To peel a tomato, place it into a pot of boiling water for about 30 seconds, then remove the tomato with tongs and immediately place it into a bowl of ice water. This quick blanch makes it easy to peel the skin off by hand.

DINNER

VEGAN COBB SALAD

An American classic with a twist, this vegan take on Cobb salad uses kidney beans and cashews for protein and seasoned coconut flakes as "fl-acon."

Makes 2 servings

COCONUT FL-ACON

3 tablespoons coconut aminos

1 tablespoon mesquite powder (see Tip)

¼ teaspoon smoked paprika

1 teaspoon ChocZero sugar-free maple syrup or pure maple syrup (I like Thrive Market)

2 cups unsweetened coconut flakes

DRESSING

2 tablespoons red wine vinegar

1 tablespoon freshly squeezed lemon juice

1 teaspoon Dijon mustard

1 teaspoon Worcestershire sauce

1 garlic clove, minced

¼ teaspoon pink Himalayan salt

¼ teaspoon freshly ground black pepper

¼ cup extra virgin olive oil

SALAD

1 romaine lettuce head

½ cup ½-inch-diced tomatoes

½ cup canned or cooked kidney beans (see page 291), drained and rinsed

½ cup diced avocado

½ cup raw unsalted cashews

1. To make the coconut fl-acon, preheat the oven to 350°F.

2. In a medium bowl, whisk the coconut aminos, mesquite powder, smoked paprika,

(continued)

and maple syrup until combined. Add the coconut flakes and toss gently to coat. Spread the flakes on a rimmed baking sheet and bake for 10 to 12 minutes, until browned.

3. To make the dressing, in a medium bowl, combine all the ingredients except the olive oil. Then, while whisking, slowly pour in the olive oil to create an emulsification.

4. To assemble the salad, combine the salad ingredients in a large bowl and toss with your preferred amount of dressing. Top with fl-acon.

TIP: Mesquite is a type of carob. It's a plant-based, gluten-free, low-glycemic superfood that comes from the seed pods of the algarrobo tree. It's high in vitamins, minerals, and fiber; contains protein and omega-3 fatty acids; and can be used as a flour or sweetener. Opt for a raw, organic brand where the only ingredient is mesquite powder. You can find options on Amazon and in select grocery stores. To get full use of what you buy, you can easily add coconut fl-acon to other salads and recipes, such as the Avocado Bean Salad (page 284), Vegan Kale Caesar (page 306), Roasted Black Bean Vegan Burgers (page 323), or any egg dish if you're vegetarian. You can also add 1 teaspoon of mesquite powder to any Fab Four Smoothie. Try it in the Triple Chocolate Crunch (page 218) or Chocolate Almond Butter Crunch (page 216).

SUNDAY SELF-CARE: Devote some time to yourself and indulge in Sunday self-care, lavishing attention on your skin, face, eyebrows, nails, and even your back! Exfoliate your skin, try a new face mask, touch up your eyebrows, book a mani-pedi, or splurge for a full massage or a session at an infrared sauna. You can also indulge in a Boosted Bath (see the Red-Carpet Ready plan, page 366). It's as simple as adding Epsom salt, magnesium flakes, or a CBD bath ball to the tub.

Day 15—Weekday

HOME HIIT: The more complicated your life becomes with a spouse, kids, or career, the harder it gets to make a workout happen. If you learn to work out at home, you'll never have an excuse not to sweat. Learn to make the time for yourself, work on that self-discipline, and hone the skill before you need it. Today, let's do an at-home HIIT workout. You don't need a gym full of equipment. I would start with a pair of dumbbells (3 or 5 pounds), one kettlebell (10, 15, or 30 pounds), and one resistance band. Then go online or use your favorite app to pick a thirty-minute HIIT workout that looks fun.

BREAKFAST: Try my Low-Sugar Açai Bowl (see the Domestic Goddess plan, page 228).

LUNCH: Revisit one of the Plant-Based Devotee salads from previous days: Ribboned Rainbow Salad over Sprouted Sunflower Seed Hummus (page 288), Brainiac Salad (page 300), Vegan Kale Caesar with Crispy Smoked Chickpeas (page 306), Asian Crunch Salad (page 311), or Mexican Chopped Salad with Cilantro Vinaigrette (page 326).

DINNER: Italian Spaghetti Squash (see the Girl on the Go plan, page 173) or Italian Butter Bean Bake (see the Domestic Goddess plan, page 208).

Day 16—Weekday

BREAKFAST

CHLOROPHYLL MINT FAB FOUR SMOOTHIE

Use the Chlorophyll Mint Water recipe from Day 4 to make this refreshing smoothie.

Vanilla protein powder containing 20 to 30 grams protein
¼ avocado
1 tablespoon chia seeds
Juice of 1 lemon
Handful of spinach
1½ cups Chlorophyll Mint Water (page 296)

Place all the ingredients in a high-speed blender and blend to your desired consistency.

LUNCH

ROMAINE WALNUT AVOCADO SALAD

This is a great recipe for those times when you have only five or ten minutes to prep, eat, and get back to your day.

Makes 2 servings

2 tablespoons extra virgin olive oil
1 tablespoon champagne vinegar
4 cups chopped romaine lettuce
1 avocado, diced

¼ cup dry-roasted walnuts

¼ cup goat cheese or soft nut cheese, such as Kite Hill ricotta

Maldon salt or other big flaky salt

In a large bowl, whisk the olive oil and vinegar until smooth. Add the romaine, avocado, and walnuts and toss to coat. Finish with cheese and a pinch of Maldon salt.

DINNER

CREAMY MUSHROOM RISOTTO

This is a clean take on the Italian classic, with nutrient-dense shiitake or oyster mushrooms and fiber-rich cauliflower rice.

Makes 2 servings

1 tablespoon extra virgin olive oil

1 shallot, minced

3 garlic cloves, minced

1½ cups shiitake or oyster mushrooms, trimmed and thinly sliced (see Tip, page 211)

½ cup Arborio rice

2 cups vegetable stock

1½ teaspoons white wine vinegar

2 cups frozen or uncooked cauliflower rice (see page 315)

2 tablespoons nutritional yeast

1 tablespoon cashew butter

1½ teaspoons roughly chopped fresh parsley

1½ teaspoons roughly chopped fresh chives

Sea salt (I like Real brand) and freshly ground black pepper

Red pepper flakes (optional)

1 tablespoon toasted hemp seeds

(continued)

1. In a large skillet over medium heat, heat the olive oil. Add the shallot and garlic and sauté until the shallot is soft, about 4 minutes. Add the mushrooms and cook for 3 to 4 minutes, until soft. Stir in the Arborio rice, stock, and vinegar and bring to a boil. Turn the heat to low and simmer for about 30 minutes, or until all the liquid has been absorbed and the rice is cooked. Add the cauliflower rice, stirring continuously, until cooked, about 5 minutes.

2. Remove the pan from the heat and stir in the nutritional yeast, cashew butter, and herbs. Season to taste with salt and pepper and (if using) the red pepper flakes. Top with the toasted hemp seeds.

EVENING STRETCH: The average American sits for ten to twelve hours per day. We've become more sedentary, and the more we sit, the more it hurts to move. Take ten or fifteen minutes tonight and stretch yourself out. The benefits include increased range of motion, better posture, and improved circulation. For some simple stretching exercises, do a quick search on YouTube, and you'll find dozens of options.

HOT SAUCE

Be aware of sugar, sodium, and artificial ingredients in the hot sauce or sriracha you buy. Ideally, you want (1) less than 4 grams of sugar, (2) less than 200 milligrams of sodium, and (3) real ingredients you recognize and can pronounce. Primal Kitchen and Siete have a delicious roster of flavors. I also like Wildbrine fermented Sriracha, Sky Valley Sriracha, and Melinda's Habanero Hot Sauce.

Day 17—Weekday

YOGA GLOW: Build on last night's stretch with a morning yoga class. Flexibility, pliability, muscle tone, and core strength are some of main benefits of yoga. If you sweat, good! And if your teacher pushes you to hold a pose for ten seconds longer than you would hold it at home, also good! Feed off the communal energy in the room, connect with your breath, and sink in to your body. You'll reap a satisfying physical and mental release afterward, also known as the post-class yoga glow.

BREAKFAST: If you have leftover mint leaves from yesterday's Chlorophyll Mint smoothie, use them to make another minty recipe, like Spa Day (see the Girl on the Go plan, page 164), Detox Winter Mint (see the Domestic Goddess plan, page 240) or Mojito (see *Body Love*).

LUNCH

VEGAN HAND ROLLS

Using nori (dried seaweed) as a wrap is a great way to mix up your leafy greens and salad routine. Try them with a dipping sauce like the Nutty Sauce from Day 4 (see page 297).

Makes 1 serving

¼ cup Spicy Cashew Spread (page 322) or ¼ cup cashew butter
1 tablespoon sriracha
2 (9-inch) nori (dried seaweed) sheets
½ cup shredded peeled carrot
½ cup thinly shredded cabbage
½ cup thinly sliced cucumber
1 avocado, thinly sliced

1. Mix the spread or cashew butter with a little sriracha to give a spicy kick.
2. Lay out a nori sheet and layer it with half of the carrot, cabbage, cucumber, avocado, and spicy filling. Roll it into a sushi hand roll and repeat with the other nori sheet.

DINNER: Try another Sheet-Pan-Roasted Vegetables recipe from Day 9 (page 316) (Vegan Teriyaki, Italian, Fajita, or Asian) and add a plant-based protein of your choice. If you use beans or grains, serve it up warm in a bowl.

EVENING MEDITATION: A simple meditation exercise is the perfect end to a day that started with yoga. Close your eyes and focus on your breath; inhale and exhale slowly through your nose. After a few breaths, begin a body scan. Starting with your toes, work your way up to your head, giving each body part between thirty and sixty seconds. With each inhale, send yourself a calm message, and as you exhale, release your body's tension. If you feel your thoughts starting to drift, calmly bring your attention back to your breath.

Day 18—Weekday

BREAKFAST

WARM TRIPLE SEED FAUXMEAL

This warming breakfast bowl is a play on oatmeal and a good source of protein and fiber to start the day. Choose the white variety of chia seeds if you want it to look more like oatmeal.

Makes 1 serving

2 cups unsweetened almond or coconut milk
Protein powder containing about 10 grams protein
3 tablespoons hemp hearts
2 tablespoons chia seeds
1 tablespoon flax meal
Optional topping: ¼ cup mixed berries, 1 tablespoon nuts, or a drizzle of nut butter

1. In a skillet, combine the almond milk and protein powder and whisk to incorporate. Add the hemp hearts, chia seeds, and flax meal and cook over medium-high heat for 3 to 5 minutes, stirring until the chia seeds have absorbed the liquid and no longer crunch.
2. Pour into a bowl and add a topping of your choice if desired.

LUNCH: Try a salad from the Domestic Goddess plan, such as the Green Goddess Salad (page 229) or the Peanut Kale Salad (page 265). You can also revisit one of the salads from earlier in this plan or skip ahead to Day 19 and make the Kale Berry Salad with Creamy Coconut Poppy Seed Dressing (page 345).

DINNER

ROASTED CURRY CAULIFLOWER

This roasted cauliflower is full of flavor, fiber, and clean cooking oils. It can be served all on its own or as a side dish. I like to assemble a trio of vegetable dishes for dinner that includes this and Sesame Broccoli and Garlic Ginger Bok Choy (page 343).

Makes 2 servings

1 tablespoon curry powder
½ teaspoon smoked paprika
½ teaspoon ground cumin
½ teaspoon ground coriander
½ teaspoon Pink Himalayan salt
1 tablespoon red wine vinegar
2 tablespoons avocado oil
3 cups cauliflower florets
3 tablespoons chopped cilantro
2 tablespoons sliced almonds

1. Preheat the oven to 425°F.
2. In a large bowl, whisk the curry powder, smoked paprika, cumin, coriander, salt, and vinegar. Continue whisking and slowly pour in the avocado oil to create an emulsification. Add the cauliflower to the bowl and toss to coat.
3. Transfer the cauliflower to a rimmed baking sheet and roast for 35 minutes, until slightly browned on the edges. Garnish with the cilantro and almonds.

SESAME BROCCOLI

If you're preparing this dish along with the curry cauliflower (see page 341), you can roast them both at the same time.

Makes 2 servings

3 cups broccoli florets
2 tablespoons avocado oil
Pink Himalayan salt
¼ cup coconut aminos
1 tablespoon cold-pressed sesame oil
1 teaspoon grated fresh ginger
2 tablespoons sesame seeds

1. Preheat the oven to 425°F.
2. In a large bowl, toss the broccoli with the avocado oil and sprinkle with a pinch of salt.
3. Transfer the broccoli to a rimmed baking sheet and roast for 15 to 20 minutes, turning it halfway through.
4. In a small bowl, whisk the coconut aminos, sesame oil, and ginger. Drizzle the sauce on the roasted broccoli and stir to coat. Top with the sesame seeds.

GARLIC GINGER BOK CHOY

If you're new to bok choy, this recipe is a tasty way to try this nutrient-dense cruciferous vegetable.

Makes 2 servings

1 tablespoon avocado oil
2 garlic cloves, minced
1 tablespoon minced fresh ginger
¼ teaspoon red pepper flakes
4 bunches baby bok choy, trimmed but left intact
1 tablespoon vegetable broth or stock

Choose a large skillet with a lid. Over medium-high heat, heat the avocado oil until it shimmers. Add the garlic, ginger, and pepper flakes and sauté for about 1 minute until fragrant. Add the bok choy and sauté for about 1 minute. Add the broth, cover the pan, and cook for 3 minutes, until the broth is absorbed. Uncover and cook until the liquid is mostly evaporated.

JOURNALING: We type and text all day, but most of us rarely take the time to write down what's really going on inside of us. It's healthy to express the thoughts, ideas, dreams, emotions, worries, fears, frustrations, and whatever else is swirling around in your head. Take some time tonight to write those things down. If you need some light guidance, buy a journal that gives you topics and questions to consider writing about. I like Maria Shriver's book *I've Been Thinking . . . The Journal* because it guides you in a positive direction, encourages you to be open and honest with yourself, and breeds the confidence needed to confront life's many challenges.

Day 19—Weekday

MORNING MOVEMENT: Let's lock in some cardio before the weekend begins. A few options: go for a brisk thirty-minute power walk, pound out a two- to three-mile run, use the elliptical machine at the gym, or pick a workout from your favorite app.

BREAKFAST

COCONUT TURMERIC FAB FOUR SMOOTHIE

This smoothie is anti-inflammatory and contains vitamin C to give you a little immunity boost.

Vanilla protein powder containing 20 to 30 grams protein
1 tablespoon coconut butter
2 tablespoons acacia fiber (I use NOW Foods)
1 tablespoon ground turmeric
Pinch of freshly ground black pepper
¼ cup frozen raspberries (optional)
1 to 2 cups unsweetened almond milk

Place all the ingredients in a high-speed blender and blend to the desired consistency.

LUNCH

KALE BERRY SALAD WITH
CREAMY COCONUT POPPY SEED DRESSING

Featuring mixed berries and leafy green kale, this salad is loaded with MCTs (medium chain triglycerides; healthy fats) that can stoke your metabolism, and the coconut yogurt adds a dairy-free probiotic boost.

Makes 1 serving

SALAD
2 cups finely sliced stemmed kale (chiffonade cut)
¼ cup fresh strawberries, hulled and sliced
¼ cup fresh blueberries
¼ cup fresh blackberries
3 tablespoons sliced almonds
¼ cup feta cheese (optional)

DRESSING
⅓ cup plain coconut yogurt
2 teaspoons apple cider vinegar
2 teaspoons poppy or chia seeds (see Reminder)
1 teaspoon honey (optional)

1. In a large bowl, combine the kale, berries, almonds, and feta cheese (if using).

2. In a medium bowl, whisk the yogurt, vinegar, poppy seeds, and honey (if using).

3. Drizzle your preferred amount of dressing onto the salad and toss.

REMINDER: Always hydrate or soak chia seeds in some manner before use. Dry chia seeds absorb bodily fluids and can greatly expand in size, which may result in intestinal blockages. If you use chia seeds in a dressing, let the chia become gelatinous before you eat it.

DINNER

VEGAN CABBAGE ROLLS STUFFED WITH EGGPLANT, MUSHROOMS, AND SPINACH

"Hearty" is one way of saying it. "Stuffed" is another. Either way, these rolls will fill you up with a colorful array of fiber and greens.

Makes 4 servings

1 large napa cabbage
2 tablespoons extra virgin olive oil
½ yellow onion, roughly chopped
2 garlic cloves, minced
2 cups ½-inch-diced zucchini
2 cups ½-inch-diced eggplant
2 cups ½-inch-diced mushrooms
4 cups frozen or uncooked cauliflower rice (see page 315)
1 teaspoon ground ginger
1 tablespoon paprika
4 cups baby spinach
1 cup diced fresh tomatoes
1 cup Tomato Soup (page 331)
½ cup Spicy Cashew Spread (page 322)
1 tablespoon chopped parsley

1. Preheat the oven to 375°F.
2. Core the cabbage, place it in a large soup pot, add enough water to cover, and bring to a boil over medium-high heat. Reduce the heat to medium, cover the pot, and cook until the cabbage is soft, 4 to 6 minutes. Peel off 8 large leaves and reserve. (The remaining cabbage can be chopped and added to a soup or sautéed with olive oil and garlic for a quick, fiber-packed side dish.)
3. In a large skillet over medium heat, heat the olive oil. Add the onion and garlic and sauté until the onion is transparent, 3 to 4 minutes. Add the zucchini,

eggplant, mushrooms, cauliflower rice, ginger, and paprika and sauté for 8 minutes, until the vegetables are crisp-tender. Remove the pan from the heat and stir in the spinach until wilted.

4. Divide the mixture into eight equal portions. In a medium bowl, stir together the diced tomatoes and tomato soup. To make the cabbage rolls, spoon a portion of the vegetable mixture and 1 tablespoon of the spread into each cabbage leaf and roll it up. Place the rolls seam side down in a baking dish. Spoon the tomato mixture over the rolls.

5. Bake for 10 minutes, until the rolls are heated through. Garnish with the parsley and serve warm.

BREAKFAST PREP FOR TOMORROW

OVERNIGHT OATS

Makes 2 servings

If you love oatmeal, try this filling variation that increases the fiber, decreases net carbs, and serves up enough protein to keep you full till lunch. Prepping this recipe the night before will save you time in the morning and allow the seeds and oats to get a good soak.

2 tablespoons hemp hearts
2 tablespoons chia seeds
2 tablespoons flaxseed meal
¼ cup organic gluten-free rolled oats
Vanilla protein powder containing 20 to 30 grams protein
1½ cups unsweetened almond milk
Topping option: 1 tablespoon nut butter of choice

1. Add the hemp hearts, chia seeds, flaxseed meal, and oats to a mason jar.

2. In a high-speed blender, blend the protein powder and almond milk for 30 seconds, then pour into the mason jar over the seed and oat mixture.

3. Tighten the lid of the mason jar and shake vigorously to incorporate.

4. Store in the refrigerator for up to 3 days.

Day 20—Weekend Day

BREAKFAST: Grab your Overnight Oats from the refrigerator, add 1 tablespoon of your favorite nut butter (if you want), and off you go.

LUNCH: Try the Peanut Kale Salad from the Domestic Goddess plan, page 265. Or if you're in the mood for something else, revisit a dish you liked from earlier in this plan.

AFTERNOON MOVEMENT: Here are a few ideas for some light weekend movement. The goal is to get outside and not turn into an all-day couch potato: (1) go for a thirty-minute walk; (2) find a bit of nature and go for a hike; or (3) be a tourist in your own city, visit a museum, or tour an up-and-coming neighborhood—those steps will add up fast.

DINNER: Make a Mediterranean plate with the falafel recipe from Day 6 (see page 303) and the Coconut Yogurt Tzatziki and Cucumber Salad from the Domestic Goddess plan, page 231.

NEGATE THE NEGATIVE: Vegetarians and vegans get hit with a lot of snide comments and remarks about their lifestyle preferences. Some people are great at letting negativity roll right off their back, while others might take it personally and get upset, especially when family or close friends challenge their decisions. A weekend day might entail a barbecue, party, or other group function where you feel put on the spot. If you feel the need to engage or respond, keep it simple and calmly explain the reason you choose to live and eat the way you do. If you're happy and healthy, what else is there to say? It can be tempting to get defensive or judge someone right back for the way they live, but take a deep breath and choose to keep the conversation positive, even if the other person is doing their best to steer it toward the negative. Remember, it's your body and your decision. What really matters isn't someone else's opinion of you; it's being true to yourself.

Day 21—Weekend Day

BREAKFAST

DARK CHOCOLATE AVOCADO MOUSSE

Let's celebrate the end of your twenty-one day journey with some sweet Fab Four fuel. This velvety and decadent dark chocolate mousse tastes like dessert, but comes packed with everything you need to start the day.

Chocolate protein powder containing 20 to 30 grams protein
2 large very ripe avocados
2 tablespoons milled chia seeds
2 tablespoons organic cacao powder (I like NOW Foods)
¼ teaspoon ground cinnamon (see Tip, page 247)
2 drops of organic liquid monk fruit
½ cup unsweetened almond milk
Pinch of pink Himalayan salt
Topping options: 1 tablespoon hemp hearts, 1 tablespoon shredded coconut, or
    ¼ cup in-season sliced fruit

In a food processor or high-speed blender, blend all the ingredients together until they reach a smooth, pudding-like consistency, about 2 minutes. Refrigerate for 1 hour and serve in a small bowl with your desired topping. Store any extra in a sealable glass container in the refrigerator for up to 3 days.

LUNCH

THAI SALAD WITH SPICY CASHEW DRESSING

*Unhealthy industrial seed oils can often sneak their way into store-bought salad dress-
ings. Like many of the other dressings in this book, I rely on avocado oil to keep things
clean. It works great in this salad. Plus, you'll have extra—save it to use as a dip for fresh
vegetables when you need a bridge snack.*

Makes 2 servings

DRESSING

1 cup unsalted dry-roasted cashews (see Tip, page 323)
½ cup packed cilantro leaves
¼ cup avocado oil
4 garlic cloves, roughly chopped
1 tablespoon tamari
1 tablespoon coconut aminos
Juice of ½ lime
1 to 2 tablespoons sriracha
1 tablespoon red pepper flakes
½ to 1 cup cold filtered water

SALAD

4 cups spinach
1 cup thinly sliced basil (chiffonade cut)
¼ cup thinly sliced red cabbage
¼ cup shredded carrot
¼ cup red cabbage microgreens (or other purple microgreens, like kohlrabi or
    radish)
2 tablespoons spicy seed mix (I like NOW Foods or Go Raw)
¼ avocado
¼ cup canned or cooked chickpeas (page 291), drained and rinsed

1. Combine all the dressing ingredients in a high-speed blender (start with 1 tablespoon sriracha and ½ cup water) and puree until a dressing consistency is reached. For thinner and/or spicier dressing, add more water and/or sriracha.
2. In a large bowl, toss all the salad ingredients with 2 tablespoons of the dressing, or more if you prefer.

DINNER

KALE DETOX SOUP

Let's end the plan with a nourishing and cleansing kale soup. And, for an accompaniment, how about a throwback from Day 21 of the Domestic Goddess plan with my Super Green Kale Chips (page 273). They're healthy chips you can dip.

Makes 3 to 4 servings

2 tablespoons extra virgin olive oil
½ yellow onion, chopped
2 garlic cloves, minced
1 small broccoli head, broken into small florets
2 cups packed chopped kale
2 cups packed chopped other greens (use your favorites: chard, spinach, or a mix)
1 zucchini, diced
2 celery stalks, roughly chopped
1½ teaspoons dried oregano
1½ teaspoons dried basil
1½ teaspoons dried thyme
½ teaspoon celery salt
6 cups vegetable broth
Pink Himalayan salt and freshly ground black pepper
Handful of fresh parsley leaves

1. In a large pot over medium heat, heat the olive oil. Add the onion and garlic and sauté until translucent, 3 to 4 minutes. *(continued)*

2. Add the broccoli, kale, greens, zucchini, celery, herbs, and celery salt and stir to coat. Add the broth, bring the mixture to a boil, and simmer for 10 minutes, until the vegetables are tender.

3. Using a hand blender, puree the vegetables until smooth.

4. Season with pink Himalayan salt and pepper to taste. Serve hot, garnished with the parsley and kale chips.

9

RED-CARPET READY

A HEALTHY REGIMEN FOR A TIGHT DEADLINE

WHAT'S YOUR RED CARPET? There are times in life when we want to look and feel our best. Maybe it's a wedding, class reunion, or big work presentation. It could be a beach vacation or bachelorette weekend. Maybe vacation *ended* six weeks ago, or you had your baby six months ago, and it's time to get back in the groove. It could even be an actual red carpet. Whatever it is, you want or need to put a deadline on your plans, either because the event is just around the corner or because you want to hold yourself more accountable during a defined time frame. Sometimes we need a healthy kick in the booty so we can confidently rock that dress, suit, or bikini. The Fab Four plan in this chapter is here to give you that body-loving boost, jump-start your progress toward a larger lifestyle goal, and help get you Red-Carpet Ready.

We won't be counting or restricting calories. We won't be juicing or cleansing for three weeks. We won't be depriving our bodies, starving ourselves, or striving for perfection. That's not what the Fab Four lifestyle, body love, or this plan is about. The Red-Carpet Ready regimen doesn't look like a crash diet. It looks like the other plans, with a few specific tools on top. So we'll nourish our body with the essential macronutrients it needs to function optimally. We'll balance blood sugar, eat to satiety, and naturally balance hunger hormones. We'll feed the strong, confident, body-loving woman inside of us. Then, we'll utilize a few key tools to propel us forward and help us meet our deadline.

Which brings me back to your red carpet. One of the first things I ask new clients is whether they have a specific goal they're trying to hit. If they have one, I ask what their time frame is. Sometimes the goal is a bit ambitious for the time we've got and where they're at healthwise. In those cases, I counsel them to set a new goal that they can more realistically achieve. The Fab Four plan in this chapter isn't about crash dieting to lose twenty-five pounds or hit a size o in three short weeks. It's about linking healthy decisions together, building on that momentum, and breeding confidence from hitting more incremental goals, such as two pounds per week. My point is that even if you're on a tight deadline, be realistic with your goals and manage your expectations accordingly.

Further, even though you might have a short-term goal, this plan will set you up for long-term, sustainable success. It will help you ditch cravings for sugar, processed foods, and alcohol. Reducing your consumption of these "Not So Fab" Four inputs can help clear brain fog, give you more energy, and help you sleep better. Further, this plan will show you the power of blood sugar balance by keeping you full and fueled *and* by helping you reach your goals. I want you to hit your goal, but I also want you to find real balance and sustainability. Just as in the other plans, my hope is that the next twenty-one days empower and inspire you to build a healthy lifestyle that's right for you in the long term. Consistently making healthy decisions adds up to vitality, longevity, and improved overall health. The Fab Four plan in this chapter can help put you on that path. When you feel the positive momentum and inner confidence growing inside you, the sky's the limit.

As with the plans in the preceding chapters, the Red-Carpet Ready plan begins on a Monday (Day 1) and ends on a Sunday (Day 21). If your deadline, event, or big occasion falls on a Monday, this exact schedule will work for you. However, if it falls on any other day of the week, you may need to adjust the schedule. For example, if your big day—let's call it Day 22—is a Saturday, you could:

- start Day 1 of the plan on a Saturday, which would result in the "weekend days" actually falling during the week on Thursdays and Fridays, but set you up for Day 22 being a Saturday
- simply skip Days 20 and 21 of the plan and, if you want, use the tools or recipes from those days earlier in the week
- start Day 1 of the plan on Monday a week *earlier* and then repeat Days 15 through 19, which would add an extra five days to the plan

These are just a few options for coordinating with your deadline, event, or big occasion. If you don't want that level of structure or you have a month (or more) to prepare, you can follow the plan in the way that's best suited to you and your personal preference.

So what exactly does the Red-Carpet Ready regimen look like? Before we get into the day-to-day, I want to highlight a few of the concepts, tools, and principles we'll be using and following.

IT STARTS WITH THE FAB FOUR. Shocker, right? Protein, fat, fiber, and greens are the foundation of the plan. We'll be eating complete meals and nourishing the body, not starving it. The daily formula will generally look like this: a Fab Four Smoothie for breakfast; a salad with clean protein, healthy fat, and raw vegetables for lunch; and a warming dinner to end the day. But we'll mix it up some, too. Also, on a couple of occasions post-weekend or midweek, we'll use a double smoothie day to give you an extra push.

Of note: all the smoothies, meals, and recipes in this plan are

WHAT'S YOUR "WHY"?

You have a deadline and a goal, but is there a deeper purpose behind it? In *Body Love*, I talked about how connecting to your "why" can increase your likelihood of success, give you inner strength, and help you overcome daily challenges. Let's use that tool before we start. Pick up a pen or pencil and journal why you picked up this book, what you're looking for, what is motivating you, what you want to do differently, and so on. Write until you discover your "why." And don't shy away from expressing the emotions, fears, or frustrations that might be inside you, too. It helps to get them out of your head and onto the page. If you have a specific weight loss or body composition goal, you can add that to your journal as well—but only *after* you've written about your deeper "why."

drawn from the other three plans in this book. If you need to substitute a plant-based option or are simply in the mood for something different for a particular meal, go for it. As I said in the introduction, use the plans in the way that's best suited to you, your lifestyle preferences, and your health and weight loss goals.

THIS ISN'T ALL-OR-NOTHING. The Fab Four lifestyle isn't about perfection. Neither is this plan. There's no starting over if you miss a workout, skip a day, or eat something that isn't on the plan. One decision—your next—is all that matters. Just pick up where you left off or move forward to the next meal or day.

WE'LL BE UTILIZING A NATURAL FORM OF INTERMITTENT FASTING. When most people hear the word *fasting*, they think it means starving themselves and not eating for days on end. We won't be doing that. We'll simply be eating three complete Fab Four meals in a more condensed eating window. We can naturally do this by eating a *slightly later* breakfast and a *slightly earlier* dinner. This is why you'll see specific eating times listed in the plan. In general, the sweet spot to get Red-Carpet Ready is an eight- to ten-hour eating window, which generally looks like this: breakfast at 8 or 9 A.M., lunch around 1 P.M., and dinner at 5 or 6 P.M. Sounds reasonable, right? Also, on a few limited occasions, we'll shrink the window to six hours to give you an extra push.

Why are we doing this? After dinner, your body will have fourteen to sixteen hours to fully digest food before breakfast. During this window, your blood sugar can return to a healthy fasting level and excess insulin can be cleared from your bloodstream. This allows you to burn fat overnight while you sleep. It also lets your body redirect energy to detoxification, decreasing inflammation, and other beautifying repairs. When you consistently eat within these windows, you can help speed up results.

Also, this method reduces snacking, which can disrupt digestion, cause the release of insulin, and turn off fat burning. Eating your meals a little closer together (roughly four hours apart) can help reduce the urge to snack. If you need an occasional bridge snack, make it a simple, whole food that's part of the Fab Four or a Fab Four Smoothie.

CALORIE DEPRIVATION OR RESTRICTION IS NOT AN OP-TION. Period. Even on days when you intermittent-fast, you eat three complete Fab Four meals.

IN FAB FOUR SMOOTHIES, WE'LL RELY ON SPECIFIC RECIPES AND MOSTLY GO FRUIT-FREE. I chose the Fab Four Smoothie recipes with the most detoxifying, hydrating, and functional ingredients. In addition, the majority of the smoothies will be fruit-free so that we can reduce sugar intake. Fruit contains fiber, vitamins, and phytochemicals, but it's also full of glucose and fructose, which will spike your blood sugar. Fructose is metabolized in the liver and turns into fat more quickly than glucose. This can also be an opportunity to try some new recipes. It's easy to become a creature of habit and make the same smoothie every day. But changing it up and reducing your fruit intake can give your body the break from insulin it may need.

SUGAR, ALCOHOL, GRAINS, GLUTEN, DAIRY, AND SOY SHOULD BE SIGNIFICANTLY CUT BACK. I support doing this in general. When you do, and you're eating the Fab Four, you should notice a difference in how you feel. Many of my clients feel more energized and clear-headed, their blood sugar doesn't spike and crash, and they tend to have better digestion and bowel movements. Reducing consumption of the "Not So Fab" Four—processed, sugary, certain starchy, and liquid carbohydrates—also gives your body a break from insulin. As for soy, I generally don't include it in my clients' Fab Four plans to begin with. As noted in chapter 1, the isoflavones and phytoestrogens in soy products have been linked to various health issues.

WE'LL SET DAILY WATER GOALS. Calculate half of your body weight and aim to drink that number in ounces. For example, if you weigh 140 pounds, aim for at least

> **WE EAT**
> I'm not a fan of intermittent fasting methods that train you to deprive yourself and restrict calories, such as the 5:2 method (eat normally five days per week and restrict to 500 calories two days per week) or the alternate day method (eat normally and restrict to 500 calories every other day). Continual caloric deprivation isn't healthy and can lead to health issues (see page 68 in chapter 2). Also, I'm not a fan of waiting until 2 P.M. to eat your first meal because it can result in late-night eating and a mismatched circadian rhythm.

MIX UP YOUR H$_2$O

To add some flavor and variety to your daily water intake, see the Plant-Based Devotee plan, page 296, where you'll find a simple formula for fruit-and-herb infused Spa Water Blends. That plan also features recipes for Matcha Limeade, Apple Cider Vinegar Lemonade, Silica ACV Lemon Water, and Chlorophyll Mint Water. You can keep them in a pitcher in the refrigerator, ready for when you need them.

70 ounces. Add 8 ounces when you work out, if you tend to overconsume caffeine, and if you're at a higher altitude. Water has too many benefits to count, and being dehydrated can derail your Red-Carpet Ready goals. If you're worried about water weight, in the two or three days leading up to your event or deadline, get a sweaty workout in or book an infrared sauna session (the plan in this chapter has both during the final week). Also, be mindful of your sodium intake; oversalting your food will cause you to retain excess water. Read the nutrition facts on your food labels. (See *Body Love* for other water-related tips.) I get a lot of questions about my skincare routine. It starts with two everyday tasks: first, drinking a lot of water and staying well hydrated, and second, eating a lot of greens, which feed my healthy gut bacteria.

WORKING OUT AND EXERCISE ARE A DAILY PRIORITY. They are central components to getting Red-Carpet Ready. I've given you one rest day per week, on Sunday. Most of the workouts are scheduled as fasted morning exercise. If the A.M. doesn't work for you, commit to finding a time that does. The key is to be consistent, hold yourself accountable, and repeat. As for the types of exercise, it's important to do both strength/weight training and cardio. I've included some ideas for both types, but you should do what's right for your body and what you like.

The goal with strength/weight training isn't to bulk up but to help tone, tighten, and build lean muscle mass. It can be weights, kettlebells, a HIIT class, yoga with weights, or even a body weight circuit, in which you're simply lifting your own body weight. The point is to get an anaerobic workout that makes your muscles sore. This can help increase insulin sensitivity, lower blood sugar levels, and increase your metabolism. All good things when you're working toward a short-term goal.

Then, to give your muscles time to recover and to balance out your week, it's important to do cardio workouts like Spin, running, walking, dance cardio, swimming, elliptical, or stairs. Cardio helps dump stored glycogen from your muscles, flushes out lactic acid, and gives your body a detoxifying sweat. When you combine strength/weight training and cardio workouts with eating the Fab Four, you can tone and tighten, all while nourishing your body from the inside out.

CREATE A BODY-LOVING BEDTIME ROUTINE. For Red-Carpet Ready clients who are feeling deadline pressure, I find that committing to a body-loving bedtime routine helps them destress, unwind, and recharge. It can be as simple as carving out twenty minutes before bedtime when they do something other than look at social media, watch television, or sit on their computer. A few options: reading, taking a warm bath or shower, meditation, breathwork, journaling, foam rolling, lying on an acupressure mat, putting on a face mask, exfoliating with a scrub, and prepping Fab Four Smoothie ingredients for the morning. Find something that works for you and use it as an opportunity to end the day on a relaxing note. It also helps to foster new habits other than snacking at night on the couch. You'll see a Bedtime 20 for every day of the plan to support your sleep hygiene.

WAIT TO WEIGH YOURSELF

The urge to step on the scale every single day or multiple times per day can be hard to resist. But I would counsel you against doing this. Body weight naturally fluctuates throughout the day and also over the course of a week. The body has a normal range or equilibrium, called homeostasis. Most people weigh less in the morning than they do at night, and many people find themselves up or down a few pounds from day to day. If you're constantly weighing yourself, you might get discouraged or frustrated by these natural fluctuations. You might also lose sight of what the scale won't show—that you're nourishing your body with the Fab Four, supporting blood sugar balance, and making strides toward a larger lifestyle goal. The scale also doesn't know the difference between muscle and fat. If you're working out and toning your lean muscle mass, the scale might not reflect the inches and fat you're losing in the process.

(continued)

If you find the scale motivating and want to check your progress while following this plan, here's how I would do it. Weigh yourself once per week—first thing in the morning—after going to the bathroom and before eating breakfast. (In the plan, I have check-in opportunities on Day 7, Day 14, and the day after finishing—Day 22.) In my practice, I actually rely more heavily on measurements than weight to track my clients' progress. Using a tape measure, I measure around their arms (at the biceps), waist (above the hips), hips, and thighs (middle). Then, at our next check-in a month later, we measure the same spots again. I can't tell you how many times the scale doesn't reflect the physical changes you can see—and, more important, feel—based on these measurements.

INSTA-INSPIRATION

Have you ever taken a screenshot of a #MondayMotivation quote on Instagram . . . and then forgotten all about it? Open your phone, scroll through your photos till you find one, write it down on a Post-it or piece of paper, and place it somewhere you see every day. If I can offer one written by yours truly:

Imagine there's a hallway in your mind.
It connects today to tomorrow.
On one wall, you frame and hang your thoughts.
On the other, moments from your past.
What would you rather walk by each day?

"I'm fat," "I'm pathetic," "I'll never do it. . . ."
Or "I'm beautiful," "I love me," "I know I can."
All your setbacks, failures, self-defeats . . .
Or all your bounce backs, breakthroughs, wins . . .

You choose what to frame.

You choose what to hang.

Choose the resilient, confident, relentless you.

Walk past her every day.

Day 1—Weekday

WORKOUT (7 A.M.): Get out of the blocks with a thirty-five- to forty-five-minute cardio workout. A few ideas: a three-mile run or power walk, a Spin class, a class on your favorite app, an upbeat Vinyasa yoga flow, lap swimming in a pool, or a stair-climbing session. If none of those are speaking to you, do what works for you and your body. Just get your blood pumping and break a good sweat.

BREAKFAST (9 A.M.): My original Spa Day Fab Four Smoothie is going to be your Monday morning go-to. It's refreshing, hydrating, and full of Fab Four fuel. See the Girl on the Go plan, page 164.

LUNCH (1 P.M.): Flaky Tuna and Toasted Walnut Salad (see the Girl on the Go plan, page 181).

DINNER (6 P.M.): Shrimp Scampi with Zoodles (see the Girl on the Go plan, page 165).

BEDTIME 20 (8 P.M.): Exfoliate and use a face mask tonight. On page 362 are a few brands I use and like. Also, for two DIY antimicrobial honey masks, see the Domestic Goddess plan, pages 256 and 257.

BODY LOVE BUDDY

Is there someone on the same deadline as you? Or who wants to start making progress toward a healthier lifestyle? Maybe he or she could be your "body love buddy" for the next twenty-one days. Whether they follow the whole plan or want to commit to only part of it (like a Fab Four Smoothie for breakfast or a daily workout), having a friend or family member at your side could be a huge source of encouragement, support, and motivation. (For them, too.) You can also help hold each other accountable if you're tempted to skip a workout or there's a bad habit one of you is trying to break. Talk, listen, vent, high-five, and cheer each other on.

BODY LOVE EVERY DAY

GO TO BED!

Can you get into bed by 10 P.M.? To hit your goal, try to make it a priority. Lack of sleep, poor sleep, and disruptions to your circadian rhythm can interfere with your hunger hormones. According to a 2017 study, "Later sleep time was associated with higher estimated insulin resistance across all groups." And according to a 2008 meta analysis of 634,511 male and female participants from around the world from age 2 to 102, there was "an increased risk of obesity among short sleepers along with an increase in appetite and caloric intake associated with reciprocal changes in leptin and ghrelin." (For more tips to help you get more beautifying shut-eye, see *Body Love*.)

Exfoliating Treatments

Goldfaden MD: Doctor's Scrub

Acure: Brilliantly Brightening Facial Scrub

MyChelle: Fruit Enzyme Scrub

Face Masks

Summer Fridays: Jet Lag Mask

Tata Harper: Resurfacing Mask

Crop Natural: Hydrating Aloe Vera or Purifying Turmeric

Éminence: Strawberry Rhubarb Masque with Hyaluronic Acid

Day 2—Weekday

WORKOUT (7 A.M.): Strength/weight training day. Choose a thirty- to sixty-minute workout that involves weight lifting, kettlebells, resistance, or strength training. A couple of class options include yoga with weights or a HIIT class. High-intensity interval training combines aerobic and anaerobic exercise over a short period of time (usually around thirty minutes). Among other benefits, it can help lower insulin resistance and improve metabolism, which are both great for weight loss. Google a well-reviewed HIIT class near you and try it out.

BREAKFAST (9 A.M.): Original Green Fab Four Smoothie (see the Girl on the Go plan, page 167).

LUNCH (1 P.M.): Ribboned Rainbow Salad over Sprouted Sunflower Seed Hummus (see the Plant-Based Devotee plan, page 288). You can either keep it plant-based or add 4 ounces of chicken.

DINNER (6 P.M.): Garlic Salmon and Brussels Sprouts (see the Domestic Goddess plan, page 263). This recipe makes 4 to 6 servings, so you should have leftovers for tomorrow's lunch.

BEDTIME 20 (8 P.M.): Try breathwork to calm your nervous system (see the Domestic Goddess plan, page 209). If it clicks for you, make it part of your daily or weekly routine.

Day 3—Weekday

PUSH DAY: To give you a midweek push, we're going to shrink your eating window to six hours today. We'll do this by delaying your Fab Four Smoothie till 11 A.M. and then eating dinner an hour earlier at 5 P.M. The purpose is to allow your body a longer break from insulin, both in the morning before breakfast and at night after dinner. If you naturally have an earlier start to your day, you can do a 10 A.M. to 4 P.M. window, or if you naturally have a later start to your day, you can also push it back to 12 P.M. to 6 P.M., but I wouldn't go later than that. If you find yourself really hungry and in need of a snack, make sure it's Fab Four: one or two hard-boiled eggs, a handful of raw nuts, celery with 1 tablespoon of almond butter, half an avocado, or half a Fab Four Smoothie.

WORKOUT (9 A.M.): Cardio day. Pound the pedals and sweat it out at a Spin class.

BREAKFAST (11 A.M.): Green Goddess Fab Four Smoothie (see the Domestic Goddess plan, page 221).

LUNCH (1 TO 2 P.M.): Leftover Garlic Salmon and Brussels Sprouts.

DINNER (5 P.M.): Coconut Tzatziki Chicken Skewers, served with Coconut Yogurt Tzatziki and Cucumber Salad (see the Domestic Goddess plan, page 230).

BEDTIME 20 (8 P.M.): Roll It Out (see the Domestic Goddess plan, page 251). Give your fasciae some love with a foam-rolling exercise. If you sit at a desk all day or have a long commute, a few minutes of foam rolling on a nightly basis can be especially beneficial.

Day 4—Weekday

WORKOUT (7 A.M.): Strength/weight training day. Find a workout that incorporates weights or kettlebells. Another HIIT workout is an option as well.

BREAKFAST (9 A.M.): Creamy Mocha Fab Four Smoothie (see the Domestic Goddess plan, page 264).

LUNCH (1 P.M.): Add a can of sardines or two soft-boiled eggs to a Brainiac Salad (see the Plant-Based Devotee plan, page 300).

DINNER (6 P.M.): Lettuce-Wrapped Pan-Fried Sliders and Roasted Root Fries (see the Domestic Goddess plan, page 269). Pair it with a big green salad and dressing of your choice.

BEDTIME 20 (8 P.M.): Give yourself some spiky stress relief by lying back on an acupressure mat (see the Girl on the Go plan, page 173).

Day 5—Weekday

WORKOUT (7 A.M.): Cardio day. If you want to mix it up with something like a boxing class, go for it. If you're looking forward to your tried-and-true, stick with it.

BREAKFAST (9 A.M.): Cookies and Cream Fab Four Smoothie (see the Girl on the Go plan, page 163).

LUNCH (1 P.M.): Asian Crunch Salad (see the Plant-Based Devotee plan, page 311). You can either keep it plant-based or add 4 ounces of chicken.

DINNER (6 P.M.): Chinese Chicken Lettuce Wraps (see the Girl on the Go plan, page 176).

BEDTIME 20 (8 P.M.): For a simple meditation exercise (see the Girl on the Go plan, page 151).

Day 6—Weekend Day

WORKOUT (7 A.M.): Light cardio day. Find nature and strike out on a ninety-minute hike. If the weather prevents you, it's not the right season, or you can't escape the city, make it a power walk at the gym or around the neighborhood.

BREAKFAST (9 A.M.): Anti-Inflammatory Vanilla Spice Fab Four Smoothie (see the Domestic Goddess plan, page 246).

LUNCH (1 P.M.): Egg Salad over Arugula with Jilz Crackerz (see the Girl on the Go plan, page 167).

DINNER (6 P.M.): Lime Cilantro Chicken and Broccoli (see the Domestic Goddess plan, page 247).

BEDTIME 20 (8 P.M.): Practice Gratitude (see the Girl on the Go plan, page 170). Everyone faces challenges in some aspect of life. One way to draw strength to meet those challenges is by tapping in to your blessings. Reflect on what you're thankful for, and use that gratitude to fuel you.

Day 7—Weekend Day

WORKOUT: Rest day. Unless you missed a day during the week, take today off to let your body rest and recover.

PUSH DAY: Today is the second push day. Just like Day 3, we're going to shrink the eating window to 6 hours.

BREAKFAST (11 A.M.): Simple Eggs and Greens (see the Girl on the Go plan, page 187).

LUNCH (1 TO 2 P.M.): Almond Bliss Fab Four Smoothie (see the Domestic Goddess plan, page 249).

DINNER (5 P.M.): Vegetable and Cauliflower Rice Soup (see the Plant-Based Devotee Plan, page 304). For protein, add 4 ounces of precooked rotisserie chicken (chopped or shredded) and swap bone broth for the vegetable broth when you make the soup.

BEDTIME 20 (8 P.M.): I love taking baths. For me, nothing is as calming or relaxing at night. It's a simple form of self-care, and I find it soothing both physically and mentally. Here are few ways to create a Boosted Bath:

- Add Epsom salt (magnesium sulfate) or magnesium flakes (100 percent pure magnesium chloride flakes), which may potentially make magnesium available for absorption through the skin.
- Add a CBD bath ball. CBD doesn't contain THC, the compound in cannabis that gets you high. **Note: Do not use CBD if you are trying to get pregnant, are currently pregnant, or are currently breastfeeding.**
- Use a body brush before the bath and a mitt while in the bath. A few I like: Aromatherapy Associates Revive Body Brush, Wholesome Beauty Dry Skin Body Brush, and the Supracor Stimulite Bath Mitt.

WEEK 1 CHECK-IN

It's the end of Week 1, which is a good time to check in with yourself.

First, take out your journal and reread your "why." Remind yourself of how the small, daily decisions you're making connect to the deeper purpose behind your goal. Then take a few minutes to write down how you're feeling physically, mentally, and emotionally. You're free to vent, give yourself a pep talk, nurture what needs love, let your confidence grow—whatever it is, express it. Sometimes we put up walls to protect ourselves. Maybe after a week of eating the Fab Four and showing yourself body love, you'll break through a wall or layer and discover another "why."

Second, if you want to step on the scale to check your weight, I would do it first thing in the morning after you've gone to the bathroom and before eating breakfast. If you measured yourself prior to starting the plan, you can also take updated arm, waist, hips, and thigh measurements to track your progress (see page 359). For some people, having a weekly goal can be a helpful way to stay motivated. For others, it can cause anxiety or lead to disappointment. Each of us has a different body with a unique body chemistry, and reaching your goals isn't always a straight-line process. Be realistic, stay positive, and remember that you're nourishing your body with the Fab Four, which goes beyond both the scale and the measuring tape.

PRACTICE MAKES PREPARED

Whatever lies at the end of your twenty-one days, you can practice and prepare for it. Below are a few ideas to help get you in prep mode.

VISUALIZE YOUR SUCCESS. Whatever the event or occasion, picture yourself being there in the moment . . . feeling confident and composed . . . savoring every second of it . . . and crushing it. While you're at it, visualize yourself calmly overcoming something unexpected. You'll be better prepared as a result.

WRITE IT, DON'T WING IT. Take the time to write down your speech or presentation. Then practice delivering it out loud to someone who will give you positive but constructive feedback. You never know what works and what doesn't until you practice. Write it, speak it, and tweak it. You'll end up with a more polished result.

THERE'S A HERO IN THE MIRROR. Too often we use the mirror to pick ourselves apart. Use it to build yourself up. Make a funny face, give yourself a steely look of grit and determination, and tell yourself you got this. Your eyes are the real you and what others connect with. Get them ready to sparkle and shine.

BODY-LOVING SELF-TALK. Positive self-talk is a habit that all of us can work on. It's also a form of preparation and practice for your mind. Optimistic thinking can inspire resiliency when adversity strikes. If you feel some negativity creeping into your head, remember you can always "turn up the volume" on your positive inner voice.

SPOTLIGHT'S ON. Some people are uncomfortable being the center of attention or having the spotlight turned on them. I've actually had a number of brides who've felt this way leading up to their wedding day. Even if that's not you, the glare might feel a little bright in certain situations. A fun way to practice being in the spotlight—literally? Grab your friends and head to a karaoke bar.

Day 8—Weekday

WORKOUT (7 A.M.): Cardio day. Choose a thirty- to sixty-minute cardio workout and start the week with a strong sweat. A few options: a sixty-minute power walk, pound out a two- to three-mile run, Spin class, use the elliptical machine at the gym, pick an upbeat workout from your favorite app, go to an up-tempo Vinyasa yoga class, or take a HIIT class.

BREAKFAST (9 A.M.): Spa Day Fab Four Smoothie (see the Girl on the Go plan, page 164).

LUNCH (1 P.M.): Brainiac Salad (see the Plant-Based Devotee plan, page 300). Add 3 to 4 ounces of the protein of your choice.

DINNER (6 P.M.): Leftover Vegetable and Cauliflower Rice Soup from yesterday.

BEDTIME 20 (8 P.M.): Brew a hot tea (see the Plant-Based Devotee plan, page 287). The ritual of sipping tea in the evening can help reduce cravings, calm the body, and support sounder sleep. If you're struck by the urge to snack, try occupying your mind with something else, like a good book or adult coloring (see the Domestic Goddess plan, page 221).

Day 9—Weekday

WORKOUT (7 A.M.): Strength/weight training day. Choose a thirty- to sixty-minute workout that involves weight lifting, kettlebells, resistance, or strength training. A couple of class options include yoga with weights or a HIIT class.

BREAKFAST (9 A.M.): Matcha Limeade Green Fab Four Smoothie (see the Plant-Based Devotee plan, page 295).

LUNCH (1 P.M.): Peanut Kale Salad (see the Domestic Goddess plan, page 265).

DINNER (6 P.M.): Steamed Fish and Vegetables (see the Girl on the Go plan, page 169).

BEDTIME 20 (8 P.M.): Tech-Free Tuesday (see the Domestic Goddess plan, page 166). Prying yourself away from your phone, television, and computer can be hard, but try to give yourself at least one night off per week.

Day 10—Weekday

WORKOUT (9 A.M.): Cardio day. Mix it up or go with your tried-and-true.

PUSH DAY: Give yourself a push over the midweek hump and shrink your eating window to six hours today.

BREAKFAST (11 A.M.): Chocolate Almond Butter Crunch Fab Four Smoothie (see the Domestic Goddess plan, page 216).

LUNCH (1 TO 2 P.M.): Ribboned Rainbow Salad over Sprouted Sunflower Seed Hummus (see the Plant-Based Devotee plan, page 288). You can either keep it plant-based or add 4 ounces of chicken.

DINNER (5 P.M.): Coconut Cauliflower Rice with Sweet Coconut Chicken and Broccoli (see the Girl on the Go plan, page 182).

BEDTIME 20 (8 P.M.): Phone a Friend (see the Domestic Goddess plan, page 248). Dopamine is released when we hear, see, or touch another person. You might be surprised how good it makes you feel to actually talk to someone on the phone again.

Day 11—Weekday

WORKOUT (7 A.M.): Strength/weight training day. Tone, tighten, and get sore. See Day 9 for a few different options.

BREAKFAST (9 A.M.): Raspberry Lemonade Fab Four Smoothie (see the Plant-Based Devotee plan, page 325).

LUNCH (1 P.M.): Shrimp Louie Salad (see the Domestic Goddess plan, page 206).

DINNER (6 P.M.): Chicken Piccata and Asparagus (see the Domestic Goddess plan, page 220).

BEDTIME 20 (8 P.M.): Using a jade roller on your face can help reduce puffiness, inflammation, and excess fluid. My friend and *Life with Me* blogger, Marianna Hewitt, has a great post explaining the benefits of jade rolling and an easy-to-follow video that shows you how to do it (see lifewithme.com/what-is-jade-rolling). You can buy a jade roller on Amazon or a beauty supply store for under twenty dollars. Give it a try tonight and make it part of your beautifying routine in the lead-up to your event or big occasion. (Marianna has other beautifying and detoxifying tips, too!)

Day 12—Weekday

WORKOUT (7 A.M.): Cardio day. See page 368 for a few options and ideas.
BREAKFAST (9 A.M.): Sweet and Savory Basil Fab Four Smoothie (see the Domestic Goddess plan, page 266).

LUNCH (1 P.M.): Thai Salad with Spicy Cashew Dressing (see the Plant-Based Devotee plan, page 350).

DINNER (6 P.M.): Steamed Fish and Vegetables (see the Girl on the Go plan, page 169).

BEDTIME 20 (8 P.M.): Too often we focus on the negative, like how we're lacking in some way, why we're not good enough, or replaying regrets over and over. Take a few minutes tonight to redirect your thoughts and emotions to a positive place. Journal the positive, like what you love about yourself, your accomplishments, the joy and laughter you bring to others. Turn on the spotlight, step onstage, and bask in some self-made shine. Tell yourself, "I love me, unconditionally."

Day 13—Weekend Day

WORKOUT (7 A.M.): Light cardio day. Walk to do your errands, find some nature and go for a hike, or be a tourist in your own city. Visit a museum, or tour an unfamiliar neighborhood—those steps will add up.

BREAKFAST (9 A.M.): Super Green Machine Fab Four Smoothie (see the Girl on the Go plan, page 174).

LUNCH (1 P.M.): Add shrimp or chicken to my Vegan Hand Rolls (see the Plant-Based Devotee plan, page 339).

DINNER (6 P.M.): Herby Italian Chicken (see the Girl on the Go plan, page 192).

BEDTIME 20 (8 P.M.): Cleanse and oil face massage. Keeping my skin well-hydrated is one of my secrets for supple skin. I avoid stripping the skin with harsh cleansers and instead use an oil-based cleanser and pure facial oil to rehydrate my face before bed. Below are few brands I like.

OIL-BASED CLEANSER
1. MyChelle Perfect C Cleansing Oil
2. Biossance Squalane + Antioxidant Cleansing Oil
3. Tata Harper Nourishing Oil Cleanser
4. Éminence Stone Crop Cleansing Oil

FACIAL OILS
1. Honest Beauty Magic Organic Facial Oil
2. NOW Foods Rosehip Seed Oil
3. Vintner's Daughter Active Botanical Serum
4. Naturopathica Carrot Seed Soothing Facial Oil
5. Éminence Calendula Oil

Day 14—Weekend Day

WORKOUT: Rest day. But if you feel the itch to be active or you missed a workout this week, go get it.

PUSH DAY: Use a six-hour eating window to finish off the week.

BREAKFAST (11 A.M.): Farmers' Market Frittata (see the Domestic Goddess plan, page 210).

LUNCH (1 TO 2 P.M.): Sweet Spiced Carrot Cake Fab Four Smoothie (see the Plant-Based Devotee plan, page 284).

DINNER (5 P.M.): Mexican Chicken Vegetable Soup (see the Girl on the Go plan, page 178).

BEDTIME 20 (6 P.M.): Treat yourself to a Sunday-evening massage. One of my favorite treats to myself every month or two is to book a sixty-minute massage on a Sunday night (we have an affordable massage parlor right around the corner). My routine is to take a shower and scrub my body *before* I go, and then I bring my own nourishing body oil for the masseuse to use. That way I can enjoy a hydrating, toxin-free experience that I don't feel the need to immediately wash off. Below are a few oils I like. Simple oils and balms are my favorite.

MY FAVORITE BODY AND MASSAGE OILS

1. NOW Foods Sweet Almond Oil
2. The Honest Company Organic Body Oil
3. African Botanicals Marula Oil (Firming Botanical or Stretchmark formulations)
4. Nucifera The Balm

WEEK 2 CHECK-IN

Time for your second self-check-in. Take out your journal and reread your "why." Then spend a few minutes writing down how you're feeling physically, mentally, and emotionally. If you want to step on the scale or take updated body measurements, you can do that as well and write down where you are. Or if you're feeling good and know you're making progress, skip the scale and the tape measure.

FINAL WEEK PUSH

During weeks 1 and 2, we used push days on Wednesdays and Sundays to intermittent-fast and shrink your eating window to six hours. During the final week before your deadline, we can use two other tools to give you a final push. First, a double smoothie day, in which you have a Fab Four Smoothie for breakfast, a complete Fab Four meal for lunch, and then another Fab Four Smoothie for dinner. Second, a double workout day, in which you add an afternoon exercise session. These are occasional tools, and I recommend using them only rarely, such as when you need a final push before your deadline. As I said in Part One, the Fab Four lifestyle isn't a smoothie diet. I also don't want you obsessively working out.

> ## JUST A FRIENDLY REMINDER . . .
>
> . . . that practice makes prepared. If you're gearing up for an event or big occasion, one way to help calm any nerves or stress is to plan, practice, and prepare in advance. You've still got a week to do all three P's! Even an hour can go a long way to making you feel ready. See page 367 for a few tips.

FINAL WEEK NERVES

If you feel nervous, anxious, or stressed out in the week leading up to your big event or deadline, you might be tempted to seek comfort in food and indulge in something unhealthy. If this happens, know that you can always bring yourself back into balance with the Fab Four at your next meal. One decision—your next—is all that matters.

If stress strikes, use a body-loving tool to help you. A few options:

- Brew a hot tea (see the Plant-Based Devotee plan, page 287).
- Practice breathwork (see the Domestic Goddess plan, page 209).
- Lead yourself through a simple meditation exercise (see the Girl on the Go plan, page 151).
- Take out your journal and write down how you're feeling (see the Plant-Based Devotee plan, page 343).

(continued)

> - Talk—no texting!—to your body love buddy (if you have one) or someone who you trust (see the Domestic Goddess plan, page 248).
> - Move your body to process the emotion physically, such as a walk around the office, the block, or a park (see the Plant-Based Devotee plan, page 329)

Day 15—Weekday

WORKOUT (7 A.M.): Cardio day. Push to a full sixty minutes today.

BREAKFAST (9 A.M.): Spa Day Fab Four Smoothie (see the Girl on the Go plan, page 164).

LUNCH (1 P.M.): Spicy Salmon Nori Burrito (see the Domestic Goddess plan, page 211).

DINNER (5 P.M.): Leftover Mexican Chicken Vegetable Soup.

BEDTIME 20 (8 P.M.): Exfoliate and put on a face mask (see Day 1, page 256).

Day 16—Weekday

PUSH DAY: Double workout day.

MORNING WORKOUT (7 A.M.): Thirty- to sixty-minute cardio workout.

BREAKFAST (9 A.M.): Original Green Fab Four Smoothie (see the Girl on the Go plan, page 167).

LUNCH (1 P.M.): Green Goddess Salad (see the Domestic Goddess plan, page 229). Add 3 to 4 ounces of protein of your choice.

AFTERNOON WORKOUT: Thirty- to sixty-minute strength/weight training workout.

TIP: You might have heard the term "backloading carbohydrates." All this means is eating your starchy carbohydrates after a workout. The benefit of doing this is it gives your body carbohydrates when your muscles are primed to accept glucose. In addition, glucose and insulin can be more efficiently cleared from the bloodstream. This can set you up for more fat burning during the day and ensure your muscles are fueled for your next hard workout.

DINNER (5 P.M.): Because you worked out twice today, we're going to eat some starchy carbohydrates at dinner. A few options: (1) add ½ cup white rice to Korean Barbecue Steak with Spicy Bok Choy from the Domestic Goddess plan, page 250; (2) serve a roast sweet potato with Vegan Kale Caesar with Crispy Smoked Chickpeas from the Plant-Based Devotee plan, page 306; or (3) Sheet Pan Mackerel and Red Potatoes from the Domestic Goddess plan, page 253.

BEDTIME 20 (8 P.M.): Try a bedtime tonic, like Natural Vitality Natural Calm (magnesium and antistress) or Four Sigmatic Reishi Mushroom Elixir Mix (supports sleep).

Day 17—Weekday

DOUBLE PUSH DAY: Double smoothie day *and* a six-hour eating window.

WORKOUT (9 A.M.): Because yesterday was a double workout day, today will be a light cardio day. Aim for a thirty-minute power walk or light run.

BREAKFAST SMOOTHIE (11 A.M.): Super Green Machine Fab Four Smoothie (see the Girl on the Go plan, page 174).

LUNCH (1 TO 2 P.M.): Greek Chicken Salad (see the Domestic Goddess plan, page 259).

TURMERIC BONE BROTH

I generally advise my clients to avoid snacking because it can disrupt fat burning and digestion. However, on double smoothie days, I've found that many clients need a bridge between lunch and dinner. A warming cup of turmeric-infused bone broth adds protein and fat and won't spike your blood sugar.

1 cup bone broth (see page 36)
1 tablespoon minced fresh ginger
1 tablespoon ground turmeric
Pinch of freshly ground black pepper
1 tablespoon extra virgin olive oil

Combine all the ingredients in a medium saucepan over medium-high heat. Simmer for 5 minutes to infuse all the flavors together. Pour through a mesh strainer (to catch the ginger) and enjoy.

DINNER SMOOTHIE (5 P.M.): Triple Chocolate Crunch Fab Four Smoothie (see the Domestic Goddess plan, page 218). On double smoothie days, I like the dinner smoothie to be something more decadent.

BEDTIME 20 (8 P.M.): Give your feet some love (see the Domestic Goddess plan, page 217). An easy form of self-care is to use a spiky foot massage ball to stimulate the nerve endings on the bottom of your feet. This can relieve tension and help you relax

TIP: Another occasion in which you can use a double smoothie day is the day after a carb-heavy or boozy weekend. It works like a quick reset and will help your fasting blood sugar and triglyceride levels return to normal.

Day 18—Weekday

WORKOUT (7 A.M.): Thirty-minute strength/weight training workout.

BREAKFAST (9 A.M.): Ginger Lemonade Fab Four Smoothie (see the Plant-Based Devotee plan, page 302).

LUNCH (1 P.M.): Wild Fish Boats (see the Girl on the Go plan, page 172).

DINNER (5 P.M.): Sausage and Pepper Skillet (see the Girl on the Go plan, page 188).

BEDTIME 20 (8 P.M.): Your choice tonight. A few options: (1) hop in a Boosted Bath (page 366); (2) exfoliate and put on a face mask (see Day 1, page 362); and/or (3) roll out your fasciae with a foam roller (see the Domestic Goddess plan, page 251).

Day 19—Weekday

WORKOUT (7 A.M.): Cardio day. Push it and go a full sixty minutes again.

BREAKFAST (9 A.M.): "Fat fast" by drinking a fat coffee for breakfast this morning (see page 76).

LUNCH (1 P.M.): Creamy Coconut Broccoli Soup with Watercress and Spicy Pepitas (see the Plant-Based Devotee plan, page 292).

DINNER (6 P.M.): Ground Beef Tostada Salad (see the Domestic Goddess plan, page 260).

BEDTIME 20 (8 P.M.): Cleanse and oil face massage (see Day 13, page 371).

Day 20—Weekend Day

WORKOUT (7 A.M.): Light cardio day, such as a nature hike or walk.

BREAKFAST (9 A.M.): Southwest Scramble (see the Domestic Goddess plan, page 239).

LUNCH (1 P.M.): Cookies and Cream Fab Four Smoothie (see the Girl on the Go plan, page 163).

DINNER (5 P.M.): Vegan Cauliflower Rice Bowl with Avocado and Crispy Harissa Chickpeas (see the Plant-Based Devotee plan, page 294).

BEDTIME 20 (8 P.M.): Tonight, I want you to write a note to yourself. Thank yourself for committing to making body-loving decisions for the past three weeks. Tell yourself how proud you are of the healthy decisions you've made so far. Remind yourself that you're making progress every day, even if it doesn't always follow a straight line. Count your blessings and be grateful for the life you live. Whether Day 22 involves a wedding, class reunion, work presentation, the start of vacation, or is simply another day, remind yourself to be present and enjoy the moment.

Day 21—Weekend Day

PUSH DAY: Use a six-hour eating window to end the week.

BREAKFAST (11 A.M.): Green Ginger Fab Four Smoothie (see the Girl on the Go plan, page 161).

LUNCH (1 TO 2 P.M.): Flaky Tuna and Toasted Walnut Salad (see the Girl on the Go plan, page 181).

SUNDAY SELF-CARE (3 P.M.): Book a forty-minute session at an infrared sauna. The infrared heat can help stimulate the production of collagen, will make you sweat and in the process detoxify, and give your metabolism a kick. Another option is to book a cryotherapy session, which has similar benefits, except using cold instead of heat.

DINNER (5 P.M.): Cowboy Skillet (see the Girl on the Go plan, page 194).

BEDTIME 20 (8 P.M.): Your choice tonight. Choose an activity (or activities) that you know will relax you and help you look and feel your best. To me, a bath, hot tea, and a face mask sounds like a good combination. Whatever you do, get in bed by 10 P.M. so you're fully rested for the next day. If your thoughts are racing or you're having trouble falling asleep, drink a glass of water, focus on your breath, and read a book if need be.

FINAL CHECK-IN

You did it! Twenty-one days of nourishment, twenty-one days of body love, and twenty-one days of healthy decisions. Congratulations on giving it your all and showing your body the love that it deserves. I'd be so excited to hear about your progress—please don't hesitate to share with me on Instagram or my website. Speaking of progress, time for your final self-check-in.

First, I want you to journal how you're feeling physically, mentally, and emotionally. Do you feel different than your first journal entry? Have you unearthed another "why" that's driving you? Has your relationship with food changed, and if so, how? Is there something from the book that's really sticking with you—a nugget of science from Part One, a tip, tool, or recipe from the other plans, a new sense of confidence or balance?

Next, if you started with a specific weight loss or body composition goal, let's see where you are. Remember to weigh yourself first thing in the morning after going to the bathroom and before eating breakfast. You can take updated body measurements at that time, too, if you want. My hope and belief is that you will have made progress toward your goal. Always remember that prioritizing the Fab Four, balancing your blood sugar, and adopting the body love mentality are rewards in and of themselves. You're living a healthy lifestyle, and your body knows it . . . trust me. I'm proud of you!

Day 22—The Big Day

How should you approach Day 22 if it entails an event or big occasion? In my experience, you feel the best when you continue to do what you've been doing. The "day of" should be a continuation of the healthy, body-loving choices you've been making during the past three weeks. First, I would encourage some type of movement in the morning. A few ideas would be a yoga class or some light cardio (such as a thirty-minute power walk). Breaking a little sweat will help you physically process any nerves or jitters. Second, I would start the day with a Fab Four Smoothie. Pick your favorite recipe or use the Spa Day recipe again. This will balance your blood sugar and calm your hunger hormones. Third, your big day isn't the time to start starving yourself. Eat! And stick to the Fab Four. One tip: if you know that beans or high-fiber cruciferous vegetables can make you feel a little bloated, opt for other options in the fiber and greens categories. Finally, if you need a confidence booster, break out the note you wrote to yourself on Day 20 and give it a read. You got this!

10
INNER PERFECTIONIST

LET GO OF PERFECT AND EMBRACE BODY LOVE

WE'VE ALL CHASED PERFECT before. Some of you might even be chasing it right now. Even if you aren't, there might be days when you battle perfectionist thoughts—when perfect seems to be chasing *you*. One picture on Instagram, one meal gone wrong, one negative interaction with someone, and our minds fill up with all the reasons we're not good enough, all the ways we lack, all the ways we could be perfect. A perfect body, with perfect abs and perfect legs. A perfect eater, who always makes the healthy decision. A perfect life, with everything always perfectly under control. It's the ultimate mind game—and the mind is where perfect lives. In reality, there's no such thing.

In my practice, I've worked with hundreds of women who've struggled with their inner perfectionist. So I've seen firsthand and in a variety of ways how perfect really is the enemy of good, how constantly striving for the unattainable prevents progress, and how over time that negative, self-defeating voice in your head can chip away at your confidence and ultimately your happiness.

When I created the Fab Four, part of my goal was to help my clients break free of a perfectionist offshoot: the all-or-nothing diet mentality. I wanted to create a livable framework for eating clean, finding balance, and reaching your goals. Perfect is rigid. The Fab Four is flexible. It's light structure that works for everyday living. In a way, it's kind of an antiplan, which I know sounds a bit ironic given all the plans in the previous chapters. But as I said in the introduction, the plans are merely four examples that you can aspire to and follow—if you want to. They're not the only ways to go about living a Fab Four lifestyle. If your inner perfectionist rears her head, remind her that this isn't all-or-nothing or just about twenty-one days; it's about balance, body love, and building a healthy lifestyle that you love.

A good long-term goal is to try to internalize the science, concepts, and tools in this book. That way you can chart your own path to food freedom and always bring yourself back into balance if you need to. When you prioritize the Fab Four, you'll be nourishing your body and fostering a more positive relationship with food. And instead of beating yourself up about having an imbalanced meal or day, you'll be building self-confidence and resilience.

This chapter is kind of an antiplan as well. Unlike the rest of Part Two, it doesn't contain a daily program to follow. It offers a few tips and tools to help manage perfectionist thoughts and embrace the body love mentality.

First, I want to share two quick stories.

I'm lucky to work with some of the most inspiring businesswomen and female entrepreneurs in Los Angeles. Perhaps none of them is more on the go than Jane, age forty-three, who took her one-woman business, built it into a brand, and turned it into a nationwide juggernaut. Jane travels nearly every week to a different part of the country and spends a lot of time in hotels. When I met her, her typical workday was sixteen hours long, and she was trying to be perfect every single minute of it. She set her expectations so high that she was only allowing herself cucumbers and hard-boiled eggs some days. This wasn't who Jane was. She grew up in the South and loved comfort food and savory dishes. Demanding perfection meant depriving herself and denying her roots. The stress of it all was too much, and she would end up eating fast food lunches to make herself feel better.

For a lifestyle to truly work, it has to be you. I asked Jane what she liked to eat growing up and what felt emotionally satisfying to her. Then we hit the aisles in the grocery store and picked out clean options that would satisfy her. We deprogrammed her diet mentality and showed her how she could eat what she loved within the light structure of the Fab Four. She was in shock when I told her she could still enjoy a beef stick (grass-fed, no added sugar) and dark chocolate (see page 232) when she needed it. As for her cucumbers and hard-boiled eggs, I encouraged her to make those part of a bridge snack when she needed one (see page 168). Jane started a new relationship with food and used the Fab Four as her framework for a healthy plate. Then she let go of perfect. She ended up losing eight pounds in six weeks.

When life does slow down a little bit, some of my clients swing from one extreme to the other. They hunker down in hermit mode and adopt a restrictive, all-or-nothing system in an attempt to hit the reset button. Mary, age twenty-seven, quickly built a large and loyal following for her restaurant review business. This has opened a lot of fun doors for her, but she's on a nonstop carousel of dinners out, late nights, and weekends away. When I met her, she was feeling out of control, unmotivated, and overwhelmed if she had back-to-back nights out. Similar to Jane, she thought "being good" meant being perfect. She would end up canceling a week's worth of events so she could hermit up and eat "perfectly." I asked her not to do that and instead to text me what she ate that was healthy when she was out. Instead of focusing on the bite of flatbread or three onion rings she might have had, we refocused her on the herb chicken or side salad or broccoli she also ate. Mary's text history with me turned into a running success story—all the positive, body-loving choices she was making, with me cheering her on. Sometimes, all it takes is one small shift in perspective to free yourself of the burden of perfection. In Mary's case, it completely changed her mentality. She felt more confident in herself and had less anxiety around food. That turned into a renewed ability to find balance even when her schedule was hectic or unpredictable.

BODY LOVE EVERY DAY

ONE DECISION DOES NOT DEFINE A DAY. I see my clients do this all the time: they'll label their entire day a failure based on one food choice. Grading yourself down like this is a form of self-sabotage. If one unhealthy decision means the whole day gets an F, you're more likely to write off whatever is left of it. You may end up snacking on junk food, bingeing after dinner, or sliding into a weekend free-for-all. We've falsely told ourselves it's all-or-nothing when it isn't and shouldn't be. It's a bad habit and takes effort to break, but every time we do, we lay another brick of resiliency in our minds. Below are two quick, easy, in-the-moment ways to snap yourself out of this mind-set.

- **GIVE YOURSELF AN A.** The moment you feel a bad grade coming, find a decision that made you happy or healthy today—you had a Fab Four Smoothie for breakfast, you worked out or took the stairs, a kind gesture or word to a friend or stranger—and give yourself an A for it. I don't want you to start an inner label war with yourself, but shifting your focus to something positive can quickly break the false narrative of failure in your mind. You will always find an A, and probably loads of them. Choose to let those moments define your day.

- **MOVE AND MOVE ON.** Labels are sticky, and bad grades weigh you down mentally. So get up and move your body to process the emotion physically. If you're at work, it's as simple as taking a quick lap around the office. When you come back to rest, write down one thing you're going to do to move on. It can be as simple as drinking a glass of water or booking a workout class for later. Convert the negative feeling into a positive action, and the moment you do, tell yourself you've moved on. Choose to move on.

FOCUS ON 33 PERCENT. This strategy can help every archetype. You might start one of the Fab Four plans in this book with the best intentions and total commitment. But if you run into an oops! moment on Day 1, 2, or 3—or all of them—I don't want you to feel like you're suddenly "off plan" and need to restart. This isn't a cleanse or elimination diet; there are no restarts. One strategy I use all the time with new clients is to focus them on the first third of the day, until healthy mornings become a habit. I focus them on an attainable goal—breakfast—rather than on executing a complete lifestyle makeover on a dime. Give 100 percent effort toward 33 percent of the day, then gain momentum and grow from there. Wake up and commit to moving for thirty minutes, then follow it with a Fab Four Smoothie, which will get you to lunch feeling great about yourself. And the 33 percent doesn't have to be breakfast. It can be lunch or dinner, too. The point is not to overwhelm yourself. It's okay to start with a smaller, more manageable chunk of the day as you ease into a healthier lifestyle.

LET NEGATIVE THOUGHTS BE. A visual that has always resonated with me is to imagine my thoughts are clouds. They float across the sky of my mind, while I sit on the ground below watching them. I am not my thoughts, and my thoughts are not me. I'm simply the observer. Some thoughts are fluffy and fun, and others are dark and gray. Whatever they are, they're just passing by. It's a way of acknowledging, and not denying, the thoughts I have each day, but also separating myself from them, because I have the power to choose which to act on and make a reality.

Sometimes negative, self-defeating thoughts will get the best of us and lead to actions we regret. But the next time they come floating by (and they will), we have a new opportunity to let them pass. Just because they got us last time doesn't mean they will today. We always have the power to choose which ones to act on. There are a lot of positive, confident clouds up there. Better yet, so is the sun.

WHAT DOES BODY LOVE MEAN TO YOU? To me, it means loving myself unconditionally. It means being grateful for all of the incredible things my body does for me every day, without me even having to think about it. It means loving and accepting my body the way it is. But it also means that I'm allowed to have goals. It means being patient with myself. It means doing things that are positive for my body and giving it the nourishment and love it deserves. It means eating real, whole, unprocessed foods that nourish me. It means exercising daily and prioritizing my health. It means knowing that my mistakes, weaknesses, and flaws don't make me a bad person; they make me human. It means believing in myself, staying positive in the face of setbacks, and breathing life into the brave me. It means accepting there will be all sorts of dark, gray clouds that float by. It means always believing the sun is about to break through. It means not taking one split second in my body for granted. It means loving myself, unconditionally.

Ask yourself the question: what does body love mean to me? In my opinion, if there's any standard to which you should hold yourself, it's not perfection—it's love.

GIRL, WASH YOUR FACE. As in the title of my client Rachel Hollis's fearless, funny, and inspiring *New York Times* bestseller. In it, she shares how she overcame myriad challenges in her life, from gut-wrenching tragedy and an abusive childhood to finding her way as a woman. I read it in a weekend and can't think of a more timely book to help you let go of perfect and become the person you were meant to be. A few other books to check out are *Perfectly Imperfect* by Baron Baptiste, *21 Days to Resilience* by Dr. Zelana Montminy, and *Judgment Detox* by Gabrielle Bernstein.

FINAL NOTE

I THRIVE ON POSITIVITY. When I step back and look at the Fab Four lifestyle as a whole, I think it embodies a spirit of positivity around food and nutrition. It's also a pretty spot-on representation of who I am and my outlook on life. I want to live it! I want to make choices, not cheats. I want to live in balance, quiet my inner perfectionist, and never feel like my goals are out of reach. I want to love the way I look and feel. I want to be proactive about my long-term health and wellness. I want to have a positive relationship with food . . . for the rest of my life.

I want for you what I want for myself. I hope that reading *Body Love Every Day* has been a positive and empowering experience for you. You have the science, the tools, the guidance, and the recipes to chart your own path to food freedom. (Plus four sample plans to aspire to and follow, if you want.) The Fab Four and body love will always be there for you, no matter where life takes you.

Be well!
All my love,
Kelly

FAB FOUR RECIPES BY CATEGORY

FAB FOUR SMOOTHIES

Remember that every single Fab Four Smoothie recipe in this book and in *Body Love* can be tailored to your lifestyle preference. All you have to do is use the animal- or plant-based protein powder of your choice. That's it. So if you're a meat-eater, don't miss out on the recipes in the Plant-Based Devotee plan. And if you're vegetarian or vegan, make sure to check out the recipes in the Girl on the Go and Domestic Goddess plans.

Fab Four Recipes by Category

FAB FOUR ROADIES

If you're out and about, these are easy ways to turn everyday coffee shop beverages into modified versions of the Fab Four Smoothie. All of these recipes are in the Girl on the Go Plan, page 150.

FAB FOUR BREAKFASTS

FAB FOUR LUNCHES

FAB FOUR DINNERS

Fab Four Recipes by Category

FAB FOUR LEMONADES AND SPA WATERS

All of the following recipes are in the Plant-Based Devotee plan, page 296:

Apple Cider Vinegar Lemonade

Chlorophyll Mint Water

Matcha Limeade

Silica ACV Lemon Water

Spa Water Blends

OTHER FAB FOUR RECIPES

Aquafaba (egg white substitute)—Plant-Based Devotee, page 309

Cauliflower Potato Salad—Domestic Goddess, page 226

Cauliflower Rice—Plant-Based Devotee, page 315

Coconut Tzatziki—Domestic Goddess, page 231

Cucumber Salad—Domestic Goddess, page 231

Curry in a Hurry Sauce—Girl on the Go, page 169

Fab Four Snack Packs (three options)—Girl on the Go, page 137

Fermented Coleslaw—Domestic Goddess, page 225

Freezer Fudge (Original, Hazelnut, Caramel Candy, and Praline)—Domestic Goddess, page 214

Garlic Ginger Bok Choy—Plant-Based Devotee, page 343

Homemade Celery Juice—Girl on the Go, page 175

Homemade Plant-Based Milks—Domestic Goddess, page 205

Lemon Butter Sauce—Girl on the Go, page 170

Lemon Tahini Dressing—Girl on the Go, page 158

My Everything Bagel Seasoning—Girl on the Go, page 172

Pressure-Cooked Dry Beans—Plant-Based Devotee, page 291

Presto Pesto (Classic Basil, Popeye, Spicy Taco, Cruciferous Punch, and Fresh Herb)—Plant-Based Devotee, page 286

Sesame Broccoli—Plant-Based Devotee, page 342

Spicy Bok Choy—Domestic Goddess, page 251

Spicy Cashew Spread—Plant-Based Devotee, page 322

Sprouted Sunflower Seed Hummus—Plant-Based Devotee, page 289

Super Green Kale Chips—Domestic Goddess, page 273

Tapioca Flour Biscuits—Domestic Goddess, page 275

Turmeric Bone Broth—Red-Carpet Ready, page 376

REFERENCES

INTRODUCTION

Lotta L, et al. (2017 Jan). Integrative genomic analysis implicates limited peripheral adipose storage capacity in the pathogenesis of human insulin resistance. *Nature Genetics* 49(1): 17–26.

Radak, Z, et al. (2008 Jan). Exercise, oxidative stress and hormesis. *Aging Research Reviews* 7(1).

PROTEIN

Halton TL, and FB Hu. (2004 Oct). The effects of high protein diets on thermogenesis, satiety and weight loss: a critical review. *Journal of the American College of Nutrition* 23(5): 373–85.

Johnstone AM, Stubbs RJ, Harbron CG. (1996 Jul). Effect of overfeeding macronutrients on day-to-day food intake in man. *European Academy of Nutritional Sciences* 50(7): 418–30.

Leidy HJ, et al. (2011 Apr). The effects of consuming frequent, higher protein meals on appetite and satiety during weight loss in overweight/obese men. *Obesity* 19(4): 818–24.

Westerterp-Plantenga MS, et al. (2004 Jan). High protein intake sustains weight maintenance after body weight loss in humans. *International Journal of Obesity and Related Metabolic Disorders* 28(1).

TRIMETHYLAMINE N-OXIDE (TMAO)

Chen ML, et al. (2016 Apr). Resveratrol attenuates trimethylamine-N-oxide (TMAO)-induced atherosclerosis by regulating TMAO synthesis and bile acid metabolism via remodeling of the gut microbiota. *Microbiology* 7(2):e02210-15. doi: 10.1128/mBio.02210-15.

De Filippis F, et al. (2016 Nov). High-level adherence to a Mediterranean diet beneficially impacts the gut microbiota and associated metabolome. *Gut* 65(11): 1812–1821.

Koeth RA, et al. (2013 May). Intestinal microbiota metabolism of L-carnitine, a nutrient in red meat, promotes atherosclerosis. *Nature Medicine* 19(5): 576–585.

Li Q, et al. (2017 Dec). Soluble dietary fiber reduces trimethylamine metabolism via gut microbiota and co-regulates host AMPK pathways. *Molecular Nutrition and Food Research* 61(12).

Obeid R., et al. (2017 Feb). Plasma trimethylamine-N-oxide following supplementation with vitamin D or D plus B vitamins. *Molecular Nutrition and Food Research* 61(2). doi: 10.1002/mnfr .201600358.

BRANCHED-CHAIN AMINO ACIDS (BCAA)

Zhang S, et al. (2017 Jan). Novel metabolic and physiological functions of branched chain amino acids: a review. *Journal of Animal Science and Biotechnology* 8:10. doi: 10.1186/s40104-016-0139-z.

References

WHEY

Salehi A, et al. (2012 May) The insulinogenic effect of whey protein is partially mediated by a direct effect of amino acids and GIP on β-cells. *Nutrition and Metabolism* 9(1): 48. doi: 10.1186/1743-7075-9-48.

COLLAGEN

Bagchi D, et al. (2002 Jan). Effects of orally administered undenatured type II collagen against arthritic inflammatory diseases: a mechanistic exploration. *International Journal of Clinical Pharmacology Research* 22(3–4): 101–110.

PEA PROTEIN

Overduin J, et al. (2015 Apr). NUTRALYS(®) pea protein: characterization of in vitro gastric digestion and in vivo gastrointestinal peptide responses relevant to satiety. *Food & Nutrition Research* 59:25622. doi: 10.3402/fnr.v59.25622.

Pownall TL, Udenigwe CC, Aluko RE. (2010 Apr). Amino acid composition and antioxidant properties of pea seed (Pisum sativum L.) enzymatic protein hydrolysate fractions. *Journal of Agricultural and Food Chemistry* 58(8): 4712–4718.

RICE

Ishikawa Y. (2015 Aug). Rice protein hydrolysates stimulate GLP-1 secretion, reduce GLP-1 degradation, and lower the glycemic response in rats. *Food & Function* 6(8): 2525–34.

Zhang H, et al. (2011 Oct). Lower weight gain and hepatic lipid content in hamsters fed high fat diets supplemented with white rice protein, brown rice protein, soy protein, and their hydrolysates. *Journal of Agricultural and Food Chemistry* 59(20): 10927–33.

FAT

Brown MJ. (2004 Aug). Carotenoid bioavailability is higher from salads ingested with full-fat than with fat-reduced salad dressings as measured with electrochemical detection. *American Journal of Clinical Nutrition* 80(2): 396–403.

Hjalmarsdottir F. (2018 Oct). 17 Science-Based Benefits of Omega-3 Fatty Acids. Healthline. https://www.healthline.com/nutrition/17-health-benefits-of-omega-3#section8.

Kaiserauer S. (1989 Apr). Nutritional, physiological, and menstrual status of distance runners. *Medicine and Science in Sports and Exercise* 21(2): 120–125.

Sanchez-Bayle M. (2008 Feb). A cross-sectional study of dietary habits and lipid profiles. The Rivas-Vaciamadrid study. *European Journal of Pediatrics* 167(2): 149–54.

Tomiyama AJ et al. (2010 May). Low calorie dieting increases cortisol. *Psychosomatic Medicine* 72(4): 357–364.

Wabitsch M et al. (1996 Oct). Insulin and cortisol promote leptin production in human fat cells. *Diabetes* 45(10) 1425–1438.

Weiss EP et al. (2008 Jun). Caloric restriction but not exercise-induced reductions in fat mass decrease plasma triiodothyronine concentrations: A randomized controlled trial. *Rejuvenation Research* 11(3): 605–609.

Williams NI et al. (2010 Sept). Estrogen and progesterone exposure is reduced in response to energy deficiency in women aged 25–40 years. *Human Reproduction* 25(9): 2328–2339.

FIBER AND GREENS

Chai W, Liebman M. (2005 Apr). Effect of different cooking methods on vegetable oxalate content. *Journal of Agriculture and Food Chemistry* 53(8): 3027–30.

Chung JH et al. (2013 May). Green tea formulations with vitamin C and xylitol on enhanced intestinal transport of green tea catechins. *Journal of Food Science* 78(5): C685–90.

Pearson KJ et al. (2008 Aug). Resveratrol delays age-related deterioration and mimics transcriptional aspects of dietary restriction without extending life span. *Cell Metabolism* 8(2): 157–68.

Shi J, Le Maguer M. (2000) Lycopene in tomatoes: chemical and physical properties affected by food processing. 20(4): 293–334.

Shoba G et al. (1998 May). Influence of piperine on the pharmacokinetics of curcumin in animals and human volunteers. *Planta Medica* 64(4): 353–6.

THE "NOT SO FAB" FOUR

Blaser MJ, Falkow S. (2009 Nov). What are the consequences of the disappearing human microbiota? *Nature Reviews Microbology* 7: 887–894. https://www.nature.com/articles/nrmicro2245.

Jackubowicz D, Maayan B, Wainstein, Froy O. (2013). High caloric intake at breakfast vs. dinner differentially influences weight loss of overweight and obese women. *Obesity* (2013) 21: 2504–2512. doi:10.1002/oby.20460.

Gardner CD et al. (2018 Feb). Effect of low-fat vs low-carbohydrate diet on 12-month weight loss in overweight adults and the association with genotype pattern or insulin secretion. *JAMA* 319(7): 667–679.

Lachat C et al. (2018 Jan). Dietary species richness as a measure of food biodiversity and nutritional quality of diets. *PNAS* 115(1): 127–132. http://www.pnas.org/content/early/2017 /12/13/1709194115.

Schnorr SL. (2014 Apr). Gut microbiome of the Hadza hunter-gatherers. *Nature Communications* 5: 3654. https://www.nature.com/articles/ncomms4654.

Spreadbury I. (2012 July). Comparison with ancestral diets suggests dense acellular carbohydrates promote an inflammatory microbiota, and may be the primary dietary cause of leptin resistance and obesity. *Diabetes Metabolic Syndrome and Obesity* 5: 175–189. https://www .ncbi.nlm.nih.gov/pmc/articles/PMC3402009/.

397

References

The lowdown on glycemic index and glycemic load: Understanding glycemic load is just as important as the glycemic index of foods. Healthbeat. Harvard Health Publishing Harvard Medical School. https://www.health.harvard.edu/diseases-and-conditions/the-lowdown-on-glycemic-index-and-glycemic-load.

IRON

Monsen ER. (1988 Jul). Iron nutrition and absorption: dietary factors which impact iron bioavailability. *Journal of the American Dietetic Association* 88(7): 786–790.

PLANT-BASED DEVOTEE

Chamikara M, Ishan M. (2016 Sept). Dietary, Anticancer and Medicinal Properties of the Phytochemicals in Chili Pepper (Capsicum spp.). *Ceylon Journal of Science (Biological Sciences)* 45(3): 5–20. https://www.researchgate.net/publication/311183215_Dietary_Anticancer_and_Medicinal_Properties_of_the_Phytochemicals_in_Chili_Pepper_Capsicum_spp.

RED-CARPET READY

Donga E et al. (2010 Jun). A single night of partial sleep deprivation induces insulin resistance in multiple metabolic pathways in healthy subjects. *Journal of Clinical Endocrinology and Metabolism* 95(6): 2963–8. https://www.ncbi.nlm.nih.gov/pubmed/20371664.

Nakamura K, Velho G, Bouby N. (2017 July). Vasopressin and metabolic disorders: translation from experimental models to clinical use. *Journal of Internal Medicine* 282(4): 298–309. https://doi.org/10.1111/joim.12649.

Pepino MY et al. (2013 Sept). Sucralose affects glycemic and hormonal responses to an oral glucose load. *Diabetes Care* 36(9): 2530–2535. https://www.ncbi.nlm.nih.gov/pmc/articles/PMC3747933/.

SLEEP

Cappucino FP et al. (2008). Meta-analysis of short sleep duration and obesity in children and adults. *Sleep* 31(5): 619–626. http://kendal-tackett.www.uppitysciencechick.com/cappuccio_sleep_dur_obesity.pdf.

Knutson KL et al. (2017 Apr). Association between sleep timing, obesity, diabetes: The Hispanic community health study/study of Latinos (HCHS/SOL) cohort study. *Sleep* 40(4). https://doi.org/10.1093/sleep/zsx014.

Potter GDM et al. (2016 Dec). Circadian rhythm and sleep disruption: Causes, metabolic consequences, and countermeasures. *Endocrine Reviews* 37(6): 584–608. https://doi.org/10.1210/er.2016–1083.

FERMENTED VEGGIES

An SY et al. (2013 Aug). Beneficial effects of fresh and fermented kimchi in prediabetic individuals. *Annals of Nutrition & Metabolism* 63(1–2): 111–9. doi: 10.1159/000353583.

Lopez HW et al. (2001 May). Prolonged fermentation of whole wheat sourdough reduces phytate level and increases soluble magnesium. *Journal of Agriculture and Food Chemistry* 49(5): 2657–62.

Parvez S, Malik KA, Ah Kang S, Kim HY. (2006 Jun). Probiotics and their fermented food products are beneficial for health. *Journal of Applied Microbiology* 100(6): 1771–85.

Scheers N, Rossander-Hulthen L, Torsdottir I, Sandberg A. (2015 Feb). Increased iron bioavailability from lactic-fermented vegetables is likely an effect of promoting the formation of ferric iron (Fe^{3+}). *European Journal of Nutrition* 55: 373–382. doi: 10.1007/s00394-015-0857-6.

POTATOES

Raben A et al. (1994 Oct). Resistant starch: the effect on postprandial glycemia, hormonal response, and satiety. *American Journal of Clinical Nutrition* 60(4): 544–51. doi: 10.1093/ajcn/60.4.544.

Muir JG, O'Dea K. (1992 July). Measurement of resistant starch: factors affecting the amount of starch escaping digestion in vitro. *American Journal of Clinical Nutrition* 56(1): 123–7.

WORKOUT

Brooks NE, Myburgh KH. (2014 Mar). Skeletal muscle wasting with disuse atrophy is multidimensional: the response and interaction of myonuclei, satellite cells and signaling pathways. *Frontiers in Physiology* 5: 99. doi: 10.3389/fphys.2014.00099.

Rebar AL et al. (2015 July). A meta-meta-analysis of the effect of physical activity on depression and anxiety in non-clinical adult populations. *Health Psychology Review* 9(3): 366–378. https://doi.org/10.1080/17437199.2015.1022901.

UNIVERSAL CONVERSION CHART

OVEN TEMPERATURE EQUIVALENTS

250°F = 120°C

275°F = 135°C

300°F = 150°C

325°F = 160°C

350°F = 180°C

375°F = 190°C

400°F = 200°C

425°F = 220°C

450°F = 230°C

475°F = 240°C

500°F = 260°C

MEASUREMENT EQUIVALENTS

Measurements should always be level unless directed otherwise.

$\frac{1}{8}$ teaspoon = 0.5 mL

$\frac{1}{4}$ teaspoon = 1 mL

$\frac{1}{2}$ teaspoon = 2 mL

1 teaspoon = 5 mL

1 tablespoon = 3 teaspoons = $\frac{1}{2}$ fluid ounce = 15 mL

2 tablespoons = $\frac{1}{8}$ cup = 1 fluid ounce = 30 mL

4 tablespoons = $\frac{1}{4}$ cup = 2 fluid ounces = 60 mL

$5\frac{1}{3}$ tablespoons = $\frac{1}{3}$ cup = 3 fluid ounces = 80 mL

8 tablespoons = $\frac{1}{2}$ cup = 4 fluid ounces = 120 mL

$10\frac{2}{3}$ tablespoons = $\frac{2}{3}$ cup = 5 fluid ounces = 160 mL

12 tablespoons = $\frac{3}{4}$ cup = 6 fluid ounces = 180 mL

16 tablespoons = 1 cup = 8 fluid ounces = 240 mL

ACKNOWLEDGMENTS

If you want to write clean, ditch your not-so-fabulous grammar, and love your healthy manuscript, Cassie Jones is the editor for you. I owe her a massive thank-you. Thank you for your patience, encouragement, and guidance. Your insightful questions and discerning edits continuously elevated the manuscript and your witty asides and wisecracks in track changes made it fun, too. Just as with *Body Love*, you were an absolute joy to work with. (Are you game for round three someday?!)

To the rest of the team at William Morrow—Kara Zauberman, Shelby Meizlik, Molly Waxman, Andrew DiCecco, Mumtaz Mustafa, Rachel Meyers, Jill Zimmerman, and Bonni Leon-Berman—thank you for helping bring *Body Love Every Day* to life! It's been a pleasure to watch you work your literary, design, and production magic and help turn my ideas into reality. A special shout-out to my eagle-eyed copyeditor, Ana Deboo, who sliced and diced my wordy ways, and who improved the manuscript at every turn.

I love my book agent, Yfat Reiss Gendell. She gets it and gets me. I have the utmost respect, gratitude, and appreciation for her and her team at Foundry. Thank you for believing in me back in 2016 and for supporting me every step of the way since then. *Body Love* and *Body Love Every Day* wouldn't exist without you. Thank you!

I'd also like to thank Matthew Morgan for shooting a beautiful cover photo for the book and my graphic designer, Amber Moon, for creating such amazing art and graphics to help bring the science and Fab Four to life.

I would be remiss if I didn't say thank you to a few groups of people who literally watched me write and type my manuscript. First, thank you to the always cheerful staff at The Larder in Brentwood, who kept the peppermint tea and good vibes coming and who let me stay after closing on countless occasions so I could keep

Acknowledgments

writing. Second, a more caffeinated thank-you to the baristas at Caffe Luxxe on Montana Avenue, who always offered me welcoming smiles, positive energy, and delectable artisanal almond milk cappuccinos—unsweetened, of course. ☺

A friendly (and professional) thank you to my friend (and manager) Antranig Balian at Mortar Media. You always take the long view, give it to me straight, and add a bit of levity to my day. Thank you for all your hard work, loyalty, and care. And to Jessica Zambrano—thank you for managing, coordinating, and everything else you tackle on a daily basis.

I'm so grateful for the rest of my BWBK team: my trusty assistant Stepfanie Villaseca, my cool-as-a-cucumber assistant Mercey Livingston, and my go-to people for all things legal—Ellie Altshuler and David Aronoff.

Thank you to my husband, Chris, for all the little things you do and for always helping me see the big picture. There's a story behind every page of this book with you in it . . . an idea or analogy to help me say something in a unique way, a silly song you were singing to Bash that made me laugh, always setting up the coffee the night before so all I had to do was push the brew button in the morning. I love you. Please don't ever stop being you. And please don't ever stop making the coffee the night before!

Last but not least, thank you to my little one, Sebastian Dume LeVeque, for making me a mom. The day you were born, my heart grew about a million sizes (roughly five million heaping tablespoons), and it hasn't stopped singing since. You're a resilient, radiant little human, Mr. Bash Man. You're my heart and soul, and I love you more than words could ever express.

INDEX

Index

Index

Index

Index

Index